AГ720394

Modern Approaches to Clinical Trials Using SAS®

Classical, Adaptive, and Bayesian Methods

Edited by
Sandeep M. Menon
Richard C. Zink

sas.
support.sas.com/bookstore

The correct bibliographic citation for this manual is as follows: Menon, Sandeep and Richard C. Zink. 2015. *Modern Approaches to Clinical Trials Using SAS®: Classical, Adaptive, and Bayesian Methods*. Cary, NC: SAS Institute Inc.

Modern Approaches to Clinical Trials Using SAS®: Classical, Adaptive, and Bayesian Methods

Copyright © 2015, SAS Institute Inc., Cary, NC, USA

ISBN 978-1-62959-385-2 (Paperback)
ISBN 978-1-63526-918-5 (Hardcover)
ISBN 978-1-62960-082-6 (EPUB)
ISBN 978-1-62960-083-3 (MOBI)
ISBN 978-1-62960-084-0 (PDF)

All Rights Reserved. Produced in the United States of America.

For a hard-copy book: No part of this publication may be reproduced, stored in a retrieval system, or transmitted, in any form or by any means, electronic, mechanical, photocopying, or otherwise, without the prior written permission of the publisher, SAS Institute Inc.

For a web download or e-book: Your use of this publication shall be governed by the terms established by the vendor at the time you acquire this publication.

The scanning, uploading, and distribution of this book via the Internet or any other means without the permission of the publisher is illegal and punishable by law. Please purchase only authorized electronic editions and do not participate in or encourage electronic piracy of copyrighted materials. Your support of others' rights is appreciated.

U.S. Government License Rights; Restricted Rights: The Software and its documentation is commercial computer software developed at private expense and is provided with RESTRICTED RIGHTS to the United States Government. Use, duplication, or disclosure of the Software by the United States Government is subject
to the license terms of this Agreement pursuant to, as applicable, FAR 12.212, DFAR 227.7202-1(a), DFAR 227.7202-3(a), and DFAR 227.7202-4, and, to the extent required under U.S. federal law, the minimum restricted rights as set out in FAR 52.227-19 (DEC 2007). If FAR 52.227-19 is applicable, this provision serves as notice under clause (c) thereof and no other notice is required to be affixed to the Software or documentation. The Government's rights in Software and documentation shall be only those set forth in this Agreement.

SAS Institute Inc., SAS Campus Drive, Cary, NC 27513-2414

July 2018

SAS® and all other SAS Institute Inc. product or service names are registered trademarks or trademarks of SAS Institute Inc. in the USA and other countries. ® indicates USA registration.

Other brand and product names are trademarks of their respective companies.

SAS software may be provided with certain third-party software, including but not limited to open-source software, which is licensed under its applicable third-party software license agreement. For license information about third-party software distributed with SAS software, refer to **http://support.sas.com/thirdpartylicenses**.

Contents

Foreword

Recent years, and perhaps particularly the past decade, have seen a rapid evolution in the statistical methodology available to be used in clinical trials, from both technical and implementation standpoints. Certain practices as they might have been performed not too far into the past might in fact now seem somewhat primitive or naïve. Much, but certainly by no means all, of the recent development is related to recent interest in adaptive trial designs. The term itself is quite broad, and encompasses a wide variety of techniques and applications. Many trial aspects are potential candidates for adaptation, including but not limited to: sample size or information requirements, dose or treatment regimen selection, targeted patient population selection, the randomization allocation scheme; and within each of these categories there may be multiple and fundamentally different technical and strategic approaches that are now available for practitioners to consider.

Classical procedures as well have undergone advancements in the statistical details of their implementation, and their usage in analysis and interpretation of trial results. Enhancements in classical approaches, and the progress made or envisioned in utilization of novel adaptive and Bayesian designs and methodologies, are reflective of the current interest in the transition to personalized medicine approaches, by which optimal therapies corresponding to particular patient characteristics are sought. A categorization of designs and methods into classical, adaptive, and Bayesian methods is by no means mutually exclusive, as a number of methodologies have aspects of more than one of these classes. Just to cite one example, group sequential designs are a familiar feature in current clinical trial practice that fall under both the classical and adaptive headings; this is also certainly an area that has seen an evolution in recent years. Aspects of clinical trial or program design such as dose finding or population enrichment may contain aspects that are adaptive, or Bayesian, or both, as is communicated well in this volume.

The interest in novel adaptive and Bayesian approaches certainly does not preclude the possibility that classical approaches will be preferred in many situations; they maintain the attributes which led to their widespread adoption in the first place. As has been pointed out by many authors, the best use of these novel approaches will be realized by a full understanding of their behavior and an objective evaluation of their advantages and relevant tradeoffs in particular situations. This point is clearly and objectively conveyed throughout this volume, as approaches of varied types are presented not to promote or endorse their casual routine use, but rather are described with sufficient explanations to help practitioners make the best choices for their situations, and of course to have the computational tools to implement them.

It seems inevitable that the availability to users of software and computational capabilities is inextricably linked with increased consideration of and interest in alternative design and analysis strategies, and ultimately their implementation. Certainly, if a novel methodology is seen as adding value in such an important arena as clinical trials, it will spur development of the computational tools necessary to implement it. However, in a cycle, the increased availability to practitioners leads to increased consideration and implementation, which spurs further interest, enables learnings from experience, perhaps motivates further research, and ultimately leads to further methodological and in-practice improvements and evolution.

Just as a simple illustration of this phenomenon: questions regarding how clinical sites should best be accounted for in main statistical analysis models had undergone some debate in past decades, with occasional flurries of literature activity, but evolution in conventional practices was limited. The introduction of SAS' **`proc mixed`** in the early 1990s provided a platform for more widespread consideration and usage of some approaches that were less commonly utilized at that time, which incorporated clinical site as a random effect in analysis models in various manners. There were implications for important related issues, such as sample size determination and targeted center-size distributions, and for certain practices that were in use at the time such as small center pooling algorithms. Given the presence of the new computational tool available to users in the form of the SAS procedure, it may not be a coincidence that by the latter part of that decade there was vigorous dialogue taking place in the literature on matters involving how best to design multicenter studies and accommodate center in analysis models, and within a relatively short period of time there were notable changes in conventional practices.

Given the extent of recent methodological advances, and the wide knowledge of and usage of SAS throughout the clinical trials community, a focused volume such as this one is particularly timely in this regard. It integrates a broad yet coherent summary of current approaches for clinical trial design and analysis, with particular emphasis on important recently developed ones, along with specific illustrations of how they can be implemented and performed in SAS. In some cases this involves relatively straightforward calls to SAS procedures; in many others, sophisticated SAS macros developed by the authors are presented. Motivating examples are described, and SAS outputs corresponding to those examples are explained to help guide readers through the most accurate understandings and interpretations. This text might well function effectively as a technical resource on state-of-the-art clinical trials methodology even if it did not contain the SAS illustrations and explanations; and it could also fit within a useful niche if it focused solely on the SAS illustrations without the methodological and practical explanations. The fact that it contains both aspects, well integrated in chapters prepared by experienced subject matter experts, makes it a particularly valuable resource. The ability that the material contained here offers to practitioners to test and compare different design and analysis options to choose the one that seems best for a given situation can help drive the most impactful usage of these new technologies; and, along the lines of the methodology-computational tools cycle described earlier, this perhaps may assist in leading to further experience-driven methodological or implementation advancements.

About This Book

Purpose

Modern Approaches to Clinical Trials Using SAS®: Classical, Adaptive, and Bayesian Methods is unique and multifaceted, covering several domains of modern clinical trial design, including classical, group sequential, adaptive, and Bayesian methods that are applicable to and widely used in various phases of pharmaceutical development. Topics covered include, but are not limited to, dose-response and dose-escalation designs; sequential methods to stop trials early for overwhelming efficacy, safety, or futility; Bayesian designs that incorporate historical data; adaptive sample size re-estimation; adaptive randomization to allocate subjects to more effective treatments; and population enrichment designs. Methods are illustrated using clinical trials from diverse therapeutic areas, including dermatology, endocrinology, infectious disease, neurology, oncology, and rheumatology. Individual chapters are authored by renowned contributors, experts, and key opinion leaders from the pharmaceutical/medical device industry or academia.

Numerous real-world examples and sample SAS code enable users to readily apply novel clinical trial design and analysis methodologies in practice.

Is This Book for You?

This book is intended for biostatisticians, pharmacometricians, clinical developers, and statistical programmers involved in the design, analysis, and interpretation of clinical trials. Further, students in graduate and post-graduate programs in statistics or biostatistics will benefit from the many practical illustrations of statistical concepts.

Prerequisites

Based on the above audience, users will benefit most from this book with some graduate training in statistics or biostatistics, and some experience or exposure to clinical trials. Some experience with simulation may be useful, though this is not required to use this book. Some experience with SAS/STAT procedures, SAS/IML, and the SAS macro language is expected.

About the Examples

Software Used to Develop the Book's Content

The output, figures, and examples presented were generated using the third maintenance release of SAS 9.4 (TS1M3), including SAS/STAT 14.1 and SAS/IML 14.1. However, the code has and is expected to generate the appropriate results using earlier releases of SAS.

Example Code and Data

Code is available for download from the companion website of this book.

Output and Graphics Used in This Book

Figures were generated using SAS and saved as TIF files. Output was captured from HTML using FullShot 9.5 Professional.

Additional Resources

SAS offers the following books for statisticians engaged in clinical trials.

1. Dmitrienko A, Molenberghs G, Chuang-Stein C & Offen W. (2005). *Analysis of Clinical Trials Using SAS®: A Practical Guide*. Cary, North Carolina: SAS Institute Inc.
2. Dmitrienko A, Chuang-Stein C & D'Agostino R. (2007). *Pharmaceutical Statistics Using SAS®: A Practical Guide*. Cary, North Carolina: SAS Institute Inc.
3. Wicklin R. (2013). *Simulating Data with SAS®*. Cary, North Carolina: SAS Institute Inc.
4. Zink RC. (2014). *Risk-Based Monitoring and Fraud Detection in Clinical Trials Using JMP® and SAS®*. Cary, North Carolina: SAS Institute Inc.

Keep in Touch

We look forward to hearing from you. We invite questions, comments, and concerns. If you want to contact us about a specific book, please include the book title in your correspondence.

To Contact the Author through SAS Press

By e-mail: saspress@sas.com

Via the Web: http://support.sas.com/author_feedback

SAS Books

For a complete list of books available through SAS, visit http://support.sas.com/bookstore.

Phone: 1-800-727-3228

Fax: 1-919-677-8166

E-mail: sasbook@sas.com

SAS Book Report

Receive up-to-date information about all new SAS publications via e-mail by subscribing to the SAS Book Report monthly eNewsletter. Visit http://support.sas.com/sbr.

Publish with SAS

SAS is recruiting authors! Are you interested in writing a book? Visit http://support.sas.com/saspress for more information.

About the Authors

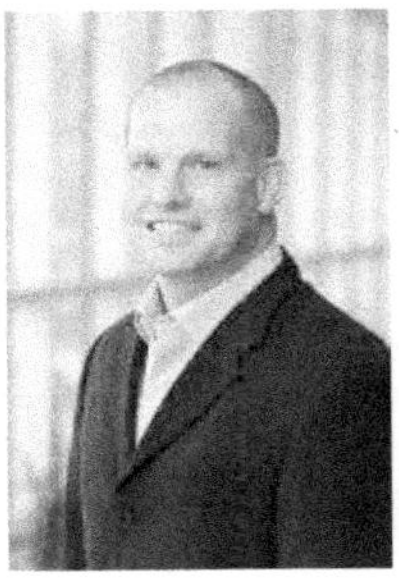

Richard C. Zink, PhD is Principal Research Statistician Developer in the JMP Life Sciences division at SAS Institute. He is currently a developer for JMP Clinical, an innovative software package designed to streamline the review of clinical trial data. He joined SAS in 2011 after eight years in the pharmaceutical industry, where he designed and analyzed clinical trials in a variety of therapeutic areas, participated in US and European drug submissions, and two FDA advisory committee hearings. He is an active member of the Biopharmaceutical Section of the American Statistical Association (ASA), serving as industry co-chair for the 2015 ASA Biopharmaceutical Section Statistics Workshop, and as a member of the Safety Scientific Working Group. He is a member of the Drug Information Association where he serves as Statistics Section Editor for Therapeutic Innovation & Regulatory Science. Richard is a member of Statisticians in the Pharmaceutical Industry, and holds a PhD in Biostatistics from the University of North Carolina at Chapel Hill, where he serves as an adjunct faculty member. He is author of Risk-Based Monitoring and Fraud Detection in Clinical Trials Using JMP® and SAS®.

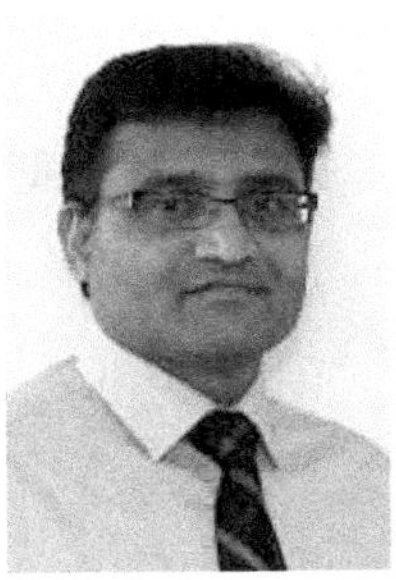

Sandeep Menon, PhD is currently the Vice President and Head of the Statistical Research and Consulting Center (SRCC) at Pfizer Inc., and he also holds adjunct faculty positions at Boston University and Tufts University School of Medicine. His group, located at different Pfizer sites globally, provides scientific and statistical leadership, and consultation to the global head of biostatistics, various quantitative groups within Pfizer, senior Pfizer management in discovery, clinical development, legal, commercial and marketing. His responsibilities also include providing a strong presence for Pfizer in regulatory and professional circles to influence content of regulatory guidelines and their interpretation in practice. Previously he held positions of responsibility and leadership where he was in charge of all the biostatistics activities for the entire portfolio in his unit, spanning from discovery (target) through proof-of-concept studies for supporting immunology and autoimmune disease, inflammation and remodeling, rare diseases, cardiovascular and metabolism, and center of therapeutic innovation. He was responsible for overseeing statistical aspects of more than 40 clinical trials, over 25 compounds, and 20 indications. He is a core member of the Global Statistics and Triad (Statistics, Clinical and Clinical Pharmacology) Leadership team. He has been in the industry for over a decade and prior to joining Pfizer he worked at Biogen Idec, Aptiv Solutions, and Harvard Clinical Research Institute. He is very passionate about adaptive designs and personalized medicine. He is the coauthor and coeditor of Clinical and Statistical Considerations in Personalized Medicine (2014). He received his medical degree from Bangalore (Karnataka) University, India, and later completed his master's and PhD in Biostatistics at Boston University.

Acknowledgments

Thanks to Stacey Hamilton, Cindy Puryear, Sian Roberts, and Shelley Sessoms at SAS Press for their excitement and encouragement. Many thanks to the reviewers for their insightful comments that improved the content and clarity of this book; John West, the copy editor who made the text consistent throughout; and Robert Harris, the graphic designer for the beautiful cover.

Richard would like to dedicate this book to SEA.

Sandeep would like to thank his parents (Mukundan and Radha Menon), his wife Shobha, brother Shashi, sister in-law Asha, little nephews (Dev and Thirth), his extended loving family in Boston and India and his colleagues at Pfizer. He would like to dedicate this book to his mentor, colleague, and friend Dr. Mark Chang from whom he has learned a lot on adaptive designs.

Contributors:

Keaven M. Anderson, Executive Director, Late Development Statistics, Merck Research Laboratories, North Wales, PA, USA.

Anindita Banerjee, Associate Director, Biotherapeutics Clinical Research, Pfizer Inc., Cambridge, MA, USA.

François Beckers, Head Global Biostatistics, Merck Serono, Inc., a subsidiary of Merck KgaA, Darmstadt, Germany.

Vladimir Bezlyak, Principal Biostatistician, Novartis, Basel, Switzerland.

Björn Bornkamp, Expert Statistical Methodologist, Novartis, Basel, Switzerland.

Frank Bretz, Global Head of the Statistical Methodology Group, Novartis, Basel, Switzerland.

Ming-Hui Chen, Professor and Director of Statistical Consulting Services, Department of Statistics, University of Connecticut, Storrs, CT, USA.

Jared Christensen, Senior Director, Biotherapeutics Clinical Research, Pfizer Inc., Cambridge, MA, USA.

Christy Chuang-Stein, Chuang-Stein Consulting, Kalamazoo, MI, USA.

Yeongjin Gwon, Graduate Assistant, Department of Statistics, University of Connecticut, Storrs, CT, USA.

Bo Huang, Director of Biostatistics, Pfizer Oncology, Pfizer Inc., Groton, CT, USA.

Joseph G. Ibrahim, Alumni Distinguished Professor, Department of Biostatistics, University of North Carolina at Chapel Hill, Chapel Hill, NC, USA.

Ruitao Lin, Ph.D. Candidate, Department of Statistics and Actuarial Science, The University of Hong Kong, Hong Kong, China.

Zorayr Manukyan, Director of Biostatistics, Biotherapeutic Research Unit, Pfizer Inc., Cambridge, MA, USA.

Sandeep Menon, Vice President and Head of Statistical Research and Consulting Center, Pfizer Inc., Cambridge, MA, USA.

Inna Perevozskaya, Senior Director, Biometrics Statistical Research and Consulting Center, Pfizer Inc., Collegeville, PA, USA.

Gaurav Sharma, Statistician, The EMMES Corporation, Rockville, MD, USA.

Oleksandr Sverdlov, Associate Director of Biostatistics, EMD Serono, Inc., a subsidiary of Merck KgaA, Rockland, MA, USA.

Naitee Ting, Senior Principal Biostatistician, Boehringer-Ingelheim Pharmaceuticals Inc., Ridgefield, CT, USA.

Jing Wang, Senior Biostatistician, Gilead Sciences, Inc., Foster City, CA, USA.

Joseph Wu, Biostatistics Manager, Global Innovative Pharma Business Unit, Pfizer Inc., Groton, CT, USA.

Guosheng Yin, Professor, Department of Statistics and Actuarial Science, The University of Hong Kong, Hong Kong, China.

Guojun Yuan, Director of Global Biostatistics, EMD Serono, Inc., a subsidiary of Merck KgaA, Billerica, MA, USA.

Richard C. Zink, Principal Research Statistician Developer, JMP Life Sciences, SAS Institute Inc, Cary, NC, USA.

Chapter 1
Overview of Clinical Trials in Support of Drug Development

1.1 Introduction

Clinical testing of a drug to support its marketing authorization is often characterized by four phases. Here, we use the word "drug" broadly for a drug or a biologic. Three of the four phases are before the drug is marketed (pre-marketing) and one is afterwards (post-marketing). During the first phase (phase I), researchers investigate what the human body will do to a drug in terms of drug absorption, distribution, metabolism and excretion. The investigation is typically conducted in healthy human volunteers, except for cytotoxic drugs. For cytotoxic drugs, phase I is often conducted in patients with very few therapeutic options due to the anticipated toxicities and uncertainty about a drug's benefits. When a drug is designed to target a receptor or induce a certain biomarker response, phase I trials can sometimes investigate what the drug does to the body. Phase I investigation usually consists of single-dose and multi-dose escalations to understand the common adverse reactions of a drug and what would be the drug's dose-limiting toxicities. If the drug's safety profile is judged to be acceptable relative to its potential (and yet to be observed) benefit at this stage, the development will progress to the second stage (phase II) with a recommended dose range. The number of volunteers included in phase I testing normally ranges between 20 and 80, but could be higher if phase I includes an assessment of the drug's mechanism of action or an early investigation of the drug's efficacy.

The second phase focuses on a drug's efficacy in patients with a targeted disorder. Clinical trials at this stage are also designed to determine dose(s), whose benefit-risk profile warrants further investigation in a confirmatory setting. Multiple doses within the dose range identified from phase I are typically studied during this phase. Occasionally, a sponsor may have to conduct more than one study if the doses chosen in the initial dose-response study are not adequate to estimate the dose-response relationship. This could occur if the doses selected initially are too high (e.g. near the plateau of the dose-response curve). To reduce the chance of having to repeat a dose-response study, it is generally recommended to include 4-7 doses in a wide dose range (the ratio of the maximum dose to the minimum dose ideally will be at least 10) in the dose-finding study. The analysis of a dose-finding study should focus on modeling the dose-response relationship instead of making pairwise comparisons between each dose and the control [1].

Phase II is typically the time when researchers first learn about the beneficial effect of a drug. It also has the highest attrition rate among the three pre-marketing phases. Therefore, if a drug is not a viable candidate, it is best to recognize this fact as soon as possible. This objective plus fewer regulatory requirements at this stage offer opportunities for out-of-the-box thinking. For example, some developers have divided phase II into two stages. The first stage tests the proof of concept (POC) of the drug, using a high dose (e.g., the maximum tolerated dose identified in phase I) to investigate a drug's efficacy. If the drug does not demonstrate a clinically meaningful efficacy compared to the control in the POC study, there will be no need to conduct a dose-response study. Otherwise, the drug will be further tested in a dose-ranging study. This two-step process is often referred to as phase IIa and phase IIb (see, for example, [2]). To streamline work that is required to initiate sites and obtain approvals from multiple institutional review boards, some sponsors combine POC and dose-response studies in one protocol with an unblinded interim analysis at the end of the POC stage. The sponsor will review results from the POC stage but use only data from the second stage to estimate the dose-response relationship. This strategy has the potential to reduce the so-called "white space" between phase IIa and phase IIb where the POC would be fully evaluated first and then the dose-response study would be planned.

Depending on the target disorders, phase II testing traditionally consists of 100-300 patients. Despite strong advocacy by researchers like [2] to use a modeling approach to analyzing dose-response data, some sponsors continue to rely on pairwise comparisons to design and analyze dose-response studies. There has been renewed emphasis that the selection of dose(s) is an estimation problem, and that this problem could be addressed more efficiently by using a modeling approach [3]. In addition, Pinheiro et al. have shown that even 300 patients in a dose-ranging study may not be enough to adequately identify the optimal dose based on a pre-set criterion [4].

If a drug meets the efficacy requirement and passes the initial benefit-risk assessment, it will be further tested to confirm its efficacy. This is the final stage of clinical testing before most drugs receive regulatory approval for marketing. This phase (phase III) enrolls a greater number of patients who are more heterogeneous in their demographic and baseline disease status. It is also at this stage that the majority of pre-marketing safety data are collected. Since a major objective of phase III is to confirm a drug's effect, analyses focus on testing pre-specified hypotheses with adequate control for the chance of making an erroneous claim of a positive drug effect. Operations at this stage require protecting a trial's integrity carefully so that trial results could be interpreted with confidence. The number of patients included at this stage typically ranges between 1,000 and 5,000. Drugs for orphan diseases will enroll much fewer patients while drugs that are designed to reduce the risk of a clinical endpoint may require thousands, if not tens of thousands of patients. In addition, more patients will be needed if the drug is developed for multiple disorders simultaneously. An example for developing multiple indications simultaneously is antibiotics.

After a drug's effect is confirmed and benefit-risk assessment supports its use in the target population, the manufacturer of the drug will file a marketing application with regulatory agencies, typically in multiple countries. Nearly all applications are for the adult population initially. If the product is expected to be used in the pediatric population, a manufacturer will often have an ongoing pediatric development program or have a plan to initiate pediatric trials at the time of the initial marketing application. The marketing application may be for a single indication or for multiple indications. If the application is approved, the drug will be commercially available to the public. A manufacturer could choose to conduct additional studies to further test the drug in the indicated population(s), or in pediatric patients with the indicated disorder(s), or comparing the drug head-to-head with an approved drug for the same disorder(s), or for additional usages. Sometimes, a manufacturer conducts post-marketing studies to meet regulatory requirements as a condition for the marketing approval. This phase is often referred to as phase IV.

Another way to characterize the four phases of drug development is by the type of studies that are conducted during these 4 phases [5]. The types of studies conducted can be described as human pharmacology studies (phase I), therapeutic exploratory studies (phase II), therapeutic confirmatory studies (phase III), and therapeutic use studies (phase IV).

There are notable exceptions to the process described above. Many cancer drugs were initially granted accelerated approval based on tumor response rates observed in phase II trials. Some of the phase II trials may be single-arm studies. A condition for the accelerated approval is that the observed efficacy in phase II needs to be confirmed in randomized phase III trials. Depending on the type of cancer, the endpoint used in phase III trials can be progression-free survival or overall survival. When overall survival is not the primary endpoint in a phase III study, regulators often require that the new drug does not compromise overall survival. Drugs used to treat rare diseases could be approved based on phase II results also. The development pathway for each drug requires careful planning with input from regulatory agencies.

On 09 July 2012, the US Congress signed the Food and Drug Administration (FDA) Safety and Innovation Act. The Act allows the FDA to designate a drug as a breakthrough therapy if (1) the drug, used alone or in combination with other drugs, is intended to treat a serious or life-threatening disease or condition; and (2) preliminary clinical evidence indicates that the drug may demonstrate substantial improvement over existing therapies on at least one clinically significant endpoint. A manufacturer can submit the breakthrough designation request to the FDA for their drug and the agency has 60 days to grant or deny the request. Once a drug is designated as a breakthrough therapy, the FDA will expedite the development and review of such drug. The breakthrough designation can be withdrawn after granting [6].

Drug development has always been a high-risk enterprise. The success rate of developing an approved drug has decreased in recent years [7-9]. In 2004, the FDA in the United States (US) issued a Critical Path Initiative Document, in which the FDA quoted a "current" success rate of around 8% and a historical success rate of 14% [10]. To help lift the stagnation around drug development, the FDA encouraged innovations in many areas of drug discovery, development, and manufacturing. In the area of clinical development, the FDA encouraged, among several things, more efficient clinical trial designs. While looking for more efficient study designs has always been an area of intense research interest for many scientists, the need to look for new design options has accelerated since 2004. A class of designs beyond the traditional group sequential design has emerged from these efforts. A common feature of these designs is to use interim data of a trial to modify certain aspects of the trial so that the trial can better address the questions it is designed to answer.

In "1.2 Evolution of Clinical Trials and the Emergence of Guidance Documents" on page 4 through "1.5 Widespread Research on Adaptive Designs Since the Turn of the 21st Century" on page 9, we discuss the evolution of clinical trials conducted to evaluate drugs. The evolution began with fixed trials, often done in a single or a few centers, to the more complex multi-center adaptive trials conducted by many manufacturers today. Group sequential design, which is an adaptive design, emerged in the early 70s. As the trial community began to embrace group sequential design in the 80s, researchers also began to develop designs using continual reassessment methods to search for the maximum tolerated dose in phase I cancer trials. Sample size re-estimation, both blinded and unblinded, was developed in the 90s and early part of the 21st century. During the first decade of the 21st century, significant efforts were dedicated to adaptive dose-ranging studies. Many of these designs are discussed in great detail in this book with companion SAS code to assist in their implementation.

As treatment became more personalized, adaptive designs have been proposed to help select the patient population for whom a new drug may be more effective. As better computational tools became more readily available, designs that incorporate information outside of the trial using Bayesian methodology have been explored and implemented. Despite the tremendous progress made over the past three decades, many challenges and opportunities in designing, conducting, and analyzing adaptive trials remain. We discuss some of them in "1.6 Opportunities and Challenges in Designing, Conducting, and Analyzing Adaptive Trials" on page 11.

We conclude this chapter with a discussion of the future adaptive trials to support drug development in "1.7 The Future of Adaptive Trials in Clinical Drug Development" on page 13.

1.2 Evolution of Clinical Trials and the Emergence of Guidance Documents

It took the pharmaceutical industry many years to reach the relatively mature state of drug development today. In 1962, the US Congress passed the Kefauver-Harris (KH) Amendment to the Federal Food, Drug, and Cosmetic Act of 1938 [11]. The amendment required drug manufacturers to prove the effectiveness and safety of their drugs in adequate and well-controlled investigations before receiving marketing approvals. Prior to the amendment, a manufacturer did not have to prove the effectiveness of a drug before marketing it.

It is not hard to imagine what drug manufacturers had to go through to comply with the KH Amendment initially. Thanks to the large polio vaccine trials in the 50s and 60s, the medical community was generally aware of the importance to randomize trial subjects in order to assess the effect of a new treatment against a comparator when the Amendment took effect. Still, the early randomized and controlled trials conducted by manufacturers were relatively simple and often took place in a single center or a few centers. It was not unusual for investigators to analyze data collected at their sites at that time. This practice began to change as drug companies began to employ statisticians in the mid 60s. Industry statisticians were initially hired to develop randomization codes and analyze data. It took several years for industry statisticians to get involved in designing drug trials. All early industry-sponsored trials used fixed designs, meaning that once a trial was started, the trial would continue until the planned number of patients was enrolled. While a trial could be stopped for safety reasons, there was no chance to stop the trial early for efficacy, for futility, or to make modifications to the trial based on unblinded interim results. The concept of a pre-specified statistical analysis plan, signed off prior to database lock, did not exist.

While drug companies took steps to develop infrastructure for adequate and well-controlled trials, the National Institutes of Health (NIH) in the US led the way in increasing the standards for the design and conduct of clinical trials. In the 60s and 70s, the National Heart Institute within the NIH launched several ambitious projects to understand and manage an individual's risk for cardiovascular events. Randomized trials launched for this goal were typically large and required enrollment at multiple sites for the trials to complete within a reasonable time period. This practical need began the era of multi-center trials. Besides recruiting at a faster pace, multi-center trials allowed trial findings to generalize more broadly to the target population because trial results came from many investigators.

Even though the NIH provided oversight to these early multi-center cardiovascular trials sponsored by the Institute, statistical leadership at the NIH realized the need for a more organized way to monitor such trials and to potentially terminate the trials early for non-safety-related reasons. For example, it would be unethical to continue a trial if interim data clearly demonstrated one treatment was much better than the other. The same statistical leaders also recognized that by looking at trial data regularly and allowing the trial to stop early to declare efficacy, one could inflate the overall type I error rate. The above thinking led to the formation of a committee to formally review, at regular intervals, accumulating data on safety, efficacy, and trial conduct. The proposed committee is the forefather of the data monitoring committee (DMC) as it is known today [12]. The experiences led to the Greenberg Report in 1967, which was subsequently published in 1988 [13]. The Greenberg Report discusses the organization, review, and administration of cooperative studies. Another document of historical importance is the report from the Coronary Drug Project Research Group on the practical aspects of decision making in clinical trials [14]. The need to control the overall type I error rate due to multiple testing of the same hypothesis motivated statistical researchers at the NIH and elsewhere to initiate research on methods to control the type I error rate in the presence of interim efficacy analyses.

Pharmaceutical companies began testing cardiovascular drugs and cancer regimens in the late 70s. Following the NIH model, drug companies recruited patients from multiple centers. It did not take long for multi-center trials to become the standard for clinical trials to evaluate drugs in other therapeutic areas also. Furthermore, it was a common practice by the 90s to have a DMC for an industry-sponsored trial with mortality or serious morbidity as the primary endpoint.

Many regulatory guidance documents were issued in the 80s and 90s. For example, the Committee for Proprietary Medicinal Products (CPMP) in Europe issued a guidance entitled "Biostatistical Methodology in Clinical Trials in Applications for Marketing Authorisations for Medicinal Products" (December, 1994). The Japanese Ministry of Health and Welfare issued "Guidelines on the Statistical Analysis of Clinical Studies" (March, 1992). The US FDA issued a guidance entitled "Guideline for the Format and Content of the Clinical and Statistical Sections of a New Drug Application" (July, 1988). To help harmonize the technical requirements for registration of pharmaceuticals for human use worldwide, regulators and representatives from the pharmaceutical industry in Europe, Japan, and the US jointly developed common scientific and technical aspects of drug registration at the beginning of the 90s. The collaboration led to the formation of the International Conference on Harmonisation (ICH) and the publication of many guidance documents on quality, safety, and efficacy pertaining to drug registration. ICH issued a guidance document on statistical principles for clinical trials (ICH E9) for adoption in all ICH regions in 1998 [15]. ICH E9 drew from the respective guidance documents in the three regions mentioned above.

At the time that ICH E9 was issued, group sequential design was the most commonly applied design that included an interim analysis. ICH E9 acknowledges that changes in inclusion and exclusion criteria may result from medical knowledge external of the trial or from interim analyses of the ongoing trial. However, E9 states that changes should be made without breaking the blind and should always be described by a protocol amendment that covers any statistical consequences arising from the changes. E9 also acknowledges the potential need to check the assumptions underlying the original sample size calculation and adjust the sample size if necessary. However, the discussion on sample size adjustment in E9 pertains to blinded sample size adjustment that does not require unblinding treatment information for individual patients.

In 2007, the Committee for Medicinal Products for Human Use (CHMP, previously the CPMP) of the European Medicines Agency published a reflection paper on adaptive designs for confirmatory trials [16]. In 2010, the US FDA issued its own draft guidance on adaptive designs [17]. Both guidances caution about operational bias and adaptation-induced type I error inflation for confirmatory trials. The US draft guidance places adaptive designs into two categories: generally "well-understood" and "less well-understood" designs. "Less well-understood" adaptive designs include dose-selection adaptation, sample size re-estimation based on observed treatment effect, population or endpoint adaptation based on observed treatment effect, adaptation of multiple design features in one study, among others. It has been more than five years since the publication of the draft guidance and much knowledge has been gained on designs originally classified as "less well-understood." As experience accumulates, we expect some of the "less well-understood" designs will become "well-understood".

1.3 Emergence of Group Sequential Designs in the 70s and 80s

While the theory of group sequential design dates back to 1969, actual application began in the 1970s [18,19]. Canner notes the early evolution of applying multiplicity-adjusted analyses along with an external monitoring board in the Coronary Drug Project (CDP) [20]. For the first two years of CDP, investigators were informed of interim data by treatment group. Subsequently, perhaps the first external data and safety monitoring committee (DSMC) was formed to be the only reviewers of data summary by treatment group for the remainder of the trial. This trial also had what we now might call an executive committee (termed the CDP Policy Board then) that was charged with acting on DSMC recommendations. While formal stopping rules were not in place, there was an awareness of multiplicity issues associated with multiple active treatment groups and analyses at multiple time points, which may have resulted in an overall type I error rate on the order of 30% to 35%, if nominal Z-value cutoff for a two-sided significance level of 0.05 had been used repeatedly.

DeMets, Furberg and Friedman note that the Greenberg Report ensured that all cooperative group studies funded by the National Heart Institute and its successors had a separate monitoring committee to review interim results [21, p5]. A commonly cited example is the BHAT trial that began in 1978 and employed an O'Brien-Fleming boundary for group sequential monitoring of efficacy every 6 months [19]. The trial was stopped in 1981 after the O'Brien-Fleming efficacy boundary was crossed at an interim analysis.

Several papers summarize the early data-monitoring practice at one of the National Cancer Institute's cooperative groups, the Southwest Oncology Group (SWOG) [22,23]. They note that prior to 1984, unblinded interim results were routinely shared with study investigators and often published. The philosophy at the time was that those responsible for the study should also be involved in the interim evaluations of safety and efficacy. Cancer researchers felt that the model of independent DMCs used in other NIH institutes was not feasible in trials conducted by the cancer cooperative groups [22]. There were noted examples where interim results were later reversed and situations where studies could not be completed due to the public sharing of interim results. As a result, starting in 1985, SWOG established a formal DMC. While toxicity was still shared with investigators in an unblinded fashion, formal group sequential stopping rules for efficacy were implemented using either Haybittle-Peto or O'Brien-Fleming bounds [24-26]. Interim efficacy results were reviewed by the DMC only.

Jennison and Turnbull provide a brief history of the theory and methods for sequential and group sequential designs, including citations for more complete histories [27, pp 5-11]. They note the work of Pocock as a key motivator for the use of group sequential designs by providing "clear guidelines for the implementation of group sequential designs attaining type I error and power requirements" [28]. The commonly used O'Brien and Fleming stopping rules came shortly thereafter, followed by developments that allow more flexible timing of interim analyses, such as the spending function methods of Lan and DeMets [26,29]. Pampallona and Tsiatis use boundary families to allow early stopping based on futility in demonstrating superiority of a new therapy over a standard [30]. Pampallona, Tsiatis and Kim extend the work of Pampallona and Tsiatis [31].

The 90s also saw aggressive pursuits of drugs to treat patients with the human immunodeficiency virus (HIV). The urgency in developing promising medicines provided a strong incentive for early monitoring of HIV trials for efficacy. This was supported by the cooperative groups and pharmaceutical industry, which was engaged in HIV trials, by patient advocacy groups, and by regulators at the FDA [32]. Finkelstein notes, for example, that the AIDS Clinical Trial Group trial #981 initiated in 1989 applied a one-sided group sequential boundary based on the Lan-DeMets spending function approximation to an O'Brien-Fleming design [33].

One of the authors of this chapter worked at Centocor in the 90s. We share two Centocor development programs as an example to illustrate the move to group sequential design by an industry sponsor. The example highlights the potential perils of inadequate documentation related to interim monitoring and benefits of group sequential design [32]. Both programs were to develop monoclonal antibodies to treat conditions that had irreversible consequences for patients. The conditions had few treatment options and, therefore, represented an urgent unmet medical need. As such, studies that investigated new treatment options merited interim monitoring to determine when study objectives had been achieved or if risk was excessive. In a first pivotal trial for one program, FDA reviewers felt that the company had not adequately documented that an interim change in the statistical analysis plan was made without incorporating information from unblinded interim results and, therefore, asked the company to perform a second pivotal trial. The second pivotal trial was unsuccessful when excess mortality was demonstrated at its first interim analysis. In a subsequent program, group sequential designs were incorporated into trials studying the effect of abciximab (a potent platelet inhibitor) to prevent acute ischemic events in patients undergoing coronary interventions. Three trials (EPIC, EPILOG, and CAPTURE) were conducted in the abciximab program. Both EPIC and EPILOG compared two abciximab-containing treatments to a standard therapy while CAPTURE was a two-arm trial [34-36]. The treatment regimens studied, particularly in the first trial (EPIC), had the potential for both substantial efficacy and substantial risk and thus merited interim monitoring for both safety and efficacy. EPIC proceeded past interim analyses and demonstrated efficacy at the final analysis. EPILOG and CAPTURE were stopped early due to demonstrated efficacy at interim analyses. These trials were all performed as industry collaborations with academic research organizations who were experienced in randomized clinical trials. All trials used independent external DMCs. Innovations to accommodate comparisons of multiple experimental arms were achieved with modifications of the freely available FORTRAN programs from the University of Wisconsin [37].

Many statisticians found career opportunities in the pharmaceutical industry in the 90s. The influx of statisticians to the industry greatly expanded in-house statistical support to clinical trials. Statisticians' presence and the establishment of ICH helped increase the rigor of industry-sponsored clinical trials. In addition to contributing to the design, conduct, analysis, and interpretation of clinical trials, pharmaceutical statisticians also engaged in methodology research to help make the drug development process more efficient.

Group sequential designs are covered extensively in Chapter 2.

1.4 Emergence of Adaptive Designs in the 90s

Sequential and group sequential designs are a special kind of adaptive designs. While group sequential designs originated in the 60s, one can probably credit Bauer's work as the origin of what some refer to today as adaptive design [38]. Bauer first described sample size adaptation based on results of an unblinded interim analysis [38]. Bauer and coauthors gave a historical overview of the history of confirmatory adaptive designs over the 25 years since 1989 [39]. They describe the early days of adaptive design research, review the key methodological concepts, and summarize regulatory and industry perspectives on adaptive designs. The overview includes an extensive list of references (178 of them) and discusses the concepts of conditional power, conditional error and combination tests as the cornerstones for many approaches. It concludes with a critical review of how expectations from the beginning of the adaptive design journey were fulfilled, and it discusses potential reasons why the expectations were not fulfilled in some cases. Another good reference for adaptive designs is the book edited by He, Pinheiro and Kuznetsova [40].

Major reasons for adaptations include: (1) adapting sample size because of uncertainties concerning design parameters (variability, background rate, treatment effect) at the planning stage; (2) choosing among multiple possible treatments; and (3) adapting to a subpopulation where study treatment is the most effective. Choosing among treatments includes selecting doses in dose-finding studies and selecting among different treatment regimens. Both types of treatment selection are covered in this book.

Initial research on adaptive designs focused heavily on modifying sample size of a clinical trial. Sample size adaptation is discussed in great detail in Chapter 3. Early methods use conditional power [38,41,42]. These approaches led to discussions regarding design efficiency, which in turn led to improvements such as the promising zone design [43,44]. While there are other techniques for sample size adaptation, not all of them have received the same level of software support as have methods based on conditional error/combination tests. Examples include optimized sample size adaptation methods [45-48].

One approach is to use information-based group sequential design to adapt sample size [49]. Wan and coauthors suggest a relatively efficient sample size adaptation allowing only one alternative sample size in order to limit potential reverse engineering that could produce an estimate for the interim treatment effect [48,50]. This strategy is implemented using the promising zone code of Chapter 3 by setting the conditional power needed to adapt very high and setting an appropriate maximum sample size.

Another class of adaptive methods that emerged early focuses on response-based adaptive randomization. Response-based adaptive randomizations such as play-the-winner or randomized play-the-winner were proposed as early as the 60s and 70s

[51,52]. This class of adaptive randomization is discussed in Chapters 9 and 10. As noted by the authors for those two chapters, response-based adaptive randomization can be particularly valuable in studies where patients have a high risk of significant short-term outcomes, allowing a study to focus on the most effective treatments. While Chapter 10 focuses on binary outcomes, it references the broader applications of adaptive randomizations in the monograph by Hu and Rosenberger [53].

1.5 Widespread Research on Adaptive Designs Since the Turn of the 21st Century

1.5.1 Early Phase Oncology Designs

For many oncology development programs, the first clinical trials in humans are in cancer patients with a primary objective to estimate the maximum tolerated dose (MTD). A review paper by Le Tourneau et al. provides an overview of dose escalation methods for phase I oncology trials [54]. A 3+3 design has traditionally been used and continues to be used to estimate the MTD by some sponsors. A 3+3 design tests 3 patients at a dose initially. If none of the 3 patients has what is referred to as a dose limiting toxicity (DLT), the next higher dose will be studied. If 2 or more out of 3 patients have a DLT, the dose is considered toxic and will be excluded from further consideration. If 1 out of the first 3 patients at a dose has a DLT, another 3 patients will be enrolled at the same dose. If no more patients among the new cohort have the DLT, the dose is considered tolerable and the study can escalate to the next dose. Otherwise, the dose is considered intolerable and will be excluded. Once an intolerable dose is identified, if the dose below it has only been studied in 3 patients, another 3 will be given the same dose. If more than 1 patient has a DLT, then the dose is considered toxic and excluded. The maximum tolerated dose is the highest dose studied that was not discontinued per the algorithm above. Once an MTD is determined, some trials employing the 3+3 design will enroll additional patients (e.g. 12 or 24) at the MTD to investigate early signs of efficacy. Dose-escalation under the 3+3 design algorithm, while safe, often escalates through doses slowly and could be ineffective in finding an MTD.

One popular approach that has been proposed to improve upon the algorithm-based 3+3 design is the continual reassessment method (CRM) [55]. This approach is covered in Chapter 5 with further developments and SAS programs to support implementation. CRM is a Bayesian dose-finding method that adapts the up-and-down dose selection during a trial based on a modeled dose-toxicity curve. Another alternative to the 3+3 design is the modified toxicity profile interval proposed by Ji at al. [56]. The latter makes dose adjustments based on a table that can be generated at the beginning of the study according to a specified target DLT rate. The dose adjustment decisions have been implemented in Excel by Ji and coauthors.

1.5.2 Multiplicity in Adaptive Designs

Multiplicity arises frequently in multi-stage trials when conclusions may be based on interim data. For confirmatory trials, it is important to strongly control the overall type I error rate over multiple hypotheses tested or the number of times a hypothesis is tested. While solutions to some of these problems appeared in the 80s and 90s [27,Ch 15 and 16], a simple way to consider this for group sequential trials is to use a generalization of graphical methods for strong type I error control [57]. The graphical approach has also been extended to adaptive group sequential designs in Sugitani, Bretz, and Maurer [58].

Multiplicity also arises when researchers attempt to identify a subpopulation that experiences a better response (or experiences less side effects) to a treatment. Subpopulations could be defined by disease state at baseline or by a proteomic or genetic biomarker. Chapter 11 offers an extensive literature review on population enrichment designs and discusses enrichment strategies from a frequentist, Bayesian or a frequentist-Bayesian hybrid perspective.

1.5.3 Formation of the Adaptive Design Working Group

The intense interest in adaptive designs during the first decade of the 21st century motivated the formation of an Adaptive Designs Working Group (ADWG) in the spring of 2005 [59]. This was a collaboration that included contributions from industry, academia and regulatory authorities. Other than the group sequential design, adaptive design was still a relatively new concept for many drug companies at that time. Operational support such as randomization and drug supply management to support adaptive trials was not available in many organizations then. Furthermore, regulatory acceptance of the new adaptive designs was generally unknown. The objectives of the ADWG were to foster and facilitate wider usage and regulatory acceptance of properly designed and executed adaptive trials to support product development through a fact-based evaluation of the benefits and challenges associated with these designs [60]. The Group was initially sponsored by the Pharmaceutical Research and Manufacturers of America (PhRMA). In order to address the many aspects related to the design and implementation of adaptive trials, ADWG initiated many workstreams to kick off a broad range of activities. The activities included sponsoring workshops, giving short courses, and publishing research and consensus papers. A workstream on regulatory interactions reached out to regulators to discuss best adaptive design practice and share experience from implementing such designs [61]. A seminal white paper on best practice for adaptive trials was published by the Group in 2009 [62]. Workstreams that completed their objectives were sunset. New workstreams were initiated to tackle emerging issues.

The sponsorship for ADWG was officially transitioned from PhRMA to the Drug Information Association (DIA) in 2010. The name of the group was changed to the Adaptive Design Scientific Working Group (ADSWG) with expanded membership.

Because new investigators continue to join the clinical trial community, there is always a need to offer education and training. A long-running education and training activity of the Group is a monthly key opinion leader lecture series. The lecture series is free to all who are interested in adaptive designs. Early lectures focused on the theory underlying adaptive designs. Over time, the lectures expanded to practice and lessons learned from implementation. Some lectures focused on adaptive trials that were used to support regulatory submissions. A recurring theme is the importance of thorough upfront planning required of adaptive trials. The lecture series was still ongoing in October 2015 when this chapter went into printing.

1.5.4 Opportunities in the Learning Phase

An equally influential working group formed about the same time as the ADWG was the Adaptive Dose Ranging Studies Working Group (ADRS WG), again under the auspices of PhRMA. ADRS WG focused on the quantitative evaluation of adaptive designs and model-based methods for estimating dose-response relationships. A major objective of ADRS WG was to recommend when adaptive dose-ranging studies could be used and how much benefit they could be expected to bring. A series of white papers was published by the ADRS WG including [4, 63]. Major recommendations from the Group include the need to place dose selection in the broader context of the overall development program, and not restrict it to only the phase IIB stage. In addition, the WG recommends evaluating the impact of the choice of dose-ranging design and analysis on the probability of success (PoS) of phase III and, ultimately, the expected net present value of a drug candidate. The ADRS WG was merged with the DIA ADSWG in early 2010. The work by the ADRS WG and continuing work by researchers on dose-response studies reminds researchers of the many opportunities to improve on how we design and analyze dose-response studies.

Thomas et al. analyzed dose-response studies conducted by a large pharmaceutical company for small molecules over a 10-year period (1998-2009) [64]. They also examined dose-response studies conducted by other drug companies [65]. They concluded that the dosing range and the number of doses tested were generally inadequate to characterize the dose-response relationship appropriately. They found that more than half of the studies they examined had a dose range (maximum dose divided by the minimum dose) less than 20. In many cases, lower doses were omitted from the original studies, causing the need for additional dose-response studies before phase III or a marketed dose to be lowered after product launch. Thomas et al. consider dose ranges less than 20-fold dubious to estimate parameters of the E_{max} model, the dose-response curve most commonly observed to fit the data. A dose range close to 100-fold would be more appropriate, in their opinion.

Dose-response is a critical stage in drug development. Getting the dose right at this stage critically impacts the chance of success in the confirmatory stage. Some simple adaptations at this stage could be useful [66]. For example, trialists could add a lower dose or a higher dose after an interim analysis. They could add a dose that is between two doses already included in the study to better estimate the sharpest part of a dose-response curve. These types of simple adaptations could help us better estimate the dose-response curve and select a dose or doses for phase III trials if the development program moves into the confirmatory phase.

More general dose-finding designs for studies outside of oncology are considered in Chapter 6 from the classical dose-finding perspective. Chapters 7 and 8 cover flexible modeling approaches.

1.5.5 Software

Since the objective of this book is to provide information as well as implementation of design and analysis of clinical trials using SAS, many SAS programs are included in this book. One other important SAS reference for adaptive design has been recently updated [67]. Chang provides some guidance on available SAS software for adaptive design (e.g., `seqdesign` and `seqtest`) as well as providing macros for many other types of adaptive designs. A good summary of other available adaptive design software can be found in Tymofyeyev [68].

1.6 Opportunities and Challenges in Designing, Conducting, and Analyzing Adaptive Trials

1.6.1 Logistics in Trial Execution

Implementing an adaptive trial requires operational support on many fronts. These include a versatile randomization system, nimble drug supply management, data monitoring support, timely access to fit-for-use data, process and documentation control. A detailed document that describes the rationale and execution of the pre-planned adaptations should be prepared in advance. The document should also describe the interim analysis plan including who will conduct the interim analysis and whether an internal or external DMC will review the interim data. For confirmatory trials, access to interim results by the sponsor should be strictly controlled. If sponsor access is foreseen as a possibility for unique circumstances, the interim plan should describe in detail who within the sponsor may have access and under what circumstances. The plan should describe steps taken to prevent additional access of information within the sponsor organization. If sponsor access did occur, it should be clearly documented in the clinical study report. In the latter case, the clinical study report should discuss steps taken to minimize potential bias that may be introduced to the trial as a result of sponsor's access to interim data.

In general, interim analysis should be conducted by a statistician independent of the study team, or by a statistician who is a member of the DMC for the study. The detailed document mentioned above should be endorsed by the DMC. When recommendations requiring actions for a confirmatory study arise, final decisions on actions are often made by the trial's executive (or steering) committee that normally includes sponsor representatives. Antonijevic et al. recommend that a single DMC with all necessary expertise be convened to monitor and execute the pre-planned adaptation(s) [69]. In other words, they advise against having a separate monitoring committee whose sole responsibility is to look after the implementation of pre-planned adaptations.

One key challenge in implementing adaptive trials is the management of drug supply if adaptions result in drug supply change. A member from the drug supply organization should be part of the clinical team that plans an adaptive trial. Manufacturing of clinical study supplies, especially when they need to be matched or blinded, is costly and can be resource intensive. In addition to upfront costs, issues such as expiry dates for existing drug must be considered. Therefore, it is important to get drug supply personnel involved in the planning of an adaptive trial as early as possible. The extent that drug supply and associated allocation (randomization) procedures can accommodate design changes is an important factor when considering an adaptive design.

Adaptive design requires timely access to fit-for-use data for interim decisions. If time-to-event endpoint requires adjudication, adjudication on the number of events required for the interim analysis needs to take place prior to the planned interim analysis. Failure in timely access to fit-for-use data could compromise the effectiveness of an adaptation plan. However, we want to point out that the need for fit-to-use data for interim analysis for an adaptive trial is the same as that needed for a trial using a traditional group sequential design.

1.6.2 Open Research Questions

There are many opportunities for continuous improvement to increase the value and acceptance of adaptive design in the next two decades. We cite 4 as examples below.

1. Statisticians have generally solved the problem of controlling the overall type I error rate for confirmatory adaptive trials although debates continue on whether simulations can sufficiently demonstrate type I error control. The challenge of estimating treatment effect in the presence of adaptations, on the other hand, remains a research question for some designs such as the promising zone design.
2. Statisticians should help set the right mindset about adaptive designs through education and training. There are many occasions when a classic fixed design is the best choice for a situation. Statisticians should work with internal and external decision makers to help lead the discussion on what are appropriate design options for a particular situation.
3. Statisticians need to be aware of the operational support needed to implement an adaptive trial. If the design is too complicated or if the infrastructure needed to support its implementation is not available, a team needs to consider carefully

whether an adaptive trial is a good choice even if the planned adaptations can result in some benefit.

4. Statisticians need to remember the assumptions underlying adaptive designs. For example, the assumption of a stationary population is critical for an adaptive trial. If some of the fundamental assumptions are in question, one needs to think hard about whether an adaptive design is appropriate for a situation.

1.7 The Future of Adaptive Trials in Clinical Drug Development

A recent study released by the Tuft's Center for the Study of Drug Development suggests that the average pre-tax industry cost to bring a new medicine to market is now around $2.56 billion USD [70]. The study included 106 investigational new drugs from 10 mid- to large-size pharmaceutical companies and the drugs were first tested in humans during 1995-2007. Cost included clinical development up to 2013. By comparison, in 2003, the cost was about $1.04 billion in the 2013 dollars.

DiMasi stated that the higher cost comes from clinical trials that are larger and more complex. In our opinion, some of the higher costs also resulted from increased regulations [70]. For example, since the FDA issued a guidance document on evaluating cardiovascular risk in new antidiabetic therapies to treat Type 2 diabetes mellitus (T2DM) in December 2008, all new drugs for T2DM approved since 2008 have been or are being evaluated in cardiovascular outcome trials [71]. In the context of these large cardiovascular trials for T2DM, Chapter 4 utilizes Bayesian methodologies to take advantage of historical information to improve trial efficiency. These outcome trials enroll thousands, if not tens of thousands, of diabetic patients who are at an increased risk for cardiovascular events. Despite the new requirement, manufacturers continue to pursue anti-diabetes drugs because as Gregg et al. predicted, lifetime risk of diagnosed diabetes from age 20 years onward is about 40%, nearly doubling the risk of those born a decade or so earlier [72]. Another factor contributing to the higher cost is a higher failure rate during the clinical development phase in recent years. For example, there has been no drug approved for Alzheimer's disease (AD) in the US since 2003 when memantine was last approved [73]. Decades of investment in AD drugs by many companies, either as symptomatic cognitive enhancing or disease-modifying agents, have failed to produce a single new approved product or a new product close to be approved as of 2015.

While drug developers have always been aware of the high risk associated with drug development, the substantial increase in development cost has begun to change the business operating models for the industry. In recent years, there has been a strategic move towards co-development between pharmaceutical companies, or to share financial burdens for product development between the private and public sectors. The high cost has also motivated many companies to look for data-driven quantitative approaches to make better decisions so that if a development program is to fail, it can be terminated earlier and more efficiently. This new direction will further increase interest in adaptive trials.

Against the backdrop of high cost for large development programs, there is also a shift for industry to invest more heavily in precision medicine or medicines for rare diseases. In 2014, the FDA approved 41 new molecular entities for marketing. According to Gulfo of Breakthrough Medical Innovations, 40% of the new molecular entities approved are for rare diseases, underscoring the industry's shift to niche products [74]. There are several reasons for this shift. First, a large number of products that are highly effective in treating common disorders (e.g. high cholesterol, high blood pressure, CNS disorders) have become generic in the past decade. It is hard to demonstrate extra value beyond what the now generic products could offer. On the other hand, value proposition is easier for rare diseases, which have received less attention in the past and continue to represent unmet medical needs. The smaller patient populations afflicted with rare diseases require out-of-box thinking and nimble applications of innovative approaches to clinical development. Carefully planned adaptive design serves this need nicely.

Another emerging trend is the use of a platform (umbrella) trial to screen multiple product candidates in a single trial. This is in contrast to traditional trials that typically investigate a new treatment (with multiple doses in some cases) in a generally homogeneous population. A platform trial could be used to investigate a product in patients with different genotypes or phenotypes (enriched subpopulations), or could also be used to investigate different treatments in one population. A more sophisticated platform trial could study multiple treatments in multiple enriched patient subpopulations. Interim analyses are conducted in platform trials to decide if a particular treatment (together with a subpopulation in some cases) could be graduated from the trial and further investigated in a confirmatory setting. Alternatively, a treatment could be dropped from the trial and a new treatment added to the trial, continuing the trial beyond the original set of treatments. Platform trials that allow the introduction of new treatments are sometimes called perpetual trials for this reason. Platform trials are also called "master protocol" trials because one protocol governs the testing of many drugs.

A well-known platform trial in the oncology area is the I-SPY 2 trial [75]. This is a phase II neoadjuvant trial for women with large primary cancers of the breast. Breast tumor is characterized by its response to three receptors (estrogen, progesterone, and HER2), resulting in 8 tumor signatures. The trial investigates multiple regimens that include investigational products from pharmaceutical companies. The primary endpoint is pathologic complete response at 6 months after treatment initiation. Within each tumor signature, adaptive randomization to regimens is employed. The trial may graduate or terminate a regimen according to a pre-specified rule based on an interim Bayesian prediction of phase III success probability for a (regimen, signature) combination. If the regimen remains in the trial after the interim decision, assignment to that regimen will continue but be capped at a pre-specified maximum number. One major advantage of a trial like I-SPY 2 is the ability to learn during the trial on what regimen benefits which patient subpopulation, and learn this by borrowing information from other (regimen, signature) combinations.

Another example is the lung-MAP (lung master protocol) trial, a multi-arm, biomarker-driven clinical trial for patients with advanced squamous cell lung cancer that was initiated in June 2014 [76]. Lung-MAP is a public-private collaboration. Lung-MAP plans to initially test five experimental drugs—four targeted therapies and an anti-PD-L1 immunotherapy. Patients will be screened for over 200 cancer-related genes for genomic alterations. The results of the test will be used to assign each patient to the trial arm that is best matched to their tumor's genomic profile. The study can test up to 5-7 drugs at one time and can be amended to test additional new drugs as current drugs exit the trial. In addition to the efficiency gain from using the same control group from the design aspect, a trial using a master protocol takes advantage of existing infrastructure and patient outreach efforts on the operational side.

The potential value of platform trials is not limited to the oncology area. Across the globe, the pace of development of new antibiotic products has slowed noticeably from its peak in the 80s, creating a public health crisis with the rapid development of drug-resistant bacteria. In the US, the President's Council of Advisors on Science and Technology (2014) published a Report to the President on Combating Antibiotic Resistance in September 2014 [77]. The Report offers practical recommendations to the US Federal government for strengthening the US's ability to combat the rise in antibiotic-resistant bacteria. In the area of clinical trials to test new antibiotics, the Report recommends increasing trial efficiency through improved infrastructure and focusing on patient populations with the most urgent need. On ways to make clinical testing more efficient, the Council suggested the formation of a robust, standing national clinical trials network for antibiotic testing. The recommended action plan for the network includes the development of platform trials for antibiotics, where multiple new agents from different sponsors can be evaluated concurrently. As the utility of platform trials for screening product candidates becomes better understood, we are likely to see more such trials in the future.

Other adaptive designs that have received increasing attention by researchers include sequential multiple assignment randomized trials (SMARTs) and sequential parallel comparison designs (SPCDs) [78, 79]. Both classes of designs involve additional randomizations, based on patients' response following the initial randomization. SPCDs are also viewed as a way to address high placebo response rates in trials involving the central nervous system. SMARTs were originally proposed to increase efficiency in behavior science trials and to investigate optimal treatment strategies, but the concept can be applied to other types of trials as well.

Elsäßer et al. examined 59 scientific advice letters given by the Scientific Advice Working Party (SAWP) of the CHMP that addressed adaptive study designs in phase II and phase III clinical trials between 01 Jan 2007 and 08 May 2012 [80]. According to the authors, the most frequently proposed adaptation was sample size re-estimation, followed by dropping of treatment arms, and population enrichment. Among the 59 proposals, 15 were accepted (25%) and 32 were conditionally accepted (54%) by CHMP/SAWP. Elsäßer and coauthors concluded that despite critical comments in some cases, a majority of the proposed adaptive clinical trials received an overall positive opinion. Among the 41 more recent cases (out of 59) with more information in the advice letters, CHMP/SAWP noted insufficient justifications of the proposed adaptations, type I error rate control, and bias in treatment effect estimate as the most frequent concerns.

By the end of the first decade in the 21st century, there was a wide-spread interest in adaptive trials in the pharmaceutical industry. In an article, Burman and Chuang-Stein asked whether the interest in adaptive designs was a short-lived fascination or a reflection that adaptive designs could become part of the future of clinical research [81]. Since 2009, the clinical trial research community has made tremendous progress in understanding when adaptive trials add value and when they do not. Some hard lessons were learned in the process. We have seen products approved using evidence from pivotal adaptive trials. Some of the adaptive features such as futility analysis and some form of sample size re-estimation have become routine features of many registration trials.

Based on our own experience, we can confidently predict that properly designed and carefully executed adaptive trials that are not overly complicated and fit well in the context of a development program will have a firm place in the clinical research. They will become important tools in our trial design armamentarium as we continue to look for more nimble and efficient strategies to develop new and valued products.

References

1. Pinheiro J. (2014). Session 2 Summary – Designs & Methods. Presentation at the European Medicines Agency/European Federation of Pharmaceutical Industries and Associations workshop on the importance of dose finding and dose selection for the successful development, licensing and lifecycle management of medicinal products. Available at: http://www.ema.europa.eu/docs/en_GB/document_library/Presentation/

2015/01/WC500179787.pdf (http://www.ema.europa.eu/docs/en_GB/document_library/Presentation/2015/01/WC500179787.pdf).

2. Sheiner LB. (1997). Learning versus confirming in clinical drug development. *Clinical Pharmacology & Therapeutics* 61: 275-291.

3. European Medicines Agency. (2014). European Medicines Agency/European Federation of Pharmaceutical Industries and Associations workshop on the importance of dose finding and dose selection for the successful development, licensing and lifecycle management of medicinal products. Available at: http://www.ema.europa.eu/docs/en_GB/document_library/Report/2015/04/WC500185864.pdf (http://www.ema.europa.eu/docs/en_GB/document_library/Report/2015/04/WC500185864.pdf).

4. Pinheiro J, Sax F, Antonijevic Z, Bornkamp B, Bretz F, Chuang-Stein C, Dragalin V, Fardipour P, Gallo P, Gillespie W, Hsu C-H, Miller F, Padmanabhan SK, Patel N, Perevozskaya I, Roy A, Sanil A & Smith JR. (2010). Adaptive and model-based dose-ranging trials: Quantitative evaluation and recommendations (with discussion). *Statistics in Biopharmaceutical Research* 2: 435-454.

5. International Conference on Harmonisation. (1997). E8: General considerations for clinical trials. Available at: http://www.ich.org/fileadmin/Public_Web_Site/ICH_Products/Guidelines/Efficacy/E8/Step4/E8_Guideline.pdf (http://www.ich.org/fileadmin/Public_Web_Site/ICH_Products/Guidelines/Efficacy/E8/Step4/E8_Guideline.pdf).

6. US Food and Drug Administration. (2014). Fact Sheet: Breakthrough Therapies. Available at: http://www.fda.gov/regulatoryinformation/legislation/significantamendmentstothefdcact/fdasia/ucm329491.htm (http://www.fda.gov/regulatoryinformation/legislation/significantamendmentstothefdcact/fdasia/ucm329491.htm) (accessed 9 Oct. 2015).

7. DiMasi JA, Hansen RW & Grabowski HG. (2003). The price of innovation: new estimates of drug development costs. *Journal of Health Economics* 22: 151-85.

8. DiMasi JA, Feldman L, Seckler A & Wilson A. (2010). Trends in risks associated with new drug development: success rates for investigational drugs. *Clinical Pharmacology & Therapeutics* 87: 272-277.

9. DiMasi JA, Reichert M, Feldman L & Malins A. (2013). Clinical approval success rates for investigational cancer drugs. *Clinical Pharmacology & Therapeutics* 94: 329-335

10. US Food and Drug Administration. (2004). Innovation or stagnation: Challenge and opportunity on the critical path to new medical products. Available at: http://www.fda.gov/ScienceResearch/SpecialTopics/CriticalPathInitiative/CriticalPathOpportunitiesReports/ucm077262.htm#fig3 (http://www.fda.gov/ScienceResearch/SpecialTopics/CriticalPathInitiative/CriticalPathOpportunitiesReports/ucm077262.htm#fig3).

11. Krantz JC. (1966). New drugs and the Kefauver-Harris amendment. *Journal of New Drugs* 6: 77-79.

12. Ellenberg S, Fleming T & DeMets D. (2002). *Data Monitoring Committees in Clinical Trials: A Practical Perspective*. Chichester, England: John Wiley & Sons.

13. Greenberg Report. (1988). Organization, review, and administration of cooperative studies. *Controlled Clinical Trials* 9: 137–148.

14. Coronary Drug Project Research Group. (1981). Practical aspects of decision making in clinical trials: the Coronary Drug Project as a case study. *Control Clinical Trials* 1: 363-376.

15. International Conference on Harmonisation. (1998). E9: Statistical principles for clinical trials. Available at: http://www.ich.org/fileadmin/Public_Web_Site/ICH_Products/Guidelines/Efficacy/E9/Step4/E9_Guideline.pdf (http://www.ich.org/fileadmin/Public_Web_Site/ICH_Products/Guidelines/Efficacy/E9/Step4/E9_Guideline.pdf).

16. Committee for Medicinal Products for Human Use. (2007). Reflection paper on methodological issues in confirmatory clinical trials planned with an adaptive design. Available at: http://www.ema.europa.eu/docs/en_GB/document_library/Scientific_guideline/2009/09/WC500003616.pdf (http://www.ema.europa.eu/docs/en_GB/document_library/Scientific_guideline/2009/09/WC500003616.pdf).

17. US Food and Drug Administration. (2010). Draft guidance for industry: Adaptive design clinical trials for drugs and biologics. Available at: http://www.fda.gov/downloads/Drugs/GuidanceComplianceRegulatoryInformation/Guidances/UCM201790.pdf (http://www.fda.gov/downloads/Drugs/GuidanceComplianceRegulatoryInformation/Guidances/UCM201790.pdf).

18. Armitage P, McPherson CK & Rowe BC. (1969). Repeated significance tests on accumulating data. *Journal of the Royal Statistics Society, Series A (Statistics in Society)* 132: 235-244.

19. DeMets DL, Hardy R, Friedman LM & Lan KKG. (1984). Statistical aspects of early termination in the Beta-Blocker Heart Attack Trial. *Controlled Clinical Trials* 5: 362-372.

20. Canner PL. (2006). Breaking new ground: Data monitoring in the Coronary Drug Project. In: DeMets DL, Furberg CD & Friedman LM, eds. *Data Monitoring in Clinical Trials: A Case Studies Approach.* New York: Springer.

21. DeMets DL, Furberg CD & Friedman LM. (2006). *Data Monitoring in Clinical Trials: A Case Studies Approach.* New York, New York: Springer.

22. Green S & Crowley J. (1993). Data monitoring committees for Southwest Oncology Group clinical trials. *Statistics in Medicine* 12: 451-455.

23. Crowley J, Green S, Liu PY & Wolf M. (1994). Data monitoring committees and early stopping guidelines. *Statistics in Medicine* 13: 1391-1399.

24. Haybittle JL. (1971). Repeated assessments of results in clinical trials of cancer treatment. *British Journal of Radiology* 44: 793-797.

25. Peto R, Pike MC, Armitage P, Breslow NE, Cox DR, Howard SV, Mantel N, McPherson K, Peto J & Smith PG. (1976). Design and analysis of randomized clinical trials requiring prolonged observation of each patient: I. Introduction and design. *British Journal of Cancer* 34: 585-612.

26. O'Brien PC & Fleming TR. (1979). A multiple testing procedure for clinical trials. *Biometrika* 35: 549-556.

27. Jennison C & Turnbull BW. (2000). *Group Sequential Methods with Applications to Clinical Trials*. Boca Raton, Florida: Chapman and Hall/CRC.

28. Pocock SJ. (1977). Group sequential methods in the design and analysis of clinical trials. *Biometrika* 64: 191–199.

29. Lan KKG & DeMets DL. (1983). Discrete sequential boundaries for clinical trials. *Biometrika* 70: 659-663.

30. Pampallona S & Tsiatis AA. (1994). Group sequential designs for one-sided and two-sided hypothesis testing with provision for early stopping in favor of the null hypothesis. *Journal of Statistical Planning and Inference* 42: 19-35.

31. Pampallona S, Tsiatis AA & Kim KM. (2001). Interim monitoring of group sequential trials using spending functions for the Type I and Type II error probabilities. *Drug Information Journal* 35: 113-121.

32. Ellenberg SS & Siegel JP. (2006). FDA and clinical trial data monitoring committees. In: DeMets DL, Furberg CD & Friedman LM, eds. *Data Monitoring in Clinical Trials: A Case Studies Approach.* New York: Springer.

33. Finkelstein D. (2006). Data monitoring in the AIDS clinical trials group study #981: Conflicting interim results. In: DeMets DL, Furberg CD & Friedman LM, eds. *Data Monitoring in Clinical Trials: A Case Studies Approach.* New York: Springer.

34. EPIC Investigators. (1994). Use of a monoclonal antibody directed against the platelet glycoprotein IIb/IIIa receptor in high-risk coronary angioplasty. *New England Journal of Medicine* 330: 956-961.

35. EPILOG Investigators. (1997). Platelet glycoprotein IIb/IIIa receptor blockade and low-dose heparin during percutaneous coronary revascularization. *New England Journal of Medicine* 336: 1689-1696.

36. CAPTURE Investigators. (1997). Randomised placebo-controlled trial of abciximab before and during coronary intervention in refractory unstable angina: the CAPTURE study. *Lancet* 349: 1429-1435.

37. Reboussin DM, DeMets DL, Kim KM, Lan KKG. (2000). Computations for group sequential boundaries using the Lan-DeMets spending function method. *Controlled Clinical Trials* 21: 190–207.

38. Bauer P. (1989). Multistage testing with adaptive designs. *Biometrie und Informatik in Medizin und Biologie* 20: 130–148.

39. Bauer P, Bretz F, Dragalin V, König F & Wassmer G. (2015). Twenty-five years of confirmatory adaptive designs: opportunities and pitfalls. *Statistics in Medicine.* Available at: http://onlinelibrary.wiley.com/doi/10.1002/sim.6472/pdf (http://onlinelibrary.wiley.com/doi/10.1002/sim.6472/pdf).

40. He W, Pinheiro J, Kuznetsova OM. (2014). *Practical Considerations for Adaptive Trial Design and Implementation.* New York, New York: Springer.

41. Bauer P & Köhne K. (1994). Evaluation of experiments with adaptive interim analyses. *Biometrics* 50: 1029–1041, correction in (1996). *Biometrics* 52: 380.

42. Proschan MA & Hunsberger SA. (1995). Designed extension of studies based on conditional power. *Biometrics* 51: 1315–1324.

43. Jennison C & Turnbull BW. (2003). Mid-course sample size modification in clinical trials based on the observed treatment effect. *Statistics in Medicine* 22: 971-993.

44. Mehta CR & Pocock SJ. (2011). Adaptive increase in sample size when interim results are promising: A practical guide with examples. *Statistics in Medicine* 30: 3267–3284.

45. Posch M, Bauer P & Brannath W. (2003). Issues in designing flexible trials. *Statistics in Medicine* 22: 953-969.

46. Lokhnygina Y & Tsiatis AA. (2008). Optimal two-stage group-sequential designs. *Journal of Statistical Planning and Inference* 138: 489-499.

47. Schmitz N. (1993). *Optimal Sequentially Planned Decision Procedures. Lecture Notes in Statistics, Volume 79.* New York, New York: Springer.

48. Wan H, Ellenberg S & Anderson KM. (2015). Stepwise two-stage sample size adaptation. *Statistics in Medicine* 34: 27-38.

49. Mehta CR & Tsiatis AA. (2001). Flexible sample size considerations using information-based interim monitoring. *Drug Information Journal* 35: 1095–1112.

50. Ellenberg SS, Golub H & Mehta C. (2006). Preface to proceedings of workshop adaptive clinical trial designs: ready for prime time? *Statistics in Medicine* 25: 3229–3230.

51. Zelen M. (1969). Play the winner rule and the controlled clinical trial. *Journal of the American Statistical Association* 64: 131-146.

52. Wei LJ & Durham S. (1978). The randomized play-the-winner rule in medical trials. *Journal of the American Statistical Association* 73: 840-843.

53. Hu F & Rosenberger WF. (2006). *The Theory of Response Adaptive Randomization in Clinical Trials*. New York, New York: John Wiley & Sons.

54. Le Tourneau C, Lee JJ & Siu LL. (2009). Dose escalation methods in phase I cancer clinical trials. *Journal of the National Cancer Institute* 101: 708-720.

55. O'Quigley J, Pepe M & Fisher L. (1990). Continual reassessment method: A practical design for phase 1 clinical trials in cancer. *Biometrics* 46: 33-48.

56. Ji Y, Liu P, Li Y & Bekele BN. (2010). A modified toxicity probability interval method for dose-finding trials. *Clinical Trials* 7: 653-663.

57. Maurer W & Bretz F. (2013). Multiple testing in group sequential trials using graphical approaches. *Statistics in Biopharmaceutical Research* 5: 311-320.

58. Sugitani T, Bretz F & Maurer W. (2014). A simple and flexible graphical approach for adaptive group-sequential clinical trials. *Journal of Biopharmaceutical Statistics* DOI: 10.1080/10543406.2014.972509.

59. Antonijevic Z, Bolognese J, Burman CF, Chuang-Stein C, Jennison C, Kimber M, Marchenko O, Patel N & Pinheiro J. (2013). A progress report from the DIA Adaptive Program Work Stream. *Biopharmaceutical Report* 20: 3-9.

60. Gallo P, Chuang-Stein C, Dragalin V, Gaydos B, Krams M & Pinheiro J. (2006). Adaptive designs in clinical drug development – An executive summary of the PhRMA Working Group. *Journal of Biopharmaceutical Statistics* 16: 275-283.

61. Chuang-Stein C, Bretz F, Komiyama O & Quinlan J. (2009). Interactions with regulatory agencies to enhance the understanding and acceptance of adaptive designs. A report by members of the PhRMA Adaptive Design Working Group. *Regulatory Focus* 14: 36-42.

62. Gaydos B, Anderson K, Berry D, Burnham N, Chuang-Stein C, Dudinak J, Fardipour P, Gallo P, Givens S, Lewis R, Maca J, Pinheiro J, Pritchett Y & Krams M. (2009). Good practices for adaptive clinical trials in pharmaceutical product development. *Drug Information Journal* 43: 539-556.

63. Bornkamp B, Bretz F, Dmitrienko A, Enas G, Gaydos B, Hsu CH, Koenig F, Krams M, Liu Q, Neuenschwander B, Parke T, Pinheiro J, Roy A, Sax R & Shen F. (2007). Innovative approaches for designing and analyzing adaptive dose-ranging trials (with discussion). *Journal of Biopharmaceutical Statistics* 17: 965–995.

64. Thomas N, Sweeney K & Somayaji V. (2014). Meta-Analysis of clinical dose–response in a large drug development portfolio. *Statistics in Biopharmaceutical Research* 6: 302-317.

65. Thomas N, Roy D, Somayaji V & Sweeney K. (2014). Meta-analyses of clinical dose response. Presentation at the European Medicines Agency/European Federation of Pharmaceutical Industries and Associations workshop on the importance of dose finding and dose selection for the successful development, licensing and lifecycle management of medicinal products. Available at: http://www.ema.europa.eu/docs/

en_GB/document_library/Presentation/2015/01/WC500179795.pdf (http://www.ema.europa.eu/docs/en_GB/document_library/Presentation/2015/01/WC500179795.pdf).

66. Milligan PA, Brown MJ, Marchant B,Martin SW van der Graaf PH, Benson N, Nucci G, Nichols DJ, Boyd RA, Mandema JW, Krishnaswami S, Zwillich S, Gruben D, Anziano RJ, Stock TC & Lalonde RL. (2013). Model-based drug development: A rational approach to efficiently accelerate drug development. *Clinical Pharmacology & Therapeutics* 93: 502-514.

67. Chang M. (2014). *Adaptive Design Theory and Implementation Using SAS and R, Second Edition.* Boca Raton, Florida: CRC Press.

68. Tymofyeyev Y. (2014). A review of available software and capabilities for adaptive designs. In: Weili H, Pinheiro J & Kuznetsova OM, eds. *Practical Considerations for Adaptive Trial Design and Implementation.* New York, New York: Springer.

69. Antonijevic Z, Gallo P, Chuang-Stein C, Dragalin V, Loewy J, Menon S, Miller E, Morgan CC & Sanchez M. (2013). Views on emerging issues pertaining to data monitoring committees for adaptive trials. *Therapeutic Innovation & Regulatory Science* 47: 495-502.

70. DiMasi J. (2014). Cost to develop a drug more than doubles to $2.56 billion. Available at: http://www.bloomberg.com/news/2014-11-18/cost-to-develop-a-drug-more-than-doubles-to-2-56-billion.html (http://www.bloomberg.com/news/2014-11-18/cost-to-develop-a-drug-more-than-doubles-to-2-56-billion.html).

71. U.S. Food and Drug Administration. (2008). Guidance to Industry: Diabetes Mellitus — Evaluating Cardiovascular Risk in New Antidiabetic Therapies to Treat Type 2 Diabetes. Available at: http://www.fda.gov/downloads/Drugs/GuidanceComplianceRegulatoryInformation/Guidances/ucm071627.pdf (http://www.fda.gov/downloads/Drugs/GuidanceComplianceRegulatoryInformation/Guidances/ucm071627.pdf).

72. Gregg EW, Zhuo X, Cheng YJ, Albright AL, Venkat Narayan KM & Thompson TJ. (2014). Trends in lifetime risk and years of life lost due to diabetes in the USA, 1985–2011: a modelling study. *The Lancet Diabetes & Endocrinology* 2: 867-874.

73. Cummings JL, Morstorf T, and Zhong K. (2014). Alzheimer's disease drug-development pipeline: few candidates, frequent failures. *Alzheimer's Research & Therapy* 6:37. Available at: http://alzres.com/content/6/4/37 (http://alzres.com/content/6/4/37).

74. Gulfo JV. (2015, January 8). FDA 2014 approvals – the message behind the numbers. The Hill. Available at: http://thehill.com/blogs/congress-blog/healthcare/228803-fda-2014-approvals-the-message-behind-the-numbers (http://thehill.com/blogs/congress-blog/healthcare/228803-fda-2014-approvals-the-message-behind-the-numbers).

75. Barker AD, Sigman CC, Kelloff GJ, Hylton NM, Berry DA & Esserman LJ. (2009). I-SPY 2: An adaptive breast cancer trial design in the setting of neoadjuvant chemotherapy. *Clinical Pharmacology & Therapeutics* 86: 97-100.

76. NCI Press Release. (2014, June 16). Lung-MAP launches: First precision medicine trial from national clinical trials network. Available at: http://www.cancer.gov/newscenter/newsfromnci/2014/LungMAPlaunch (http://www.cancer.gov/newscenter/newsfromnci/2014/LungMAPlaunch).

77. President's Council of Advisors on Science and Technology. (2014). Report to the President on Combating Antibiotic Resistance. Available at: http://www.whitehouse.gov/sites/default/files/microsites/ostp/PCAST/

pcast_carb_report_sept2014.pdf (http://www.whitehouse.gov/sites/default/files/microsites/ostp/PCAST/pcast_carb_report_sept2014.pdf).

78. Murphy SA, Oslin DW, Rush AJ, Zhu J for MCATS. (2007). Methodological challenges in constructing effective treatment sequences for chronic psychiatric disorders. *Neuropsychopharmacology* 32: 257-262.

79. Ivanova A, Qaqish B & Schoenfeld D. (2011). Optimality, sample size and power calculations for the sequential parallel comparison design. *Statistics in Medicine* 30: 2793-2803.

80. Elsäßer A, Regnstrom J, Vetter T, Koenig F, Hemmings RJ, Greco M, Papaluca-Amati M & Posch M. (2014). Adaptive clinical trial designs for European marketing authorization: a survey of scientific advice letters from the European Medicines Agency. *Trials* 15: 383. Available at http://www.trialsjournal.com/content/15/1/383 (http://www.trialsjournal.com/content/15/1/383).

81. Burman CF & Chuang-Stein C. (2009, May 21). Adaptive designs: A fad or the future of clinical research? Applied Clinical Trials. Available at: http://appliedclinicaltrialsonline.findpharma.com/appliedclinicaltrials/article/articleDetail.jsp?id=598938&sk=&date=&pageID=2 (http://appliedclinicaltrialsonline.findpharma.com/appliedclinicaltrials/article/articleDetail.jsp?id=598938&sk=&date=&pageID=2).

Authors

Christy Chuang-Stein, Chuang-Stein Consulting, Kalamazoo, MI, USA.

Keaven M. Anderson, Executive Director, Late Development Statistics, Merck Research Laboratories, North Wales, PA, USA.

Chapter 2

Designing and Monitoring Group Sequential Clinical Trials

2.1 Introduction

One of the major advances in modern clinical trials is the invention and application of sequential analysis in experimental design. This type of design is often called the group sequential design. A group sequential design consists of multiple stages and employs a repeated significance testing strategy. It is one of the most commonly used adaptive designs. The Encyclopaedic Companion to Medical Statistics [1] defines sequential analysis as "a method allowing hypothesis tests to be conducted on a number of occasions as data accumulate through the course of a trial. A trial monitored in this way is usually called a sequential trial." For example, in a phase III randomized clinical trial that has several stages; an interim analysis is planned at each stage. An interim analysis is an analysis intended to assess the treatment effect with respect to efficacy or safety based on accumulated data at a planned time prior to the completion of a clinical trial. Based on results from the interim analysis, such as when a given test statistic is compared to a given critical boundary, a decision can be made either to stop to reject the null hypothesis of no treatment effect, to accept the null hypothesis, or to continue on to the next stage.

There are three different types of group sequential designs: (1) early efficacy stopping design permitting only early claiming of efficacy, (2) early futility stopping design permitting only claiming of futility, and (3) early efficacy or futility stopping design permitting either an efficacy or futility claim. Based on prior knowledge, if we believe that the test treatment is promising, an early efficacy stopping design should be used. If we are concerned that the test treatment may not work, an early futility stopping design should be employed.

In clinical studies, there is great interest in sequential procedures for ethical, economic, and administrative reasons and the methodology has a role to play in all phases of clinical research. Therefore, this type of trial design is attractive to clinical scientists and researchers because it provides a method to add flexibility to the analysis of ongoing trial data. The most compelling reason for monitoring trial data is that, ethically, it is desirable to terminate or modify a trial when evidence has emerged concerning the particular hypothesis of interest. Armitage [2] argued that ethical considerations demand a trial be stopped as soon as there is clear evidence that one of the treatments is to be preferred and that this leads to the use of a sequential trial. For a trial with a positive result, early stopping ensures that a new drug product can be exploited sooner. If a negative result is indicated, early stopping avoids wasting resources and does not subject patients to inefficacious treatments. Sequential methods typically lead to savings in average sample size, time, and cost compared to a classical design with a fixed sample size. This is especially true if investigators are not certain of the effect size of the new treatment. If the true effect size is in fact larger, early stopping will be desirable; if the true effect size is smaller than expected, the trial may continue or may even stop for early futility.

On the other hand, there are situations when a fixed sample design may be preferred to a group sequential design. In practice, if we have good knowledge regarding the effect size, a classical design with a fixed sample size may be more efficient. In this case, it does not require periodic monitoring and can lighten the administrative burden. Also, in some trials, if safety of the test treatment was not adequately assessed in previous trials, using the group sequential design to stop early for efficacy may lead to insufficient exploration of potential safety concerns. In this case, not only is the safety population too small to answer safety questions, but if secondary outcomes are also important, early stopping for the primary efficacy outcome may not give adequate power for testing these secondary hypotheses. Also, the success of using group sequential methods necessitates that responses on the outcomes be readily measured for decision-making regarding trial termination before the recruitment of the next group of subjects, and so delayed responses may present a challenge to trial monitoring. Last, if obtaining an unbiased estimator of the effect size is one of the objectives, group sequential methods will be inadequate to achieve this goal due to shifting sampling distribution across stages. Therefore, it is important to consider these factors carefully before deciding on adopting the sequential testing approach.

If the group sequential testing strategy is appropriate, it can be executed in two phases - the design phase and the interim monitoring phase. At the design stage, the user specifies the following:

- statistical process generating the data,
- the null and alternative hypotheses being tested,
- the desired type I error,
- the power of the sequential testing procedure,
- the shape parameters for the spending functions of stopping boundaries,
- the planned number of interim looks,
- and the timing of the interim looks.

To facilitate the design, the maximum number of interim looks at the data is pre-specified. At the interim monitoring phase, the interim looks or interim analyses can be conducted at precisely equally spaced intervals or when outcomes of equal number of subjects are ascertained. During the course of a trial, many factors may influence the frequency and timing of interim analyses. If the frequency or timing of the analyses is to be substantially altered from the planned schedule then the designs described above will become inappropriate. There are two distinct approaches to monitoring: continuous and discrete. As an abstract concept, continuous monitoring refers to monitoring the test statistic on a continuous scale as a function of the continuous information fraction. In the context of clinical trial, continuous monitoring means monitoring after observing the outcome of every single subject. In practice, this is seldom performed. Discrete monitoring, however, refers to monitoring after observing the outcomes of a group of subjects. This type of sequential group monitoring is the focus of this chapter.

During the actual conduct of the group sequential trial, one may want to allow for flexibility in the analysis, while maintaining the integrity of the trial as bias may be introduced during interim examinations of accrued data. In this case, the role of a data and safety monitoring board (DSMB) should not be understated. For instance, it may be necessary to set the dates of the interim monitoring looks so as to accommodate the schedule of the DSMB. Typically, the DSMB plans to meet after equal increments of calendar time, which do not necessarily coincide with the information fractions specified at the design stage. Again, it may be necessary to alter the planned number of looks at the data, either for safety reasons or if the accrual assumptions are not met, or for some other administrative reasons. These alterations to the original plan can change the operating characteristics of the study unless suitable adjustments are made in the interim monitoring phase. Therefore, in the interim monitoring phase, adjustments by implementing the error spending function methodology are necessary. In addition, the DSMB can serve to regularly monitor whether the correct study population is being recruited and if blinding among study subjects and personnel is maintained by looking at potential inconsistency throughout the stages. Any negative impact of each interim analysis on the conduct of the trial to the next stages should also be assessed and minimized if continuation is warranted.

In a group sequential design, the control of type I error is of great importance, because repeated significant tests at a fixed level on accumulating data increase the probability of a type I error [3]. Therefore, the same critical value for a fixed sample test cannot be applied to each stage of sequential design. For example, with a fixed-sample two-sided test, the critical values ± 1.96 for a standardized statistic produce a type I error probability level $\alpha = 0.05$. But for a two-sided group sequential test with two equally spaced stages, if the same critical values are used to reject the null hypothesis at these two stages, the type I error probability level is $\alpha = 0.083$, larger than the fixed-sample α.

There are several types of methods for calculating stopping boundary values or critical values. The first type is the fixed boundary shape method which derives boundaries based on specific boundary shapes. Examples of fixed boundary shape methods are the unified family methods and the Haybittle-Peto method. The unified family methods [4] derive boundaries from specified boundary shapes. These methods include the Pocock method [5] and the O'Brien-Fleming (OBF) method [6] as special cases, among others. The Haybittle-Peto method [7, 8] uses a value of 3 for the critical values on the scale of the Z-statistic in interim stages, so the critical value at the final stage is close to the critical value for the fixed-sample design. The second type is the Whitehead method which adjusts boundaries derived for continuous monitoring so that they apply to discrete monitoring [9]. With continuous monitoring, the values for each boundary fall in a straight line when plotted on the score statistic scale. By subtracting the expected overshoot from the continuous boundary, the discrete boundary is derived to obtain the desired type I and type II error probabilities. This approach proposed by Whitehead is also known as the Christmas-tree correction. For a design with early stopping to either reject or accept the null hypothesis, the boundaries form a triangle when plotted on the score statistic scale. Therefore, it is also called the triangular test. The last type is the error (also known as α or β) spending methods. For every sequential design, the type I error α and the type II error β at each stage can be computed from the boundary values. Therefore, reversibly, you can derive the boundary values from specified errors for each stage. The error spending function approach [10] uses error spending functions to specify the errors at each stage for each boundary and then derives the boundary values accordingly. Within each type of method, you can choose approaches that create boundary values that range from conservative stopping boundary values to liberal stopping boundary values at early stages.

The control of type I and II errors is applied rigorously in later phases of clinical development and, hence, most of our examples in this chapter will be in the context of phase II or III trials. Although this methodology has been developed with reference to two-arm clinical trials, it applies with some modifications to the one-sample setting as well. For multi-arm trials in which two or more treatments arms are compared to a common control arm, the two-arm approach to control for multiple looks can still be applied if supplemented by multiple testing procedures (such as Bonferroni or Hochberg) to control for multiple comparisons. A thorough coverage of group sequential methods for clinical trials is offered in the textbook by Jennison and Turnbull, which is an excellent source of in-depth materials on sequential analysis [11]. In addition, Todd also provided a comprehensive 25-year review of the application of sequential methods [12].

In order to illustrate the practical aspects of group sequential methods, this chapter is organized in the following sections. "2.2 Examples of Classical Fixed-Sample Designs" on page 26 presents four examples of typical clinical trials that have used the fixed-sample design to calculate the total sample size. "2.3 Theories of Group Sequential Tests" on page 30 explains the distributional theories of group sequential testing with a focus on normal, binomial, and time-to-event endpoints. "2.4 Types of Stopping Boundaries" on page 37 provides more details on the derivation of stopping boundary values and their properties. Examples in SAS are given throughout this section to illustrate how the fixed sample size scenarios in "2.2 Examples of Classical Fixed-Sample Designs" on page 26 can be redesigned into a group sequential setting. "2.5 Special Issues" on page 66 briefly discusses some special issues in trial monitoring and in analysis following a sequential trial.

2.2 Examples of Classical Fixed-Sample Designs

Before we develop the theories of group sequential procedures in the next section, we will describe four examples of clinical trials that were planned using the classical fixed-sample design. However, these trials can be modified into new designs that use the group sequential methods. Detailed interpretations will accompany programming codes to introduce the different approaches and to compare designs with varying parameters. Readers can adapt these codes to further explore different design specifications.

Example 1: Pravastatin Therapy in Children with Familial Hypercholesterolemia

Familial hypercholesterolemia (FH) is a genetic disorder characterized by high cholesterol levels in the blood, specifically very high levels of low-density lipoprotein cholesterol (LDL-C). LDL-C is an undesirable type of cholesterol and therefore, FH increases the risk of early cardiovascular disease. Accumulation of LDL-C in children with FH leads to deterioration of the vascular morphology and gives rise to increased intima-media thickness (IMT) of the carotid arteries. As a result, myocardial ischemia and coronary artery stenosis have been documented in young adults with this disorder. A clinical trial was designed to answer questions regarding the long-term (2 years) efficacy and safety of a cholesterol-lowering medication, pravastatin [13].

In this clinical trial, children aged between 8 and 18 years with FH were recruited from a medical center. The intervention of interest was pravastatin 20mg taken daily for children younger than 14 years or 40mg taken daily for those who were 14 years or older. This trial was placebo-controlled and double-blinded with children randomized to either pravastatin treatment or placebo. These children were followed regularly over a period of 2 years. The primary outcome was defined as a change from baseline in mean carotid IMT, comparing pravastatin and placebo groups after 2 years follow-up. The alternative hypothesis was that the pravastatin group has a greater mean reduction in carotid IMT from baseline than the placebo group. Under a classical fixed-sample design, assuming equal allocation, we can calculate the sample size per arm as follows:

$$n_T = n_C = \frac{2\left(z_\alpha + z_\beta\right)^2 \sigma^2}{\theta^2} \quad (2.1)$$

where n_T and n_C are the sample sizes for the pravastatin and placebo groups, respectively. z_α is the $(1 - \alpha)100\%$ percentile of the standard normal distribution, and similarly is z_β. The parameter σ is the standard deviation of the primary outcome assumed known for both groups, and θ is the treatment difference in the primary outcome that we are interested in detecting. In this case, we allow a one-sided type I error rate $\alpha = 0.025$ ($z_\alpha = 1.96$) and power of 90% such that $\beta = 0.1$ ($z_\beta = 1.28$). Samples of measurements with and without FH were obtained to provide initial estimates for σ which was 0.045 mm and the treatment difference θ was 0.02mm. Therefore, the sample size per arm to achieve the target statistical power of 90% is $n_T = n_C = 106$. The results of this trial are tabulated in Table 2.1 and Example Code 2.1 below generates the total sample size for this balanced design, using the exact two-sample Student's *t*-test. In SAS, `proc power` adjusts the sample size slightly upward to $n_T = n_C = 108$ to account for the loss of degree of freedom in estimating the standard deviation in the Student's *t*-test.

Example Code 2.1 *Sample Size Calculation for Familial Hypercholesterolemia*

```
proc power;
   twosamplemeans test=diff
   meandiff=0.02 stddev=0.045
   alpha=0.025, sides=1 power=0.9 ntotal=.;
run;
```

Table 2.1 *Results of Familial Hypercholesterolemia Trial for Pravastatin on Carotid IMT*

Treatment Arm	*n*	Mean Change From Baseline, mm	SD	p-value
Pravastatin	104	-0.010	0.048	0.020
Placebo	108	0.005	0.044	---

Example 2: Anti-TNF for Treating Psoriasis

Psoriasis is a skin condition that changes the life cycle of skin cells. It causes cells to build up rapidly on the surface of the skin. The extra skin cells form thick, silvery scales and itchy, dry, red patches that are sometimes painful. The primary goal of treatment is to stop the skin cells from growing so rapidly. Biological products including fully humanized monoclonal antibodies inhibiting tumor necrosis factor have been developed and approved to treat psoriasis. A clinical trial was designed to investigate if an approved biological product is effective specifically in treating psoriasis of the feet and/or hands [14]. The primary efficacy outcome of this randomized, placebo-controlled trial was the response of achieving Physician's Global Assessment of the hands and/or feet (hfPAG) score of "clear" or "almost clear" at week 16. It has been assumed that the expected response rate for the investigational product is 40% but only 7% for placebo. Based on the superiority testing framework and the specification of Fisher's exact test, the sample sizes per arm, under a 2:1 treatment-to-placebo allocation scheme, are n_T = 50 and n_C = 25, achieving a power of 86%, as calculated below in Example Code 2.2 on page 28. The type I error was set as one-sided α=0.025. The results of this psoriasis trial are given in Table 2.2 on page 28.

Example Code 2.2 *Power Calculation for Psoriasis Trial*

```
proc power;
   twosamplefreq test=fisher
   groupproportions=(0.4 0.07) groupns=(50 25)
   alpha=0.025 sides=1 power=.;
run;
```

Table 2.2 *Results of Psoriasis Trial for an Anti-TNF on hfPGA Response*

Treatment Arm	*n*	Proportion of Responders, Week 16	p-value
Anti-TNF	49	31%	0.010
Placebo	23	4%	---

Example 3: mTOR Inhibitor for HER2-Positive Trastuzumab-Resistant Advanced Breast Carcinoma

It has been postulated that drugs that inhibit the mTOR pathway may help advanced progressive HER2-positive breast cancer patients with resistance to trastuzumab. Everolimus, as an mTOR inhibitor, has been shown to potentiate the effect of trastuzumab. Dose response of combining everolimus and trastuzumab was established in a previous phase II study with an estimated 34% clinical complete response [15]. A confirmatory randomized, placebo-controlled trial was designed to test the hypothesis that this combination therapy is indeed efficacious compared to trastuzumab alone [16]. The primary endpoint was locally assessed progression-free survival (PFS), defined as time from randomization to time of first radiologically documented tumor progression or death according to Response Evaluation Criteria In Solid Tumors (RECIST, v1.0). It could be assumed that the median PFS time for the placebo group was 6 months, while that for the treatment group was 8.25 months, about 37.5% improvement. If the trial was designed to have a total follow-up time of 2 years and an accrual time of 1 year, under the assumption of exponential survival curve and specification of log-rank test and equal allocation, the total sample size under a fixed-sample design can be approximated to be N = 508 achieving a power of 90%. The type I error was set at 0.025. Example Code 2.3 on page 28 calculates this sample size. The results of this everolimus combination therapy trial are displayed in Table 2.3 on page 29.

Example Code 2.3 *Sample Size for mTOR Inhibitor Trial*

```
proc power;
   twosamplesurvival test=logrank
```

```
    groupmedsurvtimes=(6 8.25)
    accrualtime=12
    totaltime=24
    power=0.9
    alpha=0.025 sides=1
    ntotal=.;
run;
```

Table 2.3 *Results of Trastuzumab-Resistant Breast Cancer Trial for Everolimus on PFS*

Treatment Arm	***n***	**Median PFS, months**	**HR**	**p-value**
Everolimus + Trastuzumab	284	7.00	0.88	0.0067
Trastuzumab	285	5.87	---	---

Example 4: Non-Insulin Therapy for Type 2 Diabetes Mellitus

In this example, we present some event and sample size calculations for fixed-sample, non-inferiority trials for time-to-event endpoints. This example is motivated by the recent US Food and Drug Administration (FDA) guidance on assessing cardiovascular (CV) risk for therapies used to treat type 2 diabetes mellitus (T2DM) [17]. For non-insulin T2DM therapies, the risk of major adverse cardiovascular events (MACE), which includes CV death, non-fatal myocardial infarction, and non-fatal stroke events, can be assessed in two Stages, as suggested in the guidance document. Here we capitalize "Stage" to distinguish the usage in the T2DM example from the interim analyses or "stages" that are used elsewhere in the chapter. The first Stage is a pre-market evaluation of the novel compound to placebo testing the following Stage 1 hypotheses using all accumulated pre-market trial data:

$$H_{10}\colon \frac{\lambda_T}{\lambda_C} \geq 1.8 \text{ versus } H_{11}\colon \frac{\lambda_T}{\lambda_C} < 1.8 \quad (2.2)$$

where λ_T and λ_C are the hazard rates of MACE for the novel treatment and control arms, respectively. Assuming the new drug application (NDA) is otherwise acceptable, if the CV criterion is met, the sponsor obtains full marketing approval for the new drug. In the second Stage, the sponsor must evaluate the post-marketing criteria testing Stage 2 hypotheses combining new post-market trial data and pre-market data:

$$H_{20}\colon \frac{\lambda_T}{\lambda_C} \geq 1.3 \text{ versus } H_{21}\colon \frac{\lambda_T}{\lambda_C} < 1.3 \quad (2.3)$$

This approach strikes a balance between providing evidence on cardiovascular safety to reassure patients and excessive delay of novel therapies reaching the marketplace. Each Stage is tested at a separate $\alpha = 0.05$, though if the 1.3 criteria is assessed during Stage 1, multiplicity adjustment is required for the α in Stage 2 [18].

`proc power` does not currently support non-inferiority calculations for time-to-event endpoints, but the reader can utilize **`proc seqdesign`** to calculate the number of events for a fixed trial. For Stage 1, we re-write the null hypothesis $H_{10}\colon = -\ln(\lambda_t(e)/\lambda_c(e)) + 0.5878 = -\ln(\theta) + 0.5878 \leq 0$, where $0.5878 = \ln(1.8)$. The corresponding alternative hypothesis becomes $H_{11}\colon -\ln(\theta) + 0.5878 > 0$. **`proc seqdesign`** is then used to determine the number of events for a clinical trial of fixed size (Example Code 2.4), assuming 90% power and two-sided $\alpha = 0.05$ per Stage, and equal allocation patients between the two arms. Only the hazard for the treatment arm needs to be specified in the **hazard** option. Though a two-sided test is implied by the literature, stopping boundaries can be limited to the one-sided case to test $\lambda_t(e)/\lambda_c(e) < 1.8$ by specifying **alt = upper** and **alpha = 0.025**. Running the code below shows that 122 events are required for the trial. Similar calculations can be performed for the Stage 2 hypothesis by replacing 1.8 and 0.5878 with 1.3 and 0.2624, respectively, in Example Code 2.4 on page 30, arriving at 611 events for the trial of fixed size. We illustrate toward the end of "2.4 Types of Stopping Boundaries" on page 37 how to address this trial within a group sequential testing framework.

Example Code 2.4 *Number of Events for Type 2 Diabetes Mellitus*

```
proc seqdesign;
   Stage1_Fixed: design nstages=1 alt=twosided alpha=0.05;
   samplesize model=twosamplesurv(nullhazard=1.8 1.0 hazard=1.0);
run;
```

2.3 Theories of Group Sequential Tests

2.3.1 General Framework

In this section, we define the test statistic to be monitored and specify its distributional properties. This distributional theory is presented first in terms of a general framework which is then applied to studies with normal, binomial, and time-to-failure outcomes.

In the simplest situation, if we consider a two-arm randomized clinical trial comparing a test treatment with a control treatment, we can denote the treatment difference by a parameter θ, which is also sometimes known as the effect metric. Depending on the stochastic model one chooses for the endpoint of interest, the choice of the parameter θ will also be different. For example, if a normal endpoint is considered, then θ represents the difference of means. For a binomial endpoint, θ will be a difference of proportions, a ratio of proportions, an odds ratio, or a log odds ratio. For a survival endpoint, θ may represent a difference of medians, a difference of survival rates for a given time point, a hazard ratio, or a log hazard ratio. In general, we can also consider θ as the coefficient of the treatment effect in a regression model, such as linear regression, logistic regression or Cox proportional hazard models. Further, we assume to design a trial with interim monitoring up to a maximum of J stages and data are analyzed cumulatively at the end of each stage. Therefore, we are collecting sequentially $I_1, I_2, \ldots, I_J$ units of statistical information about θ. Sometimes, I_J is also called the Fisher information at the jth stage. Since I_J is the maximum information that we can obtain from the planned trial, we can also denote the information fraction by $t_j = I_j/I_J$. For normal or binomial endpoint, I_J is proportional to n_j which is the total number of subjects accrued by the jth monitoring stage, and similarly, $t_j = n_j/n_J$. However, for survival endpoint, I_J is approximately proportional to d_j, the total number of events of interest observed by the $H_0: \theta = 0$.th monitoring stage. It is apparent that $H_0: \theta = 0$.. This information fraction is therefore necessarily bounded such that $t_j \in [0, 1]$ during the entire course of the trial.

At each interim monitoring time point, t_j, we can obtain an estimator $\widehat{\theta}(t_j)$ for the effect parameter θ and another estimator $Var\left[\widehat{\theta}(t_j)\right]$ for the variance of $\widehat{\theta}(t_j)$. We assume that the sample size at time point t_j is large enough that these estimators are consistent so that

$$\frac{1}{I_j} \approx Var\left[\hat{\theta}(t_j)\right].$$

If these estimators are maximum likelihood estimators, they are also asymptotically normal and efficient. The estimates produced by most SAS procedures are maximum likelihood estimators and they are efficient. Scharfstein, Tsiatis, and Robins have shown that, under the above conditions, if we are interested in testing the following general hypothesis,

$$H_0\colon \theta = \theta_0,$$

the joint distribution of the Wald statistics

$$Z(t_j) = \frac{\hat{\theta}(t_j) - \theta_0}{\sqrt{Var\left[\hat{\theta}(t_j)\right]}},\ j = 1, \ldots J$$

computed sequentially at information fractions $t_1, t_2, \ldots, t_J$, is asymptotically multivariate normal with

$$E\left[Z(t_j)\right] = \eta\sqrt{t_j},\ Var\left[Z(t_j)\right] = 1$$

and for $t_{j1} < t_{j2}$,

$$Cov\left[Z(t_{j1}),\ Z(t_{j2})\right] = \sqrt{\frac{I_{j1}}{I_{j2}}}$$

where $\eta = (\theta - \theta_0)\sqrt{I_J}$ is known as the drift parameter [19]. In this parameterization, the expectation of the Wald statistic is simply proportional to the square root of the information fraction.

An alternative parameterization is to express the same result in terms of stochastic process increments. We can define

$$S(t_j) = \sqrt{t_j}Z(t_j),$$

then the joint distribution of $\{S(t_1),\ S(t_2),\ \ldots,\ S(t_J)\}$ is asymptotically multivariate normal with

$$E\left[S(t_j)\right] = \eta t_j,\ Var\left[S(t_j)\right] = t_j$$

and for $t_{j1} < t_{j2}$,

$$Cov\left[S(t_{j1}),\ S(t_{j2})\right] = t_{j1}.$$

We can readily see that for $t_{j1} < t_{j2}$, the random variables $S(t_{j1})$ and the increment, $S(t_{j2}) - S(t_{j1})$ are independent.

There are a few important implications following from this result. First, in most clinical trials that use normal, binomial, or survival endpoint, the test statistic $Z(t_j)$ is often utilized. Therefore, by the above theorem, the distributional structure of these test statistics after applying the transformation above is asymptotically the same as $S(t_j)$'s. Therefore, one can construct group sequential stopping boundaries for the $S(t_j)$ stochastic process using the property that the overall probability of crossing a boundary is limited to the desired type I error rate, α, under the null hypothesis $H_0\colon \theta = \theta_0$ or equivalently when $\eta = 0$. These efficacy or rejection boundaries will then be applied to the test statistics developed to monitor trials with normal, binomial, or survival endpoint, or even more general endpoints. More details on boundary construction will be given in "2.4 Types of Stopping Boundaries" on page 37.

Second, having generated the appropriate boundaries, one may compute efficacy boundary crossing probabilities for the stochastic process $S(t_j)$ under the alternative hypothesis $H_1 : \theta = \theta_1$ or equivalently when $\eta = \eta_1$, where $\eta_1 = (\theta_1 - \theta_0)\sqrt{I_J}$. One can, therefore, search for the value of η_1 at which the overall boundary crossing probability equals the desired power, $1 - \beta$. By substituting this value of η_1 into equation

$$I_J = \left[\frac{\eta_1}{\theta_1 - \theta_0}\right]^2,$$

one can estimate I_J and hence n_J, the maximum sample size needed to attain the desired power, $1 - \beta$, at any pre-specified clinically meaningful treatment difference $\theta = \theta_1$.

Third, due to the structure of independent increments for $S(t_j)$'s, it is possible to perform the actual computations that lead to these group sequential stopping boundaries and their crossing probabilities by the technique or recursive integration [3].

We have just developed the general distribution theory which can be applicable to any data generated from any arbitrary probability model in which a single parameter θ characterizes the relationship under investigation. In the following sections, we will consider two-arm randomized clinical trials with normal, binomial, or time-to-event endpoints as examples to illustrate that different models provide us with a test statistic whose distributional structure is asymptotically the same as that of the stochastic process statistic $S(t_j)$. In addition, when testing for superiority of one treatment over the other, it is customary to assume that $\theta_0 = 0$, but when testing for non-inferiority of one treatment to other, θ_0 is often referred to as the non-inferiority margin, usually taking on a negative value.

2.3.2 Normal Endpoint

We can consider a randomized clinical trial designed to compare a test treatment, T, to a standard control treatment, C. The efficacy endpoint of interest is assumed to be a normally distributed random variable, X. For the test treatment, we assume the model for test treatment, $X_T \sim N(\mu_T, \sigma^2)$, and for control treatment, $X_C \sim N(\mu_C, \sigma^2)$, so that they have a common variance. If the investigators are interested in designing this trial as a group sequential trial with J monitoring stages with cumulative samples of $n_1, n_2, \ldots, n_J$ patients, then the information fraction at the end of the jth stage is given by $t_j = n_j/n_J$. If the treatment effect is denoted as

$$\theta = \mu_T - \mu_C.$$

The null hypothesis can be constructed as

$$H_0 : \theta = 0.$$

We want to construct a J-stage group sequential level-α test of H_0 having $1 - \beta$ power at the alternative hypothesis

$$H_1 : \theta = \theta_1.$$

We can let $\bar{X}_T(t_j)$ and $\bar{X}_C(t_j)$ be the sample mean responses of the treatment and control groups, respectively, at time t_j. If we further assume that r is the proportion of sample allocated to treatment T then

$$\hat{\theta}(t_j) = \bar{X}_T(t_j) - \bar{X}_C(t_j)$$

$$Var\left[\hat{\theta}(t_j)\right] = \frac{\sigma^2}{r(1-r)n_j}.$$

Therefore, using the parameterization of stochastic process,

$$S(t_j) = \sqrt{t_j}\frac{\bar{X}_T(t_j) - \bar{X}_C(t_j)}{\sqrt{\frac{\sigma^2}{r(1-r)n_j}}}$$

where $j = 1,2,\ldots,J$, and $S(t_j)$ is distributed as $N(\eta t_j, t_j)$. η is the drift parameter such that $\eta = 0$ under null hypothesis but $\eta = \eta_1$, where $\eta_1 = \theta_1\sqrt{I_J}$ under the alternative hypothesis.

If this trial is a non-inferiority trial, then the null hypothesis is constructed as

$$H_0 : \theta \le \theta_0$$

where θ_0 is the non-inferiority margin. Then, using the same notation, the stochastic process

$$S(t_j) = \sqrt{t_j}\frac{\bar{X}_T(t_j) - \bar{X}_C(t_j) - \theta_0}{\sqrt{\frac{\sigma^2}{r(1-r)n_j}}}$$

follows $N(\eta t_j, t_j)$ with $\eta = 0$ under the null hypothesis but $\eta = \eta_1$ where $\eta_1 = (\theta_1 - \theta_0)\sqrt{I_J}$ under the alternative hypothesis.

In both superiority and non-inferiority testing cases, we can search for the value of η_1 and hence I_J such that the power is $1 - \beta$. From the previous section, we know that

$$n_J = \frac{\sigma^2 I_J}{r(1-r)}.$$

We can use this formula to convert the maximum information I_J needed to achieve a target power into the maximum sample size n_J needed. However, we note that in order to make the translation, we need to know the value of σ^2 which is the nuisance parameter. The value of this nuisance parameter is typically unknown. In practice, we usually replace σ^2 with its sample variance $s^2(t_j)$ at each interim monitoring time point t_j when the endpoint is assumed to be normally distributed. Therefore, we cannot track the path traced by these statistics in the course of a clinical trial, and we cannot know for sure if these statistics have crossed the stopping boundaries. However, under a large sample condition, the operating characteristics of this sequential testing by tracking the modified test statistics will be the same as those that would have been obtained by tracking the original statistics.

2.3.3 Binomial Endpoint

In this section, we consider a randomized clinical trial comparing a test treatment, T, to a standard control treatment, C. We assume that the efficacy endpoint is now a binary response variable, X, which takes on the value of 1 if the response occurs but 0 otherwise, such that $P(X_T = 1) = \pi_T$ and $P(X_C = 1) = \pi_C$ where X_T and X_C are the response variables for the experimental and control treatments, respectively. We want to monitor the trial up to J times after accruing $n_1, n_2, \ldots, n_J$ patients. The information fraction at the jth stage is given by $t_j = n_j/n_J$. We let r be the fraction of subjects allocated to the experimental treatment.

Similarly, we define the treatment effect to be the difference in probabilities

$$\theta = \pi_T - \pi_C .$$

Other parameters such as an odds ratio can also be used and its logarithm (i.e. logit) is usually assumed to be normally distributed when the sample size is sufficiently large. The null hypothesis of interest is

$$H_0 : \theta = 0 .$$

We want to construct a J-stage group sequential level-α test having desired power of $1 - \beta$ at the alternative hypothesis

$$H_1 : \theta = \theta_1$$

We can further let $\hat{\pi}_T(t_j)$ and $\hat{\pi}_C(t_j)$ be the sample means, which are also the maximum likelihood estimators of π_T and π_C respectively, at time t_j such that

$$\hat{\theta}(t_j) = \hat{\pi}_T(t_j) - \hat{\pi}_C(t_j)$$

$$Var\left[\hat{\theta}(t_j)\right] = \frac{\pi_T(1-\pi_T)}{n_j r} + \frac{\pi_C(1-\pi_C)}{n_j(1-r)} .$$

Therefore, the stochastic process statistic

$$S_0(t_j) = \sqrt{t_j}\frac{\hat{\pi}_T(t_j) - \hat{\pi}_C(t_j)}{\sqrt{\frac{\pi_C(1-\pi_C)}{n_j r(1-r)}}}$$

follows $N(0, t_j)$ with independent increments under the null hypothesis. Under the alternative hypothesis, the stochastic process statistic

$$S_1(t_j) = \sqrt{t_j}\frac{\hat{\pi}_T(t_j) - \hat{\pi}_C(t_j)}{\sqrt{\frac{(\pi_C+\theta_1)(1-\pi_C-\theta_1)}{n_j r} + \frac{\pi_C(1-\pi_C)}{n_j(1-r)}}}$$

follows $N(\eta t_j, t_j)$ where $\eta = \theta_1\sqrt{I_J}$ is known as the drift parameter. Similarly, we have

$$n_J = \left\{\frac{(\pi_C+\theta_1)(1-\pi_C-\theta_1)}{r} + \frac{\pi_C(1-\pi_C)}{(1-r)}\right\} I_J$$

and for a given target power, we can search for the value of η_1 and use it to estimate the maximum information I_J needed. Using the above formula, we can find the needed maximum sample size n_J. During the planning stage of the trial, we do not know the true value of π_C which is considered a nuisance parameter. Sometimes, a pilot sample is used to provide an initial estimate of π_C.

Again, if it is a non-inferiority trial design having a non-inferiority margin of θ_0 with sequential monitoring in J stages, the stochastic process statistic will be

$$S_0(t_j) = \sqrt{t_j}\frac{\hat{\pi}_T(t_j) - \hat{\pi}_C(t_j) - \theta_0}{\sqrt{\frac{(\pi_C + \theta_0)(1 - \pi_C - \theta_0)}{n_j r} + \frac{\pi_C(1 - \pi_C)}{n_j(1 - r)}}}$$

following $N(0,\ t_j)$ under the null hypothesis. But, under the alternative hypothesis,

$$S_1(t_j) = \sqrt{t_j}\frac{\hat{\pi}_T(t_j) - \hat{\pi}_C(t_j) - \theta_0}{\sqrt{\frac{(\pi_C + \theta_1)(1 - \pi_C - \theta_1)}{n_j r} + \frac{\pi_C(1 - \pi_C)}{n_j(1 - r)}}}$$

follows $N(\eta t_j, t_j)$ where $\eta = (\theta_1 - \theta_0)\sqrt{I_J}$ is the drift parameter.

2.3.4 Survival Endpoint

Adopting similar notations as in normal and binomial endpoints, we design a sequential trial that uses a time-to-event endpoint and monitor it up to J interim stages. We denote the monitoring calendar times as $c_1, c_2, \ldots, c_J$. At calendar time c_j, we observe f_j failures or events of interest, with their corresponding event times (on patients' follow-up time-scale, not calendar time-scale) denoted by $e_1(c_j), e_2(c_j), \ldots, e_{f_j}(c_j)$.

We further let $d_T(e_i(c_j))$ be the number of events on treatment T and $n_T(e_i(c_j))$ be the number of subjects at risk of failure on the treatment arm T where $i = 1, 2, \ldots, f_j$. As for the control arm, C, $d_C(e_i(c_j))$ and $n_C(e_i(c_j))$ are defined similarly. We also let $d(e_i(c_j)) = d_T(e_i(c_j)) + d_C(e_i(c_j))$ be the total number of events observed in both arms, and $n(e_i(c_j)) = n_T(e_i(c_j)) + n_C(e_i(c_j))$ be the total number of subjects at risk for failure in both arms, all at calendar time c_j.

Then the log-rank score statistic $L(c_j)$, observed at calendar time c_j is given by summing up the observed number of events in treatment arm T minus the expected number of events in treatment arm T, as follows:

$$L(c_j) = -\sum_{i=1}^{f_j}\left\{d_T(e_i(c_j)) - \frac{n_T(e_i(c_j))d(e_i(c_j))}{n(e_i(c_j))}\right\}$$

If treatments T and C have the same underlying distribution, as in null hypothesis, it is well-known [11] that the marginal distribution of $L(c_j)$ is asymptotically normal with a mean of zero and with variance of

$$Var[L(c_j)] = \sum_{i=1}^{f_j}\frac{n_T(e_i(c_j))\,n_C(e_i(c_j))\,d(e_i(c_j))\,[n(e_i(c_j)) - d(e_i(c_j))]}{[n(e_i(c_j))]^2[n(e_i(c_j)) - 1]}.$$

Since this variance term cannot be estimated a priori, we need to make an additional assumption of proportional hazard, that is, if $\lambda_T(e)$ and $\lambda_C(e)$ are the hazard functions for treatment T and C respectively, then the log of ratio of the hazard functions

$$\theta = -\ln\frac{\lambda_T(e)}{\lambda_C(e)}$$

is constant for all values of e. If we let $D(c_j) = \sum_{i=1}^{f_j} d(e_i(c_j))$ be the total number of events observed at calendar time c_j and r be the fraction of patients randomized to treatment T, then $L(c_j)$ is asymptotically normal with the following mean and variance

$$E[L(c_j)] = \theta D(c_j)r(1-r),$$

$$Var[L(c_j)] = D(c_j)r(1-r).$$

It can be shown that the sequential log-rank score statistics, $L(c_1),\ L(c_2),\ \ldots,\ L(c_J)$ have independent increments, that is, if $j_1 < j_2$, then $L(c_{j1})$, and $L(c_{j2}) - L(c_{j1})$ are independent [20].

Similarly, if we define the treatment effect to be the log of ratio of hazard functions above, then the null hypothesis is

$$H_0 : \theta = 0$$

and the alternative hypothesis is

$$H_1 : \theta = \theta_1.$$

Instead of defining the information fraction on sample sizes as before, we define it as the ratio of the total number of events at c_j to that at c_J

$$t_j = \frac{D(c_j)}{D(c_J)}$$

In addition, we have the stochastic increment statistic as

$$S(t_j) = \frac{L(c_j)}{\sqrt{D(c_J)r(1-r)}}$$

and

$$D(c_J) = \frac{I_j}{r(1-r)},$$

such that $S(t_j)$ follows $N(\eta t_j, t_j)$ where $\eta = \theta_1\sqrt{I_J}$ under the alternative hypothesis. Under the null hypothesis, $S(t_j)$ will follow $N(0,\ t_j)$. In trials that use time-to-event outcomes such as progression-free survival (PFS) or overall survival (OS), the maximum number of events $D(c_J)$ is important to the determination the study's statistical power, instead of the maximum sample sizes n_J as in trials using normal or binomial outcome. For more practical details in the theories of sequential testing, readers are encouraged to consult the *SAS/STATUser's Guide* [21] for fuller explanations.

2.4 Types of Stopping Boundaries

2.4.1 Calculation of Stopping Boundaries

We have provided an overview of the distributional theory of sequential testing in the previous section. This section focuses on the calculation of stopping boundaries. Based on the specified hypotheses, stopping boundaries can be either one-sided or two-sided. In addition, depending on the prospective outlook of the trial, investigators can specify if the set of boundaries is to (1) reject the null hypothesis (H_0: $\theta = \theta_0$), (2) reject either the null hypothesis (H_0: $\theta = \theta_0$), or the alternative hypothesis ($H_1 : \theta = \theta_1$), or (3) reject the alternative hypothesis ($H_1 : \theta = \theta_1$) only. In the first case, we call this set of boundaries efficacy boundaries while for the third case, we call it futility boundaries. We can consider planning a clinical trial with a maximum of J monitoring interim stages with information fractions denoted by $t_1, t_2, ..., t_J$. If the sequential testing procedure is set at the desired α-level, then the stopping boundaries should reflect this control of type I error. In addition, if we want to achieve a target power of $1 - \beta$ under the alternative hypothesis ($H_1 : \theta = \theta_1$), then we can find the maximum information needed I_J and hence the maximum sample size n_J or number of events $D(c_J)$ needed.

As we have seen earlier, there are two ways to specify the test statistics, the Wald statistic $Z(t_j)$ or the stochastic process statistic $S(t_j)$. Because of the property of independent increments for the stochastic process statistic $S(t_j)$, it will be easier to illustrate the stopping boundaries using this scale. Since a relationship exists between the two, $S(t_j) = Z(t_j)\sqrt{t_j}$, the corresponding stopping boundaries for the Wald statistics can be easily obtained by appropriate transformations. In the most general form, we know that $S(t_j) \sim N(\eta t_j, t_j)$ where $\eta = (\theta_1 - \theta_0)\sqrt{I_J}$. In the following sections, we will look into three commonly used types of stopping boundaries. They are (1) p-value method, which is also known as the Haybittle-Peto boundaries, (2) unified family (power) methods, which include the Wang-Tsiatis boundaries [22], the Pampallona-Tsiatis boundaries [23], and the triangular method proposed by Kittelson & Emerson [4], and (3) Error Spending methods, which include the Lan-DeMets [10], the Gamma [24] and the Rho [25] boundaries. Brief descriptions of these methods can be found in Table 2.4 on page 38.

As discussed briefly in "2.1 Introduction" on page 23, the choice of boundary calculation method, number of stages, inclusion of futility analysis, etc., should take into account the objectives of the trials, the chosen primary and/or secondary endpoints, the initial assumptions of the effect size, subject recruitment, and others. If the effect size, although uncertain, is expected to be large, a boundary set that favors stopping early can be used, such as the Pocock boundary. If monitoring safety is important, then stopping too early may not be desirable and in such case, fewer stages or boundary options that discourage early stopping, such as the OBF method, can be used. Increasing the number of stages will certainly increase administrative costs and the chances that bias can creep into the trial. Sequential trials with too many stages are therefore not encouraged. When flexibility is needed, the α spending approach allows obvious comparison of the operating characteristics by simply adjusting the parameter of the spending functions. This is often useful when advocating and explaining a proposed group sequential method to the clinical team.

Table 2.4 *Methods of Deriving Stopping Boundaries*

Methods	**Boundaries**	**Descriptions**
P-value	Haybittle-Pelo	This is a type of fixed boundary method that fixes a constant p-value (or critical value) for the first $J - 1$ stages.
Unified Family (Power)	Wang-Tsiatis Pampallona-Tsiatis Triangular Method	These are also types of fixed boundary methods. The Pocock and the OBF methods are special cases of unified family boundaries.
Error Spending	Lan-DeMets Gamma Rho	These methods use a monotonic α spending function defined on the unit interval to control type I error, and/or a monotonic β spending function to simultaneously control type II error.

2.4.2 P-value or Haybittle-Peto Boundaries

The P-value or Haybittle-Peto boundaries are used for early rejection of the null hypothesis. It was first proposed by Haybittle [7]. These boundaries are calculated by pre-specifying a fixed rejection boundary value for the p-value or the Z-statistic for the first $J - 1$ stages. For example, we can specify a very small p-value p_1 for the first $J - 1$ analyses as a stopping criterion. If the first observed p-value in the sequence of the first $J - 1$ p-values appears to be smaller than p_1, then the trial will be stopped to declare rejection of the null hypothesis. Otherwise, the trial will go to the final stage (i.e. Jth stage) and a final p-value, p_2 is computed in such a way that the overall type I error is controlled at the α level. If we denote the upper pth quantile of the standard normal distribution as z_p, then we know $1 - \Phi(z_p) = p$. In the one-sided setting, the trial will be stopped at the jth interim stage if $Z(t_j) \geq z_{p_1}$ or if $(t_j) \geq \sqrt{t_j} z_{p_1}$. Otherwise, the trial can be successful at the final stage only if $Z(t_J) \geq z_{p_2}$ or if $(t_J) \geq \sqrt{t_J} z_{p_2}$. Given the pre-specified p_1, the value of p_2 needs to preserve the type I error and it can be obtained by solving the following equation:

$$1 - P_{\eta = 0}\left(S(t_1) < \sqrt{t_1} z_{p_1}, \ \ldots, \ S(t_{J-1}) < \sqrt{t_{J-1}} z_{p_1}, \ S(t_J) < \sqrt{t_J} z_{p_2}\right) = \alpha$$

where $P_{\eta = 0}(\cdot)$ represents the probability evaluated under the null joint distribution, that is, the distribution when $\eta = 0$. The solution of p_2 can be obtained using a numerical method for recursive integration. Once the value of p_2 is determined, the maximum information I_J needed is obtained by invoking the same numerical method to solve for the drift parameter η_1 in the following equation under the specified target power of $1 - \beta$:

$$P_{\eta = \eta_1}\left(S(t_1) < \sqrt{t_1} z_{p_1}, \ \ldots, \ S(t_{J-1}) < \sqrt{t_{J-1}} z_{p_1}, \ S(t_J) < \sqrt{t_J} z_{p_2}\right) = \beta.$$

Using this value of drift parameter η_1, evaluated under alternative hypothesis, we can evaluate I_J using

$$I_J = \left[\frac{\eta_1}{\theta_1 - \theta_0}\right]^2.$$

In turn, we can estimate the needed maximum sample size n_J if we are using the normal or binomial endpoint, or the maximum number of events $D(c_J)$ for the survival endpoint. In the two-sided hypothesis setting, there are upper and lower rejection boundary values, thus we can simply replace $S(t_j)$ in the above equations with its absolute value $|S(t_j)|$. It can be noted that this p-value method can be generalized to unequal p-values instead of constant p_1 at each of the first $J - 1$ stages.

Example: Redesigning the Familial Hypercholesterolemia Trial Using Haybittle-Peto Method

In SAS, the procedure we use to derive the operating characteristics of group sequential design is **proc seqdesign** and the procedure used to monitor ongoing sequential trial is **proc seqtest**. We will illustrate their applications using the examples discussed in "2.2 Examples of Classical Fixed-Sample Designs" on page 26. Here, we show a simple use of **proc seqdesign** to generate a Haybittle-Peto sequential design as a modified design for the pediatric FH trial.

Example Code 2.5 *Haybittle-Peto Design for Familial Hypercholesterolemia Trial*

```
proc seqdesign altref=0.02 errspend stopprob;
   hpdesignforfh: design nstages=5 method=peto(z=3) alt=upper stop=reject
   alpha=0.025 beta=0.1;
   samplesize model=twosamplemean (stddev=0.045);
run;
```

Example Code 2.5 on page 39 generates a 5-stage design with a user-created label of **hpdesignforfh**. In the **design** statement, we specify the use of the Haybittle-Peto method on the scale of the Z-statistic using **method=peto(z=3)** to set the boundary constant at 3 for the first four stages. This is the default setting. Alternatively, for the example discussed earlier, one can specify a fixed p-value using **method=peto(pvalue=0.001)** to set $p_1 = 0.001$ for the first four stages. The number of stages is indicated using **nstages=5**. The alternative hypothesis is the upper one-sided (**alt=upper**), but if one wants to change it to the default two-sided, then one can leave this out or modify it to **alt=twosided**. This design allows for stopping early only to reject the null hypothesis as indicated in **stop=reject** which is the default setting. This is known as an early stopping for efficacy only type of boundary. If one wants to allow the trial to stop early for efficacy or futility (i.e. to reject or to retain the null hypothesis), then it can be replaced with **stop=both**. The type I error allowable is specified by **alpha=0.025** while type II error is given by **beta=0.1**. The alternative mean difference θ_1 is assumed to be 0.02mm, which is the treatment difference in mean change from baseline in carotid IMT and it is specified in **altref=0.02**. Alternatively, this treatment difference can also be stated as **meandiff=0.02** inside the parentheses in the **samplesize** statement. In this **samplesize** statement, we invoke the **model=twosamplemean** option since we are testing two sample means with assumed common standard deviation of 0.045mm (**stddev=0.045**). The remaining two output options are used to request specific output tables. **stopprob** requests the display of expected stopping stages and cumulative stopping probability to reject the null hypothesis at each stage under various hypothetical treatment effect sizes. In the output below, reference (**CRef**) effect size ranged from zero to 1.5 times the effect size under alternative hypothesis. The **errspend** statement displays the cumulative error spending at each stage. The design is hereby fully specified and the SAS output for this program is shown below.

Figure 2.1 *Output for Example Code 2.5*

The SEQDESIGN Procedure
Design: hpdesignforfh

Design Information	
Statistic Distribution	Normal
Boundary Scale	Standardized Z
Alternative Hypothesis	Upper
Early Stop	Reject Null
Method	Haybittle-Peto
Boundary Key	Both
Alternative Reference	0.02
Number of Stages	5
Alpha	0.025
Beta	0.1
Power	0.9
Max Information (Percent of Fixed Sample)	101.3932
Max Information	26634.54
Null Ref ASN (Percent of Fixed Sample)	101.1638
Alt Ref ASN (Percent of Fixed Sample)	78.75909

Expected Cumulative Stopping Probabilities
Reference = CRef * (Alt Reference)

CRef	Expected Stopping Stage	Source	Stopping Probabilities				
			Stage_1	Stage_2	Stage_3	Stage_4	Stage_5
0.0000	4.989	Reject Null	0.00135	0.00246	0.00337	0.00413	0.02500
0.5000	4.814	Reject Null	0.01160	0.03112	0.05645	0.08639	0.36488
1.0000	3.884	Reject Null	0.06175	0.19161	0.35211	0.51070	0.90000
1.5000	2.504	Reject Null	0.20985	0.55578	0.80410	0.92702	0.99820

Boundary Information (Standardized Z Scale)
Null Reference = 0

Stage	Information Level			Alternative Reference	Boundary Values
					Upper
	Proportion	Actual	N	Upper	Alpha
1	0.2000	5326.909	43.14796	1.45971	3.00000
2	0.4000	10653.82	86.29592	2.06435	3.00000
3	0.6000	15980.73	129.4439	2.52830	3.00000
4	0.8000	21307.64	172.5918	2.91943	3.00000
5	1.0000	26634.54	215.7398	3.26402	1.99005

Error Spending Information

Stage	Information Level	Cumulative Error Spending	
		Upper	
	Proportion	Beta	Alpha
1	0.2000	0.00000	0.00135
2	0.4000	0.00000	0.00246
3	0.6000	0.00000	0.00337
4	0.8000	0.00000	0.00413
5	1.0000	0.10000	0.02500

Sample Sizes (N)
Two-Sample Z Test for Mean Difference

Stage	Fractional N				Ceiling N			
	N	N(Grp 1)	N(Grp 2)	Information	N	N(Grp 1)	N(Grp 2)	Information
1	43.15	21.57	21.57	5326.9	44	22	22	5432.1
2	86.30	43.15	43.15	10653.8	88	44	44	10864.2
3	129.44	64.72	64.72	15980.7	130	65	65	16049.4
4	172.59	86.30	86.30	21307.6	174	87	87	21481.5
5	215.74	107.87	107.87	26634.5	216	108	108	26666.7

The first table in Figure 2.1 on page 41 describes the design aspects of this trial. The maximum information percentage is 101.4% which is also known as the inflation factor, indicating a small 1.4% increase from total sample size N=212 in fixed-sample design (see "2.2 Examples of Classical Fixed-Sample Designs" on page 26) to about N=216 here. It can be noted that **`proc seqdesign`**, unlike **`proc power`**, uses the stated standard deviation as a known parameter in calculating the information without adjustment to loss of degree of freedom. Under the specified alternative hypothesis, the expected sample size in this sequential trial is only 78.8% of the fixed total sample size, due to early stopping for efficacy. The second table (**`StopProb`**) shows the expected cumulative stopping probabilities under four hypothetical true treatment effect scenarios. Parameter **`CRef`** represents a fraction of the originally specified alternative hypothesis effect size (i.e. $\theta_1 = 0.02$). For example, if c = 0 it makes the first scenario $c^*\theta_1 = 0$ identical to the null situation. Under the null scenario, the cumulative stopping probability at the final stage is 0.025. If c = 1.5, it makes $c^*\theta_1 = 0.03$. Under this treatment effect scenario, the design can achieve a cumulative power of greater than 80% (0.8041) as early as at the third stage. In addition, it can be expected under this optimistic alternative situation that the trial can stop at stage 2.5, on average, meaning that this trial is likely to stop before reaching the third stage. The next default table (**`Boundary`**) summarizes the alternative references and boundary values under the default boundary Z scale. The alternative reference (also known as the drift) for the first stage is calculated as T and so on. Using the Haybittle-Peto method, the boundary values of the first four stages are set to a constant at 3 and that for the final stage is 1.99. The next table (**`ErrSpend`**) displays the cumulative error spending by stage under the null hypothesis. The last two tables as requested by the **`samplesize`** statement, show a summary of sample size calculation and the total sample size required rounded up to 216, as well as the cumulative sample size by stage and treatment arm. Saving in patient recruitment occurs if this sequential trial is able to stop early to declare efficacy.

However, a major critique of re-designing this pediatric FH trial into a sequential framework is that it has a long follow-up period of 2 years. It implies that subjects may still be steadily recruited while we wait for the responses of an earlier group of subjects to be measured and analyzed. This happens if the recruitment rate is faster than the rate at which the outcomes are ascertained and this situation is called "overrunning." Unless the recruitment rate is slow, re-designing a trial with a long follow-up period into a sequential trial may not reap additional benefits compared to a fixed-stage design. As a general rule of thumb, if the calculated recruitment period is four times longer than the treatment follow-up period, then a group sequential or adaptive design that has up to four interim stages can be more beneficial.

2.4.3 Unified Family Boundaries

The unified family method is also known as the power method, in which a power or shape parameter ϕ is adjusted. A good example is the Wang-Tsiatis boundaries [22]. This set of boundaries is used for early rejection of the null hypothesis. Generally, on the scale of the score statistic, it takes the following form:

$$c(t_j) = C(\phi,\ \alpha,\ J)t_j^{\phi},$$

for $j = 1, 2, \ldots, J$ and ϕ is a shape parameter that characterizes the boundary shape. $C(\phi,\ \alpha,\ J)$ is a positive constant indexed by ϕ, α, and J. If $\phi = 0$ then we get the OBF [6] stopping boundaries while if $\phi = 0.5$, we yield the Pocock [5] stopping boundaries. For a one-sided setting, the trial stops at the jth interim look if $S(t_j) \geq c(t_j)$. Therefore, in order to preserve the type I error, the boundary set must satisfy the following equation:

$1 - P_0\{\bigcap_{j=1}^{J} S(t_j) < c(t_j)\} = \alpha$. (2.4)

Since the stopping boundaries $c(t_1),\ c(t_2),\ \ldots,\ c(t_J)$ are completely specified by the single constant defined earlier, this constant can then be evaluated by numerical method of recursive integration. Once the boundaries have been determined, the maximum information I_J needed can be estimated. But this time, its corresponding η_1 needs to satisfy the following equation with pre-specified target power of $1 - \beta$:

$P_{\eta_1}\{\bigcap_{j=1}^{J} S(t_j) < c(t_j)\} = \beta$. (2.5)

Using this evaluated drift parameter η_1, we can get the I_J using

$$I_J = \left[\frac{\eta_1}{\theta_1 - \theta_0}\right]^2.$$

With evaluated I_J, we can estimate the needed maximum sample size n_J if we are using the normal or binomial endpoint, but the maximum number of events $D(c_J)$ if survival endpoint. In the two-sided setting, we simply replace $S(t_j)$ in the above equations with $|S(t_j)|$.

On the other hand, the Pampallona-Tsiatis boundaries [23] allow for early rejection of either the null or alternative hypothesis. That means we additionally include the possibility of stopping the trial based on convincing evidence of futility. Therefore, at each of the first $J - 1$ stages, we have two stopping boundaries, the upper stopping boundary for early rejection of the null hypothesis and a lower stopping boundary for early rejection of the alternative hypothesis. In the one-sided setting, we can denote these boundaries as C_U and C_L respectively which satisfy

$$S(t_j) \geq C_U(\phi_U,\ \alpha,\ \beta,\ J)t_j^{\phi_U}$$

$$S(t_j) - \eta t_j < -C_L(\phi_L,\ \alpha,\ \beta,\ J)t_j^{\phi_L}.$$

We emphasize that both C_U and C_L are positive constants, and indexed by shape parameters of ϕ_U and ϕ_L, that may take on different values. We also impose one more constraint

$$C_U(\phi_U,\ \alpha,\ \beta,\ J) = \eta - C_L(\phi_L,\ \alpha,\ \beta,\ J),$$

so that the boundaries at the last interim look at t_J will be the same, thereby ensuring that a decision is made to reject either of the two hypotheses. In order to calculate the stopping boundaries, a numerical method can be applied to solve for the boundary values using a set of two equations

$$P_0(S(t_1) \geq u_1) + P_0(l_1 < S(t_1) < u_1,\ S(t_2) \geq u_2) + \ldots + P_0$$
$$(l_1 < S(t_1) < u_1,\ l_2 < S(t_2) < u_2, \ldots, l_{J-1} < S(t_{J-1}) < u_{J-1},\ S(t_J) \geq u_J) = \alpha$$

$$P_{\eta_1}(S(t_1) \leq l_1) + P_{\eta_1}(l_1 < S(t_1) < u_1,\ S(t_2) \leq l_2) + \ldots + P_{\eta_1}$$
$$(l_1 < S(t_1) < u_1,\ l_2 < S(t_2) < u_2, \ldots, l_{J-1} < S(t_{J-1}) < u_{J-1},\ S(t_J) \leq l_J) = \beta$$

where

$$u_j = C_U(\phi_U,\ \alpha,\ \beta,\ J)t_j^{\phi_U}$$

and

$$l_j = \eta_1 t_j - C_L(\phi_L, \alpha, \beta, J) t_j^{\phi_L}$$

for $j = 1, 2, \ldots, J$. The parameter η_1 is determined simultaneously along with $C_U(\phi_U, \alpha, \beta, J)$ and $C_L(\phi_L, \alpha, \beta, J)$ through the relationship

$$\eta_1 = C_U(\phi_U, \alpha, \beta, J) + C_L(\phi_L, \alpha, \beta, J).$$

Similarly, the maximum information I_J and hence the maximum sample size n_J or the maximum number of events $D(c_J)$ can be estimated accordingly for a given value of η_1. For the two-sided setting, for the rejection of the null hypothesis, the boundaries will be a set of top outer boundaries and bottom outer boundaries, while for the rejection of the alternative hypothesis, the boundaries will be a set of inner wedge boundaries.

Another approach that is different from using the power or shape parameter on t_j is the triangular boundary method proposed by Kittelson and Emerson [4]. This boundary set takes on the following shape

$$c(t_j) = C(\phi, \alpha, J)\left(1 + \tau \frac{t_j}{I_J}\right).$$

The boundary function is a linear function on t_j with a variable slope parameter of τ. When a trial is testing a one-sided hypothesis, with an early decision to stop to reject or to accept the null hypothesis, this method produces a triangular continuation region on the scale of the score statistic $S(t_j)$.

Example: Redesigning Familial Hypercholesterolemia Trial Using Pocock and O'Brien-Fleming Methods

In this example, we want to re-create two one-sided sequential trials using Pocock and OBF approaches for the children FH trial using multiple design statements.

Example Code 2.6 *Pocock and O'Brien-Fleming Designs for Familial Hypercholesterolemia Trial*

```
ods graphics on;
proc seqdesign pss stopprob errspend;
   pocdesignforfh: design nstages=4 method=poc alt=upper alpha=0.025;
   obfdesignforfh: design nstages=4 method=obf alt=upper alpha=0.025;
   samplesize model=twosamplemean (stddev=0.045 meandiff=0.02 weight=1);
run;
ods graphics off;
```

Each of these two designs in Example Code 2.6 on page 44 requires a separate design statement but the same **samplesize** statement. A user-specified label can be given to each of the designs, but they have to be valid SAS names. For the first design, a label of **pocdesignforfh** is given, and **nstages=4** suggests that it has four stages. The option **method=poc** specifies that we are calling for the Pocock boundaries. For the second design, a label of **obfdesignforfh** is given, and it too has four stages. The option **method=obf** indicates that we are asking for the OBF boundaries. The **samplesize** statement returns the required sample sizes for the sequential designs that are specified in each design statement. In the **twosamplemean** option, the default **weight=1** option indicates equal allocation between the two treatment arms. The standard deviation is given such that sample size can be calculated in this design. Default standard deviation is 1 if not specified. In addition to the two other display options discussed earlier, the option **pss** displays power and sample size under various hypothetical references. Note that these options are included by default if not specified:

alpha=0.05, **beta=0.1**, **alt=twosided** and **stop=reject**. The graphical option can be turned on using **ods graphics on/off**, but this is sometimes not required in recent releases of SAS as graphical output is already generated by default. It is assumed that in the following programs, the graphical option is always turned on.

Figure 2.2 *Output for Pocock Boundaries for Example Code 2.6*

The SEQDESIGN Procedure
Design: pocdesignforfh

Design Information	
Statistic Distribution	Normal
Boundary Scale	Standardized Z
Alternative Hypothesis	Upper
Early Stop	Reject Null
Method	Pocock
Boundary Key	Both
Alternative Reference	0.02
Number of Stages	4
Alpha	0.025
Beta	0.1
Power	0.9
Max Information (Percent of Fixed Sample)	118.3135
Max Information	31079.17
Null Ref ASN (Percent of Fixed Sample)	116.9601
Alt Ref ASN (Percent of Fixed Sample)	69.74955

Powers and Expected Sample Sizes Reference = CRef * (Alt Reference)		
		Sample Size
CRef	Power	Percent Fixed-Sample
0.0000	0.02500	116.9601
0.5000	0.34252	104.1213
1.0000	0.90000	69.7495
1.5000	0.99869	43.6600

Sample Size Summary	
Test	Two-Sample Means
Mean Difference	0.02
Standard Deviation	0.045
Max Sample Size	251.7413
Expected Sample Size (Null Ref)	248.8616
Expected Sample Size (Alt Ref)	148.4095
Weight (Group A)	1
Weight (Group B)	1

Figure 2.3 *Output for O'Brien-Fleming Boundaries for Example Code 2.6*

The SEQDESIGN Procedure
Design: obfdesignforfh

Design Information	
Statistic Distribution	Normal
Boundary Scale	Standardized Z
Alternative Hypothesis	Upper
Early Stop	Reject Null
Method	O'Brien-Fleming
Boundary Key	Both
Alternative Reference	0.02
Number of Stages	4
Alpha	0.025
Beta	0.1
Power	0.9
Max Information (Percent of Fixed Sample)	102.2163
Max Information	26850.73
Null Ref ASN (Percent of Fixed Sample)	101.8945
Alt Ref ASN (Percent of Fixed Sample)	76.73971

Powers and Expected Sample Sizes Reference = CRef * (Alt Reference)		
		Sample Size
CRef	Power	Percent Fixed-Sample
0.0000	0.02500	101.8945
0.5000	0.36495	96.3719
1.0000	0.90000	76.7397
1.5000	0.99821	57.2590

Sample Size Summary	
Test	Two-Sample Means
Mean Difference	0.02
Standard Deviation	0.045
Max Sample Size	217.4909
Expected Sample Size (Null Ref)	216.8062
Expected Sample Size (Alt Ref)	163.283
Weight (Group A)	1
Weight (Group B)	1

The partial output for these two redesigned trials (Figure 2.2 on page 45 and Figure 2.3 on page 46) shows a summary of the design information. The OBF method has a smaller maximum information (or inflation factor) of 102.2% than the Pocock method with 118.3%. However, the Pocock method has a smaller average sample number (ASN) in percentage of the total sample size from fixed-sample design under the alternative hypothesis, 69.7% compared to 76.7% in the OBF design. This is due to their differences in stage-wise stopping probabilities and monitoring patterns. In this example, the Pocock design is more likely to stop the trial for efficacy in an earlier stage than the OBF design, although it requires more stage-wise samples. The Powers and Expected Sample Sizes tables generated by the `pss` option show their respective powers under four hypothetical alternative situations. If c = 0.5, meaning the alternative situation is only half of the assumed original alternative reference, the OBF design will have a power of 36.5%, but the Pocock design has a slightly smaller power of 34.3%. The reverse is true for **c = 1.5**. Therefore, investigators will have to weigh in the benefits of the two designs in terms of time and resources, as well as their business preferences, before deciding which boundary approach best meets the study objectives.

Example Code 2.7 *Requesting Plots for Summary Statistics of Sequential Designs*

```
proc seqdesign plots=boundary(hscale=samplesize) boundaryscale=mle;
   pocdesignforfh: design nstages=4 method=poc alt=upper alpha=0.025;
   obfdesignforfh: design nstages=4 method=obf alt=upper alpha=0.025;
   samplesize model=twosamplemean (stddev=0.045 meandiff=0.02 weight=1);
run;

proc seqdesign plots=boundary(hscale=samplesize) boundaryscale=score;
   triangularforfh: design nstages=4 alt=upper alpha=0.025 beta=0.1 stop=both
   method(alpha)=tri(tau=1) method(beta)=tri(tau=1);
   samplesize model=twosamplemean (stddev=0.045 meandiff=0.02 weight=1);
run;
```

In the updated SAS program in Example Code 2.7 on page 47, the option **plots=boundary (hscale=samplesize** produces a user-specified graphical display of the detailed boundaries. These boundary plots include the rejection region and the acceptance region. With the option for horizontal scale **hscale=samplesize**, the boundary plot is given with sample size accrued plotted on the horizontal axis. The other option **boundaryscale=mle** indicates that the vertical axis uses the maximum likelihood estimator (MLE). Both Figure 2.4 on page 48 and Figure 2.5 on page 49 show the boundary plots of the redesigned 4-stage children FH trial using the Pocock and OBF boundaries, respectively. As seen in the figure, the MLE represents the estimated mean difference in change from baseline carotid IMT (mm) and the Pocock boundary allows a more lenient early stopping in early stages than the OBF's. Though not shown here, it is possible to design a group sequential trial with asymmetric boundaries for two-sided hypotheses to take advantage of the properties of the Pocock and OBF boundaries. For example, a two-sided hypothesis can be tested using an OBF boundary in the direction the test treatment shows benefit and a Pocock boundary in the direction the test treatment shows harm (compared to the control arm). This would allow the trial to stop quickly for a safety issue, while providing a higher hurdle for benefit.

Figure 2.4 *Pocock Boundary Plot for Familial Hypercholesterolemia Trial*

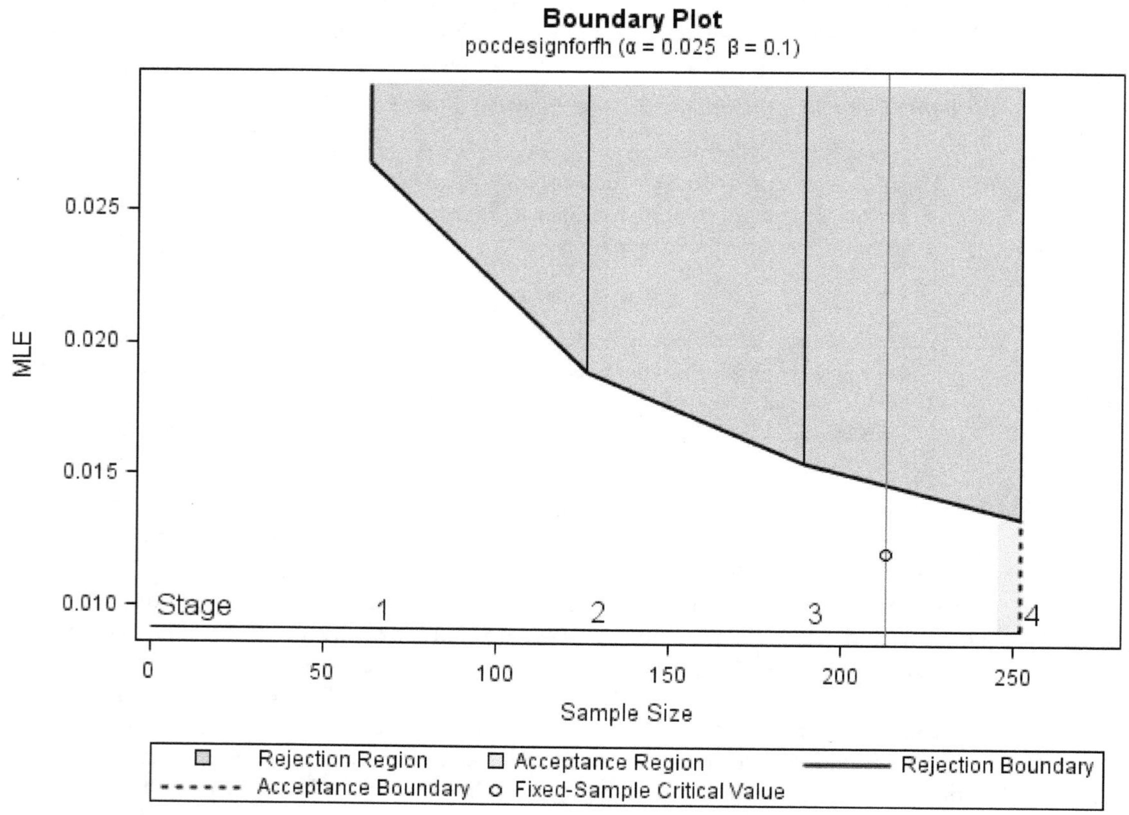

Figure 2.5 *O'Brien-Fleming Boundary Plot for Familial Hypercholesterolemia Trial*

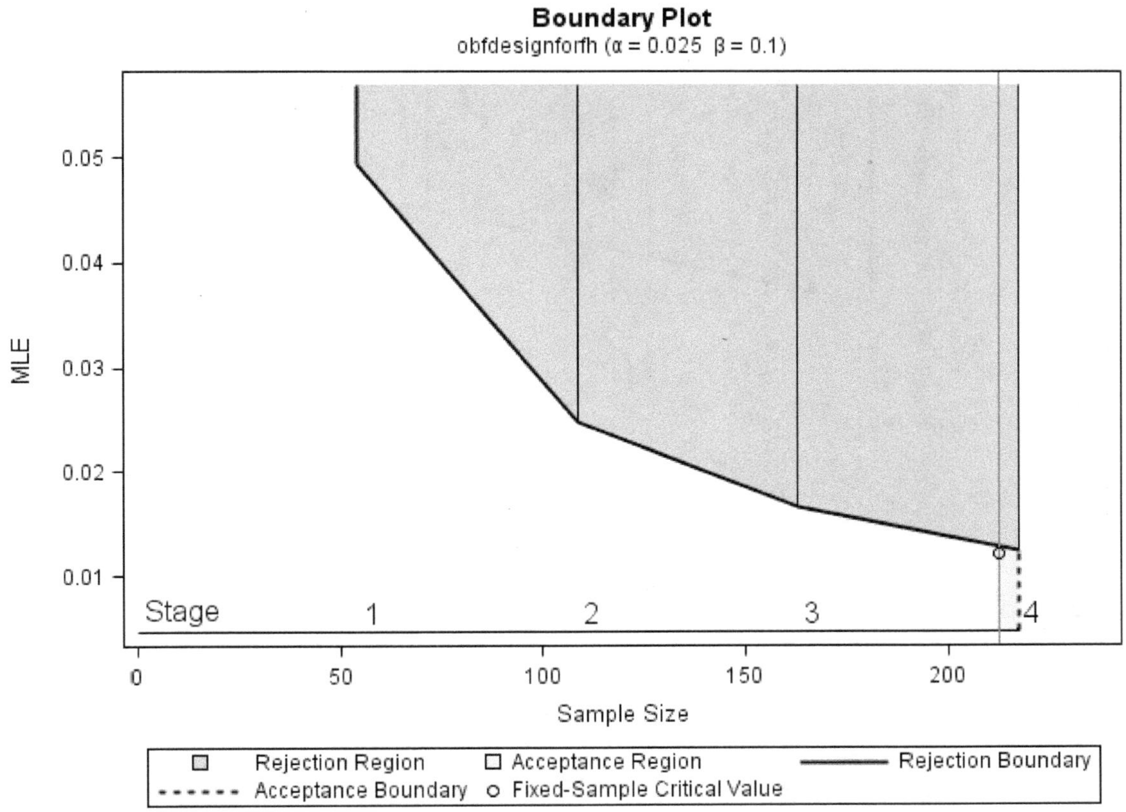

In the second part of Example Code 2.7 on page 47, another sequential design labeled **triangularforfh** is presented with early stopping to either reject or accept the null hypothesis **(stop=both)**. The rejection boundary is monitored using the triangular method with slope parameter $\tau = 1$ (**method(alpha)=tri(tau=1)**), and futility is monitored by the same method (**method(beta)=tri(tau=1)**). The continuation region has a triangular shape on the score statistic (see Figure 2.6 on page 50).

Figure 2.6 *Triangular Method Boundary Plot for Familial Hypercholesterolemia Trial*

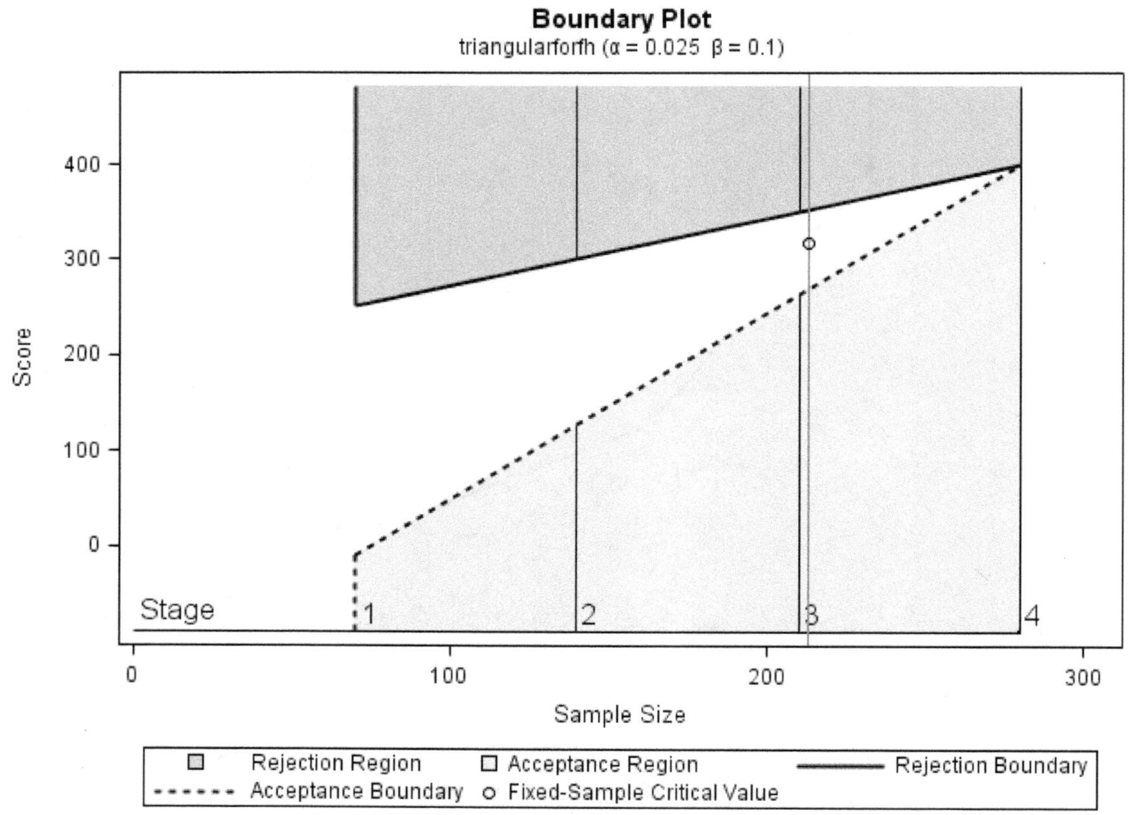

Example: Redesigning the Psoriasis Trial Allowing Both Efficacy and Futility Stopping

In this example, we want to illustrate the redesign of the psoriasis trial to test the difference between two proportions. In addition, we want to allow the trial to stop for either claiming early efficacy or futility, knowing that if the treatment is discovered to be inefficacious early, we do not want to continue exposing patients to the ineffective treatment. We also want to demonstrate how one can monitor the trial using `proc seqtest` and make necessary adjustments to the trial designs as it goes along during its course.

Example Code 2.8 *Efficacy and Futility Boundaries for the Psoriasis Trial*

```
proc seqdesign boundaryscale=mle plots=all;
   pocobfdesignforpso: design nstages=4 alt=upper alpha=0.025 beta=0.14 stop=both
   method(alpha)=poc method(beta)=obf;
   samplesize model=twosamplefreq (nullprop=0.07 prop=0.4 test=prop weight=2);
   ods output Boundary=boundaryinfo1;
run;

proc print data=stage1data; run;

proc genmod data=stage1data;
   model outcome=trt;
   ods output ParameterEstimates=paraest;
run;
```

```
data paraest1;
   set paraest;
   if parameter='trt';
   _scale_='MLE';
   _stage_=1;
   keep _scale_ _stage_ parameter estimate stderr;
run;

proc print data=paraest1; run;

proc seqtest boundary=boundaryinfo1 parms(testvar=trt)=paraest1
   infoadj=none boundaryscale=mle errspend plots=errspend;
   ods output Test=boundaryinfo2;
run;

/* stage2data contains cumulative data up to end of stage 2 */
proc genmod data=stage2data;
   model outcome=trt;
   ods output ParameterEstimates=paraest;
run;

data paraest2;
   set paraest;
   if parameter='trt';
   _scale_='MLE';
   _stage_=2;
   keep _scale_ _stage_ parameter estimate stderr;
run;

proc print data=paraest2; run;

proc seqtest boundary=boundaryinfo2 parms(testvar=trt)=paraest2
   infoadj=none boundaryscale=mle;
   ods output Test=boundaryinfo3;
run;
```

In Example Code 2.8 on page 50, we have a sequential trial designed with the objective of comparing the anti-TNF treatment to a placebo. The clinical outcome is a binary response. In the design statement, this newly modified design has four stages with power set at 86% (**beta=0.14**) as in the fixed-sample design. Additionally, we want to conduct a trial with options for early rejection or acceptance of the null hypothesis; therefore, the option **stop=both** is used. However, the monitoring approach for stopping for efficacy is based on the Pocock boundary while that for futility is based on the OBF boundary: **method(alpha)=poc** and **method(beta)=obf**, respectively. In the **samplesize** statement, we specify the **twosamplefreq** option for testing two proportions with a null proportion of 7% and an alternative proportion at 40%. The test available in **proc seqdesign** is the binomial test (**test=prop**), which relies on normal approximation to the binomial distribution. Fisher's exact test is not available in sequential design because it does not follow canonical multivariate distribution and it usually requires a larger sample size. Group-sequential methodology based on exact binomial distribution is described in Chapter 12 in [11] but it is not available in SAS at the present time. Consequently, it is beyond the scope of this chapter.

For our example above, the 2:1 allocation ratio is specified in **weight=2**, meaning that the treatment group will receive patients double that of the placebo group. The **plots=all** option requests all plots available in the procedure: boundary plot, average sample size (ASN) plot, error spending plot and power plot (see Figure 2.7 on page

52). Again, we have chosen the MLE scale for the vertical axis, but other options exist: **score** (score statistics), **stdz** (default, standardized normal Z statistics), and **pvalue** (p-values). Lastly, **ods output Boundary=boundaryinfo1** requests the output of the boundary information to a data set named **boundaryinfo1,** which can be used for monitoring the clinical trials using **proc seqtest**.

Figure 2.7 *Plots for the Redesigned Psoriasis Trial with Efficacy and Futility Boundaries*

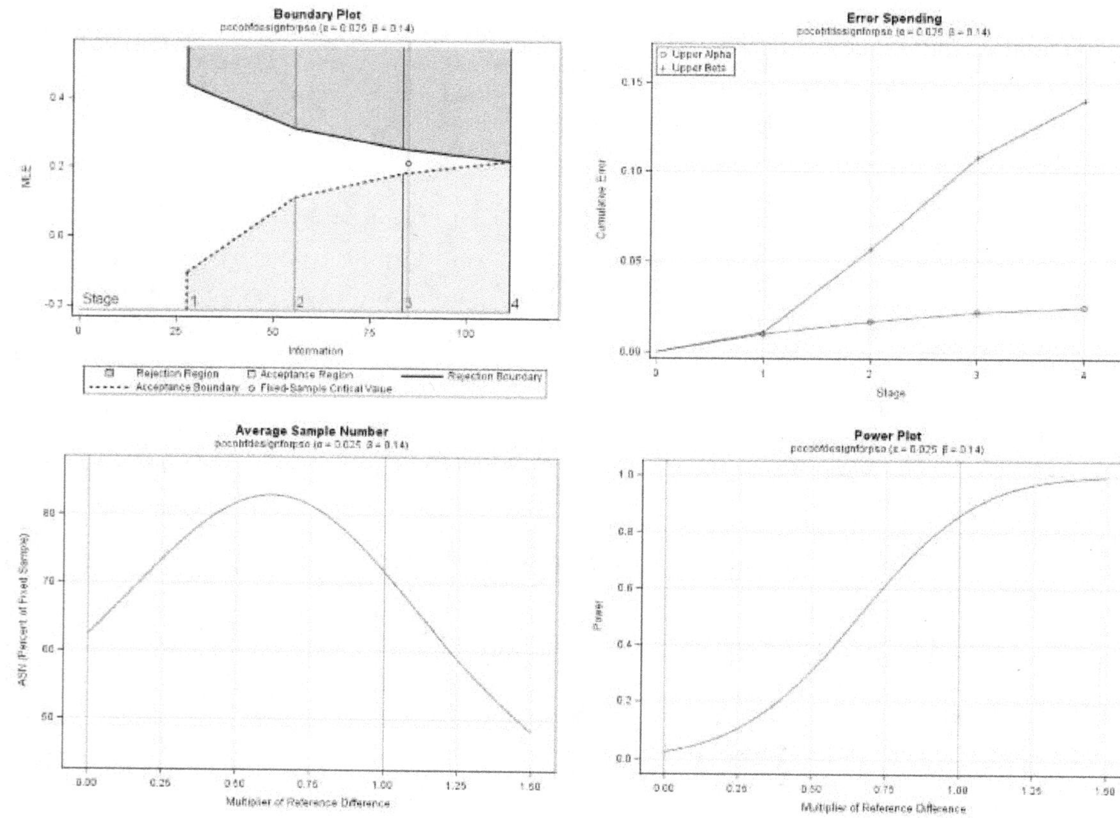

Figure 2.8 *Output for Example Code 2.8*

The SEQDESIGN Procedure
Design: pocobfdesignforpso

Design Information	
Statistic Distribution	Normal
Boundary Scale	MLE
Alternative Hypothesis	Upper
Early Stop	Accept/Reject Null
Method	Unified Family
Boundary Key	Both
Alternative Reference	0.33
Number of Stages	4
Alpha	0.025
Beta	0.14
Power	0.86
Max Information (Percent of Fixed Sample)	130.9114
Max Information	111.1162
Null Ref ASN (Percent of Fixed Sample)	62.35328
Alt Ref ASN (Percent of Fixed Sample)	71.69203

Boundary Information (MLE Scale)
Null Reference = 0

				Alternative	Boundary Values	
	Information Level			Reference	Upper	
Stage	Proportion	Actual	N	Upper	Beta	Alpha
1	0.2500	27.77906	15.42571	0.33000	-0.10446	0.44277
2	0.5000	55.55812	30.85142	0.33000	0.11277	0.31309
3	0.7500	83.33718	46.27714	0.33000	0.18518	0.25563
4	1.0000	111.1162	61.70285	0.33000	0.22139	0.22139

Sample Sizes (N)
Two-Sample Z Test for Proportion Difference

	Fractional N				Ceiling N			
Stage	N	N(Grp 1)	N(Grp 2)	Information	N	N(Grp 1)	N(Grp 2)	Information
1	15.43	10.28	5.14	27.7791	17	11	6	30.6108
2	30.85	20.57	10.28	55.5581	32	21	11	57.6477
3	46.28	30.85	15.43	83.3372	47	31	16	84.6691
4	61.70	41.14	20.57	111.1	63	42	21	113.5

Figure 2.9 *Output for Example Code 2.8, continued*

The PRINT Procedure

Obs	Parameter	Estimate	StdErr	_scale_	_stage_
1	trt	0.3788	0.2323	MLE	1

The SEQTEST Procedure

Design Information	
BOUNDARY Data Set	WORK.BOUNDARYINFO1
Data Set	WORK.PARAEST1
Statistic Distribution	Normal
Boundary Scale	MLE
Alternative Hypothesis	Upper
Early Stop	Accept/Reject Null
Number of Stages	4
Alpha	0.025
Beta	0.13882
Power	0.86118
Max Information (Percent of Fixed Sample)	130.4524
Max Information	111.116243
Null Ref ASN (Percent of Fixed Sample)	65.05767
Alt Ref ASN (Percent of Fixed Sample)	73.73526

Test Information (MLE Scale)
Null Reference = 0

			Alternative	Boundary Values		Test	
	Information Level		Reference	Upper		trt	
Stage	Proportion	Actual	Upper	Beta	Alpha	Estimate	Action
1	0.1668	18.53617	0.33000	-0.23737	0.57635	0.37879	Continue
2	0.5000	55.55812	0.33000	0.11273	0.30345	.	
3	0.7500	83.33718	0.33000	0.18431	0.25444	.	
4	1.0000	111.1162	0.33000	0.22093	0.22093	.	

The PRINT Procedure

Obs	Parameter	Estimate	StdErr	_scale_	_stage_
1	trt	0.4805	0.1619	MLE	2

The SEQTEST Procedure

Test Information (MLE Scale)
Null Reference = 0

			Alternative	Boundary Values		Test	
	Information Level		Reference	Upper		trt	
Stage	Proportion	Actual	Upper	Beta	Alpha	Estimate	Action
1	0.1668	18.53617	0.33000	-0.23737	0.57635	0.37879	Continue
2	0.3435	38.16953	0.33000	0.02274	0.39635	0.48052	Reject Null
3	0.7500	83.33718	0.33000	0.18525	0.24326	.	
4	1.0000	111.1162	0.33000	0.21909	0.21909	.	

The partial output in Figure 2.8 on page 53 and Figure 2.9 on page 54 summarizes the design and sample sizes for this redesigned psoriasis trial. For the first interim stage, a total number of 15.43 factional patients would be needed, as specified by the timing of the 1st interim look. However, because the number of patients actually used in the trial has to be rounded up to an integer in both treatment groups, the resulting (**ceiling**) sample size at the time of the first interim look will be $N = 17$. This first stage with $N = 17$ patients total corresponds to 30.6, a bit more than 27.8 corresponding to 15.43 fractional patients. On the MLE scale, based on the originally planned fractional sample sizes, the upper boundary value for rejection of null hypothesis is 0.4428 and the lower boundary for the acceptance of null hypothesis is -0.1045. The boundary values for the subsequent stages are adjusted as in the tables. This program output also prints out the simulated outcomes on the primary binary endpoint for the first 17 patients for both treatment groups, where **trt=0** refers to the placebo and **trt=1** refers to the anti-TNF group. The simulated outcomes can be viewed by downloading the SAS code from the companion website.

Next, **proc genmod** is invoked to produce the MLE parameter estimates on the data generated from the first interim stage and then **proc seqtest** is invoked with the sequential design's boundary information that is stored in **boundaryinfo1,** and the MLE parameter estimates in **paraest1** are imported as indicated by **boundary=boundaryinfo1 params(textvar=trt)=paraest1**. It is important to remember that **paraest1** must have the two variables and corresponding values: **_scale_='MLE'** and **_stage_=1** to match with the information from the boundary data set of the first interim analysis. To calculate the information level, the value supplied for the standard error (**stderr**) is used, as described in "2.3.1 General Framework" on page 30. Alternatively, one can use the number of observations to derive the information level, and in this case, one should use **parms(infovar=Nobs)=paraest1**. The data set **paraest1** must have the variable **Nobs** and the number of observations for the stage supplied. The option **infoadj=none** serves to maintain the information levels at future interim stages. This is sometimes desirable if making changes to pre-planned subject recruitment is logistically difficult; it is easier to stay with the planned information in subsequent stages. If subject recruitment occurs at a steady rate and can be flexibly modified, default **infoadj=prop** can be used to produce proportionally adjusted information and boundary values. The result of the first testing stage (**Test**) is saved into a new boundary data set named **boundaryinfo2 ,** which displays if the trial can be stopped for efficacy or futility or if it should continue.

The partial output continues to display the result of the **proc genmod** step. The MLE estimate of the treatment effect is 0.3788 which will be compared to the revised MLE boundary values for the first stage (-0.2374, 0.5764). Since it is within the stopping boundaries, the trial will continue to the second stage with the accrual of an additional 15 patients to a total of 32 according to the original design plan. It is important to note that the boundary values for the subsequent stages have been updated in **boundaryinfo2** based on the same information levels suggested by **infoadj=none**. After the collecting data on the second cohort, the second interim analysis produces a new MLE estimate of 0.4805. When compared to the MLE boundary values (0.0227, 0.3964), it is determined that the MLE estimate has crossed the upper boundary; therefore, the null hypothesis will be rejected and no more patients will need to be recruited in this trial. This psoriasis trial is declared a success, meaning that the investigational anti-TNF product is superior to the placebo in improving the hfPAG outcome.

2.4.4 Spending Function Boundaries

Error spending functions are the most flexible and general way of deriving the stopping boundaries. The α-spending functions where the α level is pre-specified are used to control the type I error in the trial. They are monotonic functions that are defined on the unit interval with $\alpha(t = 0) = 0$ and $\alpha(t = 1) = \alpha$. Similarly, the β-spending functions, with pre-specified β level, are used to control the type II error. They are defined on the unit interval with $\beta(t = 0) = 0$ and $\beta(t = 1) = \beta$. This idea of using an error spending function was first introduced by Lan and DeMets [10]. One can use either the α or the β spending function singly or combine both of them in sequentially monitoring a single trial. They can be used for either one-sided or two-sided hypotheses, and produce either symmetric or asymmetric boundaries.

There are numerous proposed error spending functions, and we will briefly describe only three of the most commonly used spending functions and their properties. The forms of the functions are expressed as $\alpha(t)$ and $\beta(t)$ where $t(0 < t < 1)$ is the information fraction. Here we illustrate the α-spending function, but it can apply also to the β-spending function.

1. The Lan-DeMets spending function has two possible forms. The first one closely resembles the OBF boundaries:

$\alpha(t) = 2 - 2\Phi\left(\frac{z_{\alpha/2}}{\sqrt{t}}\right)$ for one-sided tests, and

$\alpha(t) = 4 - 4\Phi\left(\frac{z_{\alpha/4}}{\sqrt{t}}\right)$ for two-sided tests.

The second one closely resembles the Pocock boundaries:

$\alpha(t) = \alpha \ln\{1 + (e - 1)t\}$

2. The Gamma spending function was first proposed by Hwang, Shih and DeCani [24]. The functional form is

$$\alpha(t) = \begin{cases} \alpha\frac{\left(1 - e^{-\gamma t}\right)}{\left(1 - e^{-\gamma}\right)}, & \gamma \neq 0 \\ \alpha(t) = \alpha t, & \gamma = 0 \end{cases}.$$

Negative values of γ yield convex spending functions that make stopping early more difficult as γ decreases. Positive values of γ yield concave spending functions that favor stopping early as γ increases. The choice of $\gamma = 0$ spends the error linearly. When $\gamma = -4$, it resembles the OBF boundaries, while $\gamma = 1$ produces boundaries that resemble those of Pocock.

3. The Rho spending function was first proposed by Kim and DeMets [25], and was further generalized. The functional form is simply represented as

$\alpha(t) = \alpha t^{\rho}, \ \rho > 0.$

When $\rho = 1$, the corresponding stopping boundaries resemble the Pocock stopping boundaries, but when $\rho = 3$, the boundaries resemble the OBF boundaries. Large values of ρ yield boundaries make early stopping more difficult, while $0 < \rho < 1$ favors early stopping.

Here we want to illustrate using an example that will derive boundaries for early rejection of either the null or the alternative hypothesis given the one-sided setting. There are two sets of stopping boundaries for this design. The upper boundary set corresponds to the early rejection of the null hypothesis, while the lower boundary set refers to the early rejection of the alternative hypothesis. If at the jth interim stage, the test statistic crosses the upper boundary, then the trial will be stopped for efficacy, but if it crosses the lower boundary, the trial is stopped for futility. We impose the constraint that the upper and lower boundaries should meet at t_J at the end of the trial, in order to ensure that a decision is made to reject either of the hypotheses. The upper and lower boundaries therefore form a triangular continuation region.

We further specify that these stopping boundaries will be able to preserve the type I error at the α level under the null hypothesis when $\theta = 0$, but they can offer a target power of $1 - \beta$ under the alternative hypothesis when $\theta = \theta_1$ or when the drift parameter is η_1, therefore, protecting this trial from the type II error of β. We let the upper boundary at the jth interim stage as u_j and the lower boundary as l_j for $j = 1, 2, \ldots, J$. Again, we will be able to use a numerical method to evaluate the set of boundaries which should satisfy the following equations at t_1

$$P_0(S(t_1) \geq u_1) = \alpha(t_1),$$

$$P_{\eta_1}(S(t_1) \leq l_1) = \beta(t_1).$$

Similar conditions are evaluated subsequently at $t_2, t_3, \ldots, t_J$ as follows. If we have calculated the pair of stopping boundaries up to t_{j-1}, (l_{j-1}, u_{j-1}), then we can find (l_j, u_j) using the following equation and numerical method

$$P_0(l_1 < S(t_1) < u_1, l_2 < S(t_2) < u_2, \ldots, l_{j-1} < S(t_{j-1}) < u_{j-1}, S(t_j) \geq u_j) = \alpha(t_j) - \alpha(t_{j-1})$$

$$P_{\eta_1}(l_1 < S(t_1) < u_1, l_2 < S(t_2) < u_2, \ldots, l_{j-1} < S(t_{j-1}) < u_{j-1}, S(t_j) \leq l_j) = \beta(t_j). - \beta(t_{j-1})$$

For the final stage at t_J, we set $u_J = l_J$, so that they meet and a definitive decision at the end of a trial is guaranteed. Then the desired maximum information I_J can be evaluated and then translated into the maximum sample size n_J or the maximum number of events $D(c_J)$ (in case of a survival endpoint). The two-sided testing can be similarly derived by replacing $S(t_J)$ with $|S(t_J)|$ which gives symmetric boundaries. In other cases, we may be interested in asymmetric boundaries. When deriving asymmetric boundaries, the α will be split into two parts such that $\alpha_U + \alpha_L = \alpha$ and two different α-spending functions can be specified, $\alpha_U(t)$ and $\alpha_L(t)$. Similarly, this can also be applied to β spending functions.

Example: Redesigning the Psoriasis Trial Using Gamma Spending Functions

Example Code 2.9 on page 57 demonstrates the use of the gamma spending function in testing the two proportions in the psoriasis trial.

Example Code 2.9 *Psoriasis Trial Using Gamma Spending Functions*

```
proc seqdesign boundaryscale=mle plots=all;
   gammadesignforpso: design nstages=4 alt=upper alpha=0.025 beta=0.14
   stop=both method(alpha)=errfuncgamma(gamma=0.5)
   method(beta)=errfuncgamma(gamma=1.5);
   samplesize model=twosamplefreq (nullprop=0.07 prop=0.4 test=prop weight=2);
run;
```

In this case, the type I error is monitored using the gamma function with $\gamma = 0.5$ which is close to linear error spending, while type II error is monitored using $\gamma = 1.5$ which is closer to the Pocock boundary, allowing more aggressive stopping due to futility in early stages.

Figure 2.10 *Output for Example Code 2.9*

The SEQDESIGN Procedure
Design: gammadesignforpso

Design Information	
Statistic Distribution	Normal
Boundary Scale	MLE
Alternative Hypothesis	Upper
Early Stop	Accept/Reject Null
Method	Error Spending
Boundary Key	Both
Alternative Reference	0.33
Number of Stages	4
Alpha	0.025
Beta	0.14
Power	0.86
Max Information (Percent of Fixed Sample)	134.5514
Max Information	114.2059
Null Ref ASN (Percent of Fixed Sample)	53.29816
Alt Ref ASN (Percent of Fixed Sample)	71.62607

Sample Size Summary	
Test	Two-Sample Proportions
Null Proportion	0.07
Proportion (Group A)	0.4
Test Statistic	Z for Proportion
Reference Proportions	Alt Ref
Max Sample Size	63.41851
Expected Sample Size (Null Ref)	25.12118
Expected Sample Size (Alt Ref)	33.75972
Weight (Group A)	2
Weight (Group B)	1

This new sequential design (Figure 2.10 on page 58) requires similar expected sample sizes ASN=33.8 compared to the previous design defined in Example Code 2.8 on page 50 (output not shown here). Figure 2.11 on page 59 provides the plots that can be used to compare to the previous design in Figure 2.7 on page 52. Using the plots, we can see that the design using the gamma spending function allows more aggressive beta spending in early stages. This can be appropriate if there is a concern that the treatment is not as efficacious as the placebo, then it is more ethical to allow stopping for futility as early as possible.

Figure 2.11 *Flots for the Psoriasis Trial Using Gamma Spending Functions*

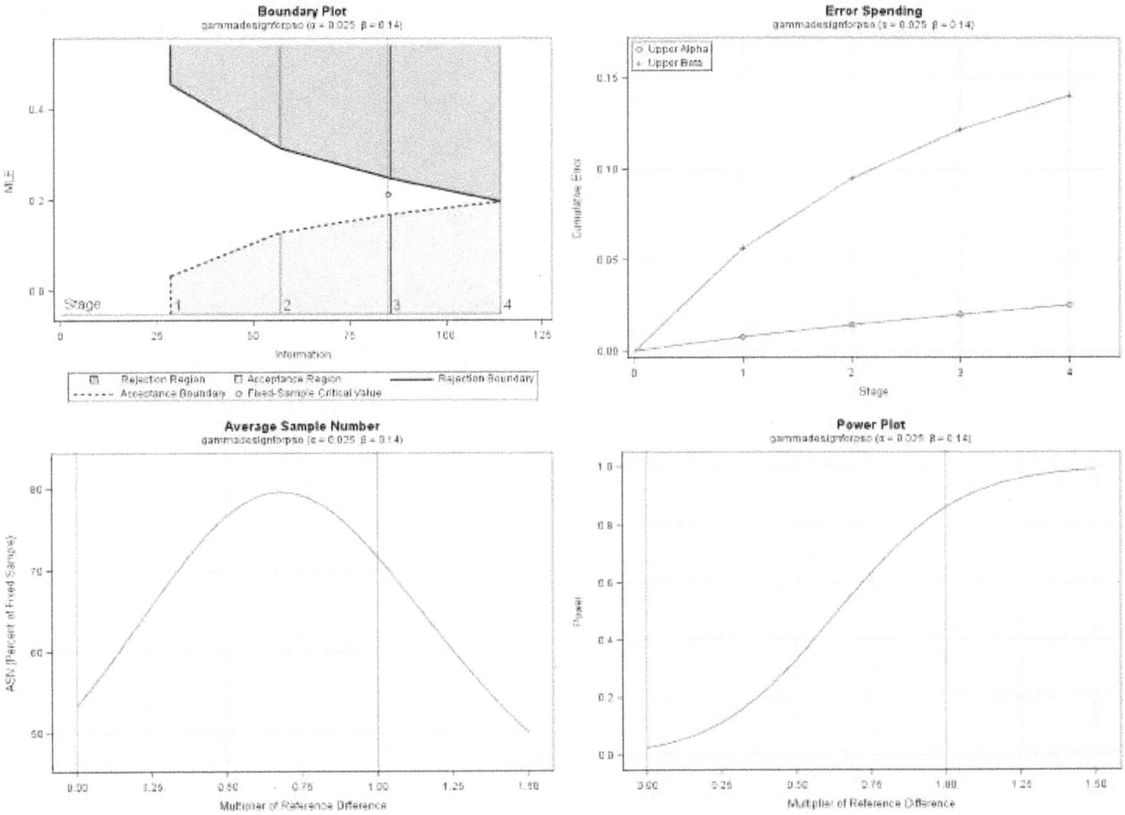

Example: Redesigning the Advanced Breast Cancer Trial Using Power Spending Functions

When designing a sequential clinical trial, one of the important aspects is to compare a number of possible designs to see if any one of them appears to be most suitable to the trial objectives. Example Code 2.10 on page 59 illustrates the modification of the breast cancer trial comparing trastuzumab alone to a combination therapy with everolimus. We want to make a design comparison in the use of the power spending function in testing the two survival distributions given the non-parametric log-rank test. In the trial design phase, investigators may be interested in comparing designs with varying values of ρ such as 0.3, 0.9, or 1.5 in the power spending function. Graphical comparison becomes an important tool in this investigation.

Example Code 2.10 *Advanced Breast Cancer Trial Using Power Spending Functions*

```
proc seqdesign boundaryscale=stdz plots=all;
   rhodesignforcan1: design nstages=4 method=errfuncpow(rho=0.3) alt=upper
   stop=reject alpha=0.025 beta=0.1;
   rhodesignforcan2: design nstages=4 method=errfuncpow(rho=0.9) alt=upper
   stop=reject alpha=0.025 beta=0.1;
   rhodesignforcan3: design nstages=4 method=errfuncpow(rho=1.5) alt=upper
   stop=reject alpha=0.025 beta=0.1;
   samplesize model=twosamplesurvival (nullmedsurvtime=6 medsurvtime=8.25
   acctime=12 totaltime=24);
run;
```

In these three 4-stage designs, the standardized Z-statistic scale is chosen using the log-rank statistic (**`boundaryscale=stdz`**). In the **`samplesize`** statement, we have used

model=twosamplesurvival to test two survival curves assumed to have a median survival time of 6 months in the null distribution, but 8.25 months in the alternative distribution. This is based on an exponential survival distribution assumption. The accrual time is set to be 12 months while the total time is 24 months.

Figure 2.12 *Output for Example Code 2.10*

The SEQDESIGN Procedure
Design: rhodesignforcan1

Design Information	
Statistic Distribution	Normal
Boundary Scale	Standardized Z
Alternative Hypothesis	Upper
Early Stop	Reject Null
Method	Error Spending
Boundary Key	Both
Alternative Reference	0.318454
Number of Stages	4
Alpha	0.025
Beta	0.1
Power	0.9
Max Information (Percent of Fixed Sample)	131.9093
Max Information	136.6716
Null Ref ASN (Percent of Fixed Sample)	129.9394
Alt Ref ASN (Percent of Fixed Sample)	72.39565

Numbers of Events (D) and Sample Sizes (N)
Two-Sample Log-Rank Test

	Fractional Time								Ceiling Time							
Stage	D	D(Grp 1)	D(Grp 2)	Time	N	N(Grp 1)	N(Grp 2)	Information	D	D(Grp 1)	D(Grp 2)	Time	N	N(Grp 1)	N(Grp 2)	Information
1	136.67	59.99	76.68	7.9546	443.32	221.66	221.66	34.1679	138.05	60.61	77.44	8	445.85	222.92	222.92	34.5131
2	273.34	121.96	151.38	11.8994	663.17	331.58	331.58	68.3358	277.22	123.74	153.48	12	668.77	334.39	334.39	69.3044
3	410.01	186.68	223.34	16.2245	668.77	334.39	334.39	102.5	428.85	195.99	232.86	17	668.77	334.39	334.39	107.2
4	546.69	257.53	289.16	24.0000	668.77	334.39	334.39	136.7	546.69	257.53	289.16	24	668.77	334.39	334.39	136.7

This partial output in Figure 2.12 on page 60 shows only the first design **rhodesignforcan1** using $\rho = 0.3$. The inflation factor is 131.9%, but under the specified alternative reference, it is 72.4%. The number of events needed for the trastuzumab (Group 2: null distribution) is listed under **D(Grp 2)** and that for the combination therapy group (Group 1: alternative distribution) under **D(Grp 1)** with the corresponding required stage-wise information in the last column. The first interim analysis can be performed by the team after observing a total of about 138 events in both groups, corresponding to information of 34.5. Based on the default uniform accrual rate and specified accrual time and total trial time (**acctime=12** and **totaltime=24**), a sample size of 446 subjects are needed for the first stage. The calendar times for observing the needed events for interim analyses are 8, 12, 17, and 24 months, calculated based on the accrual information supplied. SAS provides two accrual models: uniform as default (**accrual=uniform**) and parametric truncated exponential (**accrual=exp(parm=<>)**) with optional loss to follow-up models to calculate the sample sizes and approximate calendar times of analyses. If the study team believes that these accrual models are not applicable to their situation, they will have to specify their own accrual model and to estimate the required sample sizes and calendar times on their own. Therefore, if this accrual information is not supplied in the SAS program, only the number of events required are displayed, but the required sample sizes and calendar times will not be displayed. Interim analyses are still required to follow the number of events derived.

We also request all plots to combine the three stopping boundary sets together for visual comparison using **plots=all**. Figure 2.13 on page 61 and Figure 2.14 on page 62, as examples, are the combined boundary and ASN plots, respectively. As we can see, the first design with $\rho = 0.3$, allows for aggressive stopping for efficacy in the first stage while the other two designs ($\rho = 0.9,\ 1.5$) are conservative in the early stages. Unless one strongly believes that the two survival curves diverge markedly in the early stage, it is more desirable to approach early stopping conservatively in the beginning of this trial.

However, it is important to emphasize that in the examples with futility stopping boundaries discussed so far, the assumption was that the futility boundary cannot be overruled. In other words, if the test statistic crosses the futility boundary, the trial must be terminated, or else the type I error will be inflated. This is called a "binding futility boundary". It is because, when calculating the efficacy boundaries, the presence of the binding futility boundary will pull the efficacy boundary down, thus making it easier to cross under the null hypothesis, i.e. potentially inflating the type I error when the binding futility boundary is ignored at the interim. This binding futility is usually not desirable to sponsors of the trial because futility decisions are not always clear-cut. For that reason, a methodology is available to construct a non-binding futility boundary, analogous to examples discussed in previous sections. Non-binding futility boundary allows trial continuation even if such boundary is crossed without inflation of the type I error because the corresponding efficacy boundary is adjusted accordingly. It results in pushing up the efficacy boundary, as well as increasing the overall sample size compared to the binding futility boundary although the impact may be small. In this case, in order to change the default setting where `stop=both(betaboundary=binding)` one can opt to use `stop=both(betaboundary=nonbinding)` to construct a non-binding futility boundary. In "2.5 Special Issues" on page 66, we will return to the issue of monitoring and briefly introduce some additional monitoring tools besides binding and non-binding futility boundaries.

Figure 2.13 *Combined Boundary Plot for Breast Cancer Trial Using 3 Different Power Spending Functions*

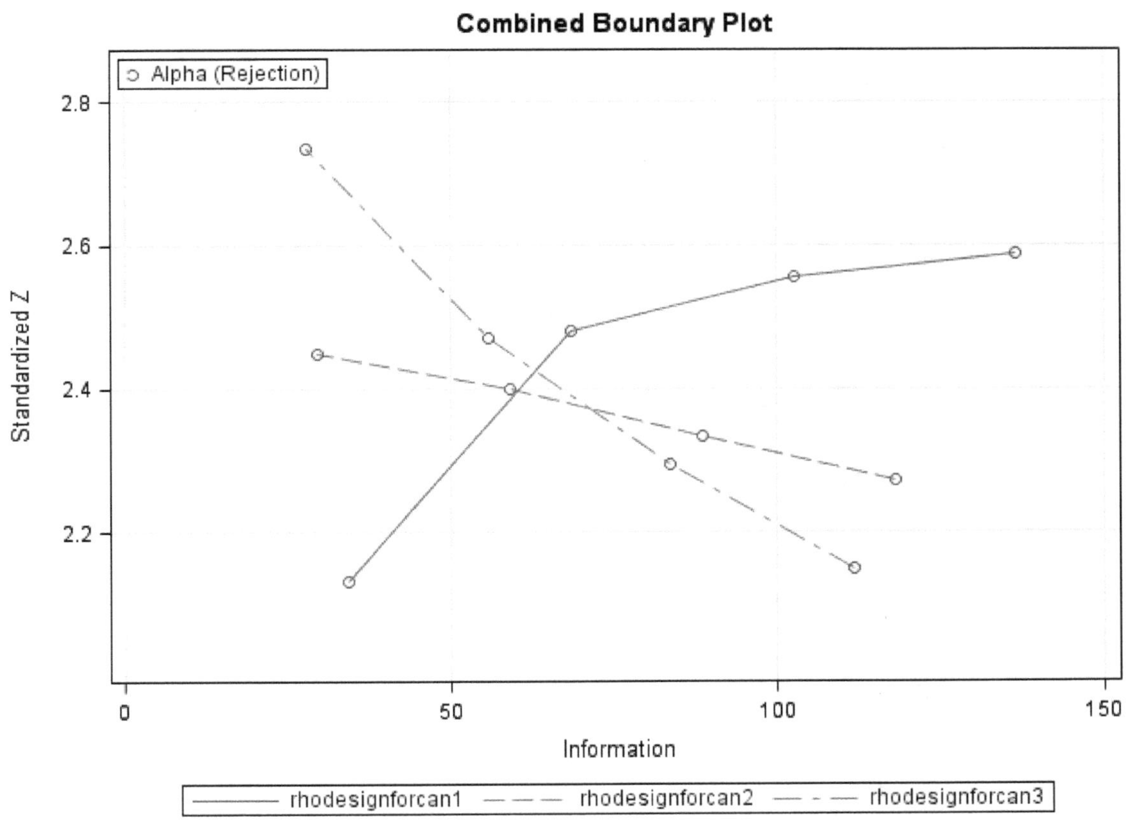

Figure 2.14 *Combined Average Sample Size Plot for Breast Cancer Trial Using 3 Different Power Spending Functions*

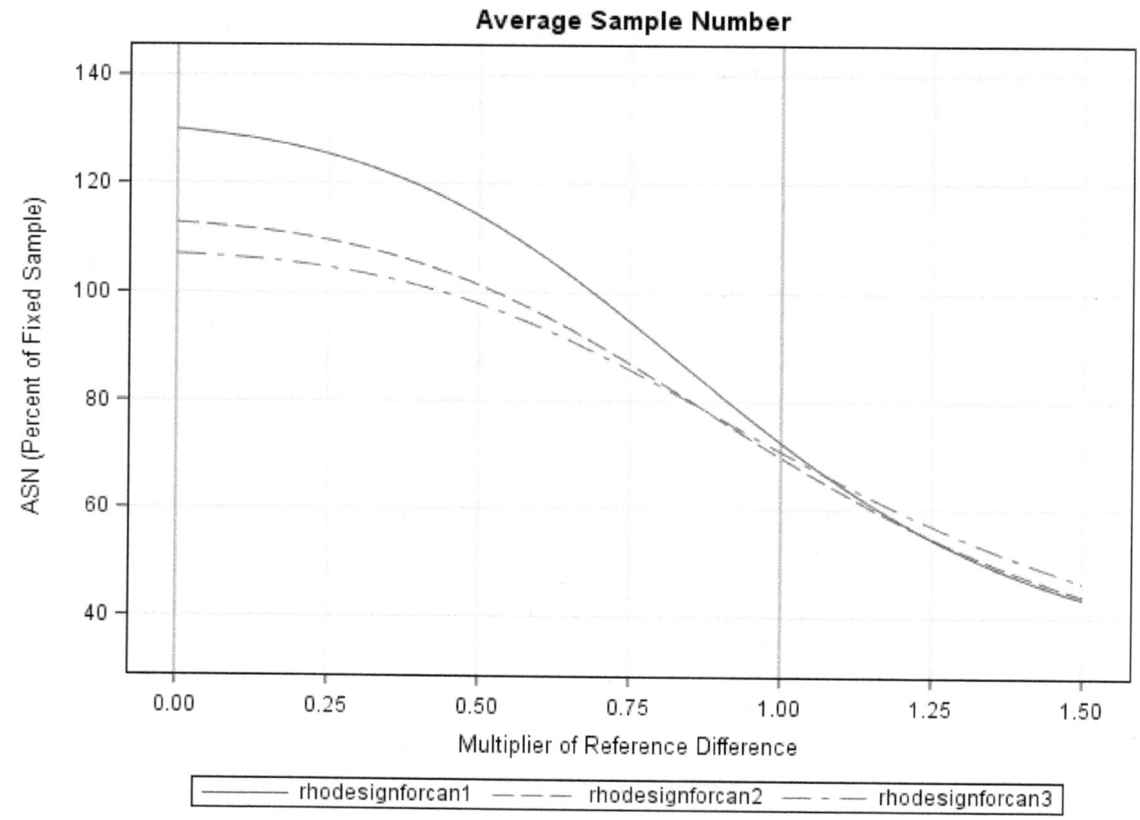

Example: Designing Sequential Tests for Assessing Cardiovascular Risk for Type 2 Diabetes Mellitus

When evaluating CV risk for T2DM, many development options are possible; we limit our focus to a single cardiovascular outcomes trial (CVOT) to further illustrate the methods used for group sequential designs. The pros and cons of various approaches to assess CV risk for T2DM are discussed elsewhere [26, 27]. As described above, for Stage 1 we can re-write the non-inferiority null hypothesis as $H_{10}: \theta \leq 0$ where $\theta = -\ln(\lambda_T / \lambda_C) + 0.5878$ and $\ln(1.8) = 0.5878$. The corresponding alternative hypothesis becomes $H_{11}: \theta > 0$. This is the preferred parameterization in SAS and Example Code 2.11 on page 62 is used to illustrate this example.

Example Code 2.11 *Sequential Analysis for Cardiovascular Outcome Trial of Type 2 Diabetes Mellitus*

```
/* Fixed-sample design for Stage 1 testing, default: beta=0.1 */
proc seqdesign;
   stage1fixed: design nstages=1 alt=twosided alpha=0.05;
   samplesize model=twosamplesurv(nullhazard=1.8 1.0 hazard=1.0);
run;

/* Three-stage sequential design for Stage 1 testing 1.8 criterion */
proc seqdesign errspend pss stopprob boundaryscale=mle plots=all;
   stage1power: design nstages=3 method=errfuncpow(rho=3) alt=twosided
   alpha=0.05 info=cum(0.5 0.75 1);
   samplesize model=twosamplesurv(nullhazard=1.8 1.0 hazard=1.0);
```

```
   ods output Boundary=test_interim1;
run;

/* Analysis of Stage 1 data */
proc phreg data=T2DM;
   model weeks*event(0)=treatment;
   ods output ParameterEstimates=parms_interim1;
run;

data parms_interim1;
   set parms_interim1;
   where parameter='Treatment';
   parameter=-parameter+0.5878;
   _scale_='MLE';
   _stage_=1;
   keep _scale_ _stage_ parameter estimate stderr;
run;

proc seqtest boundary=test_interim1 parms(testvar=treatment)=parms_interim1
   infoadj=none boundaryscale=mle;
   ods output Test=test_interim2;
run;

/* Interim analysis of 1.3 criterion at end of Stage 1 (20% info)
   and interim analyses at 50% and 75% for Stage 2 */
proc seqdesign errspend pss stopprob boundaryscale=mle plots=all;
   stage2power: design nstages=4 method=errfuncpow(rho=3) alt=twosided
   alpha=0.05 info=cum(0.2 0.5 0.75 1);
   samplesize model=twosamplesurv(nullhazard=1.3 1.0 hazard=1.0);
   ods output Boundary=combtest_interim1;
run;
```

The first set of codes allows **proc seqdesign** to determine the number of events for a clinical trial of fixed size. By setting **nstages=1** and leaving out the specification of method, it corresponds to the fixed-sample design. Under the null hypothesis, the hazard rates for treatment T and control C arms are specified in this order: **nullhazard: 1.8 1.0** so that their ratio is 1.8. Under the alternative hypothesis, we only need to specify the hazard rate for treatment T since that for control C is assumed to be the same, i.e. 1.0, such that **hazard=1.0** for T. Alternatively, we can use **hazardratio=1.0**. Although the output for a fixed trial is not shown, the required number of events needed is 122. Similar coding can be used for Stage 2, by replacing 1.8 and 0.5878 with 1.3 and 0.2624, respectively; 611 events are required for the trial of fixed size.

In a large long-term trial designed to assess cardiovascular safety, it is appropriate to schedule one or more interim analyses to allow an independent DSMB to review trial data to ensure the well-being of the study participants. Further, as described above, these interim analyses may allow for early stopping of the trial if safety thresholds have been met. For Stage 1, we can design a group sequential trial with two interim analyses planned when 50% and 75% of the trial information is available as suggested in [18]. To provide greater flexibility for the timing and frequency of interim analyses, the design **stage1power** in the second set of code makes use of the power error spending function with $\rho = 3$ to provide OBF-like boundaries in **pr oc seqdesign**. The option **info=cum(0.5 0.75 1)** allows three unequally spaced monitoring that corresponds to 50%, 75%, and 100% of information accrued. **boundary=mle** requests the boundary values to be on the MLE scale for θ defined earlier and stores them in **test_interim1**.

Figure 2.15 *Output for Stage 1 of Example Code 2.11*

The SEQDESIGN Procedure
Design: stage1power

Design Information	
Statistic Distribution	Normal
Boundary Scale	MLE
Alternative Hypothesis	Two-Sided
Early Stop	Reject Null
Method	Error Spending
Boundary Key	Both
Alternative Reference	0.587787
Number of Stages	3
Alpha	0.05
Beta	0.1
Power	0.9
Max Information (Percent of Fixed Sample)	102.4384
Max Information	31.15446
Null Ref ASN (Percent of Fixed Sample)	101.7382
Alt Ref ASN (Percent of Fixed Sample)	75.98826

Expected Cumulative Stopping Probabilities
Reference = CRef * (Alt Reference)

			Stopping Probabilities		
CRef	Expected Stopping Stage	Source	Stage_1	Stage_2	Stage_3
0.0000	2.973	Reject Null	0.00625	0.02109	0.05000
0.5000	2.759	Reject Null	0.05774	0.18281	0.36479
1.0000	1.967	Reject Null	0.33926	0.69357	0.90000
1.5000	1.255	Reject Null	0.77200	0.97265	0.99822

Boundary Information (MLE Scale)
Null Reference = 0

				Alternative		Boundary Values	
	Information Level			Reference		Lower	Upper
Stage	Proportion	Actual	Events	Lower	Upper	Alpha	Alpha
1	0.5000	15.57723	62.30892	-0.58779	0.58779	-0.69281	0.69281
2	0.7500	23.36585	93.46338	-0.58779	0.58779	-0.48757	0.48757
3	1.0000	31.15446	124.6178	-0.58779	0.58779	-0.36343	0.36343

Error Spending Information

	Information Level	Cumulative Error Spending			
		Lower		Upper	
Stage	Proportion	Alpha	Beta	Beta	Alpha
1	0.5000	0.00313	0.00000	0.00000	0.00313
2	0.7500	0.01055	0.00000	0.00000	0.01055
3	1.0000	0.02500	0.10000	0.10000	0.02500

Numbers of Events (D)
Two-Sample Log-Rank Test

Stage	D	Information
1	62.31	15.5772
2	93.46	23.3658
3	124.62	31.1545

From the partial output in Figure 2.15 on page 64, we can determine that the maximum number of events for the trial has increased to 125, a relatively minor increase for the added flexibility in the design. Under the specified alternative hypothesis, the expected number of events is approximately 76% of the fixed design (or 93 events), with a 69.4% chance of rejecting the null hypothesis at or before the second interim analysis.

Whenever the first interim analysis occurs, assuming a Cox proportional hazard model is appropriate, the output from **proc phreg** can be used to evaluate whether the boundary has been crossed. For example, **treatment=1** for the experimental treatment *T* and **event=1** if the patient experienced a MACE outcome, **event=0** otherwise. Subjects were censored at their current follow-up time as measured in weeks when **event=0**. Since in SAS, the null hypothesis is always in the form of H_0: $\theta = 0$, the parameter estimate is adjusted in the **parms_interim1** DATA step to account for the non-inferiority hypothesis, and passed to **proc seqtest** to determine whether a boundary has been crossed. Additional interim analyses can be accommodated as needed. For example, a second interim analysis would use **test_interim2** as the input boundary data set for a second call to **proc seqtest**.

Interim analyses for Stage 2 can be developed in a similar manner as described above for Stage 1. This requires a separate call to **proc seqdesign**. The last call to **proc seqdesign** in the program adds an additional interim analysis at (122/611)*100 = 20% of the information available for 611 events. Here, the data available for the last stage of the 1.8 boundary of Stage 1 (using the remainder of the first $\alpha = 0.05$) would also serve as the first analysis of the 1.3 boundary for Stage 2 (using the initial part of the second $\alpha = 0.05$). A subsequent call to **proc seqtest** would analyze Stage 2 data (not shown). The output for this design **stage2power** is partially shown in Figure 2.16 on page 66.

Figure 2.16 *Output for Stage 2 of Example Code 2.11*

The SEQDESIGN Procedure
Design: stage2power

Design Information	
Statistic Distribution	Normal
Boundary Scale	MLE
Alternative Hypothesis	Two-Sided
Early Stop	Reject Null
Method	Error Spending
Boundary Key	Both
Alternative Reference	0.262364
Number of Stages	4
Alpha	0.05
Beta	0.1
Power	0.9
Max Information (Percent of Fixed Sample)	102.4747
Max Information	156.4242
Null Ref ASN (Percent of Fixed Sample)	101.7618
Alt Ref ASN (Percent of Fixed Sample)	75.53034

Numbers of Events (D)
Two-Sample Log-Rank Test

Stage	D	Information
1	125.14	31.2848
2	312.85	78.2121
3	469.27	117.3
4	625.70	156.4

As described above, this analysis approach is to strike a balance between providing evidence on CV safety to reassure patients and excessive delay of novel therapies reaching the marketplace. An important point for any analysis strategy, one that utilizes sequential methodologies or not, is to maintain confidentiality of the CV results at the end of Stage 1 to minimize bias for the ongoing or additional trials needed to assess cardiovascular safety at the 1.3 margin. This includes the public, because knowledge of the point estimates and confidence intervals may affect the enrollment of current or future trials, but also includes sponsor personnel, since trial integrity may be compromised. It is recommended that unblinded sponsor personnel be independent of the study team, and limited to those individuals needed to initiate activities. Additional details on the confidentiality of interim results of CVOT trials for T2DM are available in [27, 28].

2.5 Special Issues

So far, we have demonstrated some statistical implementation of group sequential methods to clinical trials with different primary objectives. The validity of the trial that uses the sequential testing procedures relies heavily on strict adherence to the pre-specified stopping rules. In practice, deviations from the rules during the trial are common, and as a result, may compromise the integrity and interpretability of the final results. The rigidity of adhering to the rule presents challenges to investigators when deviations are ethically necessary and justified. Recent research on clinical trial monitoring introduces the use of conditional power and predictive power within the Bayesian paradigm. As discussed earlier, due to possible inflation of type I error, binding futility extends no flexibility in continuing the trial even when futility boundary is crossed, while non-binding futility offers flexibility but may increase sample size. Conditional power [29] and predictive power [30] become additional monitoring tools for sequential design that stops early only to reject the null hypothesis. Conditional power at the *j*th interim stage is defined as the total probability of rejecting the null hypothesis at any future stages given the observed statistic at stage *j*. A small conditional power ($\ll 0.5$) signals a small probability of declaring a successful trial given the current observed evidences. The trial can be stopped to accept the null hypothesis. Predictive power is the posterior probability that the test statistic at the final stage would exceed the rejection critical value given the observed data and a prior distribution of the hypothetical reference. Usually, a non-controversial non-informative prior is used in calculating the predictive power. The following SAS code updates the previous example on monitoring the psoriasis trial.

Example Code 2.12 *Conditional and Predictive Power for the Psoriasis Trial*

```
proc seqdesign boundaryscale=mle plots=all;
   pocobfdesignforpso: design nstages=4 alt=upper alpha=0.025 beta=0.14 stop=reject
   method(alpha)=poc;
   samplesize model=twosamplefreq (nullprop=0.07 prop=0.4 test=prop weight=2);
   ods output Boundary=boundaryinfo1;
run;
proc seqtest boundary=boundaryinfo1 parms(testvar=trt)=paraest1
   infoadj=none boundaryscale=mle condpower(cref=0.5, 1, 1.25)
   predpower plots=condpower;
   ods output Test=boundaryinfo2;
run;
proc seqtest boundary=boundaryinfo2 parms(testvar=trt)=paraest2
   infoadj=none boundaryscale=mle condpower(cref=0.5, 1, 1.25)
   predpower plots=condpower;
   ods output Test=boundaryinfo3;
run;
```

In the first part of Example Code 2.12 on page 67, **proc seqdesign** is updated to remove futility monitoring and uses **stop=reject** only. This allows the rejection boundary not be affected by a decision on the futility assessed based on conditional or predictive power. The option **condpower(cref=0.5,1,1.25)** generates the conditional powers for rejecting the null at all future stages (default) under different hypothetical references: **c=0.5, 1, 1.25** times the original reference. The partial output is given below in Figure 2.17 on page 68. A conditional power plot is requested using **plots=condpower** (Figure 2.18 on page 69). As for the predictive power of the final stage, **predpower** is used and since only predictive power for the final stage is calculated, no plot for predictive power is generated.

Figure 2.17 *Output for Example Code 2.12*

Conditional Power Information Reference = CRef * (Alt Reference)				
		Reference		
Stopping Stage	MLE	Ref	CRef	Conditional Power
1	0.37879	MLE	1.1478	0.96019
1	0.37879		0.5000	0.46577
1	0.37879	Alternative	1.0000	0.90756
1	0.37879		1.2500	0.97980

Predictive Power Information		
Stopping Stage	MLE	Predictive Power
1	0.37879	0.75409

Test Information (MLE Scale) Null Reference = 0						
			Alternative	Boundary Values	Test	
	Information Level		Reference	Upper	trt	
Stage	Proportion	Actual	Upper	Alpha	Estimate	Action
1	0.1833	18.53617	0.33000	0.57469	0.37879	Continue
2	0.3774	38.16953	0.33000	0.39557	0.48052	Reject Null
3	0.7500	75.851	0.33000	0.26119	.	
4	1.0000	101.1347	0.33000	0.23326	.	

Parameter Estimates Stagewise Ordering					
Parameter	Stopping Stage	MLE	p-Value for H0:Parm=0	Median Estimate	Lower 95% CL
trt	2	0.480519	0.0076	0.454397	0.15835

Figure 2.18 Conditional Power Plot for the Psoriasis Trial Based on Observed Stage 1 Data

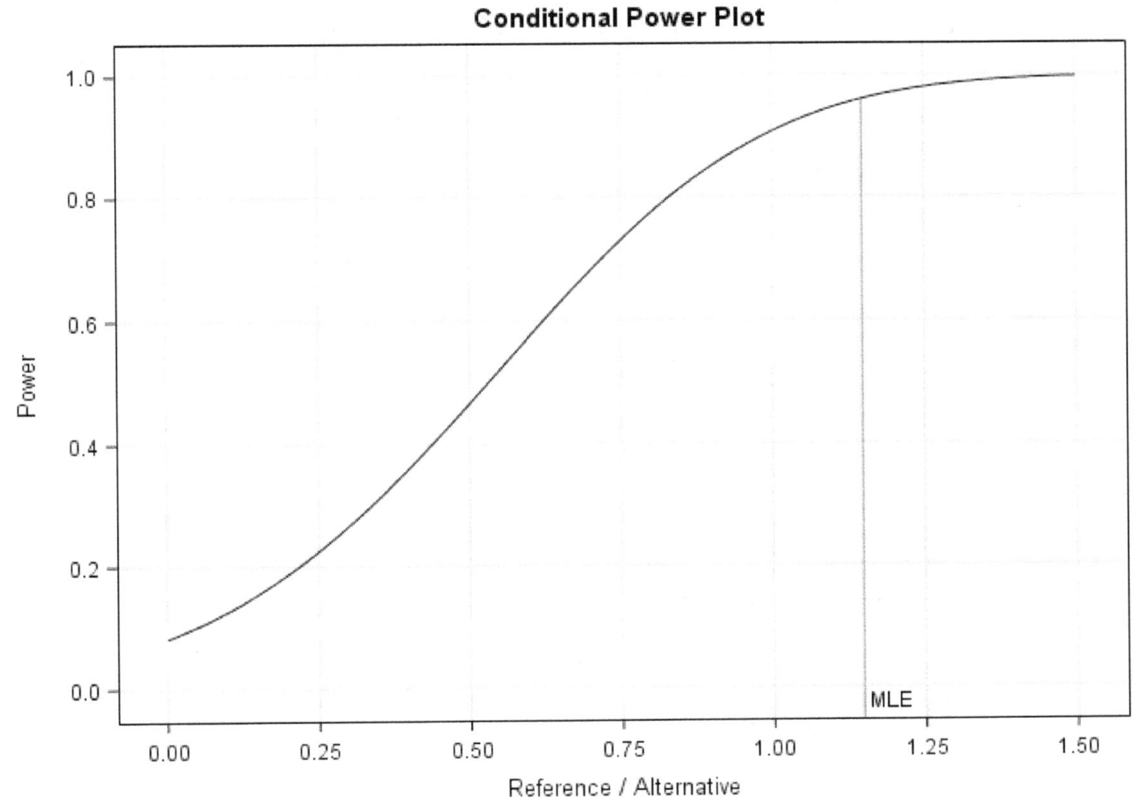

The conditional power of 96.02% refers to the hypothetical reference when it is the observed MLE. Since the MLE in the first stage is 0.3788, slightly larger than the original reference of 0.4-0.07=0.33, therefore the calculated $c = 0.3788/0.33 = 1.1478$. If the hypothetical reference is 1.25*0.33 = 0.4125, the conditional power is 97.98%. These estimated conditional powers suggest strong evidence of continuing the trial to the next stage. The predictive power of 75.41%, although smaller than the conditional powers, still implies strong evidence to continue. The next table is the same as before, displaying the rejection of the null hypothesis at the second stage and therefore, neither conditional nor predictive power needs to be calculated.

Another important issue that arises from sequential testing is the provision of unbiased estimation of the mean effect size of an experimental drug. For a fixed-sample design without interim analyses for early termination, it is possible to achieve unbiased quantitative evaluation of treatment difference. However, under sequential design, the usual maximum likelihood estimator for the mean usually produces over-estimation because of the choice of stopping rules and therefore the sampling distribution of the test statistic is no longer the same as the one from fixed-sample design. Jennison and Turnbull [11] gave a brief exposition of this issue. Methods have been proposed to adjust for this bias and this topic is beyond the scope of this chapter. However, as for median, an unbiased median estimator can be available in SAS. The last table of the output displays the unbiased median estimator of 0.4548 based on default stagewise ordering. The corresponding p-value of the trial is 0.0075 based on the data collected at the end of the second stage.

Occasionally, some clinical trials will include multiple groups such as multiple doses of an investigational drug. In this case, futility analysis plays an important role to drop doses that do not exhibit clear evidence of efficacy, however, since multiple comparisons are being conducted, measures to control the inflation of type I error must be in place to account for multiplicity. In fact, dropping doses cannot be addressed in a classical group-sequential framework and requires completely different methodology, similar to the one described in Chapter 3, "Sample Size Re-estimation." The latter extends the distributional theory and methods of preserving type 1 error that we have just reviewed to situations when a trial's total maximum information can be adjusted upward as well as downward during the interim analysis. This flexibility in direction of adjustment is unique to unblinded sample size re-estimation and is often used to contrast it with the group sequential methods discussed here: the group-sequential method can only adjust the sample size downward by stopping early.

2.6 Summary

Over the last couple of decades, the theories of group sequential testing have been well-established, particularly in the context of clinical trials. The US Food and Drug Administration (FDA) released a draft guidance for industry on "Adaptive Design Clinical Trials for Drugs and Biologics" in 2010 [31] and stated that "group sequential designs are among the other adaptive designs considered well-understood designs, offering valid approaches to clinical trial implementation." This chapter has provided an exposition of both theoretical and practical aspects of designing and monitoring a clinical trial adopting the sequential testing procedure. The sequential testing methodologies we have surveyed are able to preserve the type I error under nominal α level. With an independent DSMB, it is possible to maintain study integrity during the course of a trial. The SAS procedures and the examples discussed in this chapter provide a solid introduction to the sequential testing framework and programming tools for scientists, clinicians, statisticians, and programmers to investigate if group sequential methods can be effectively used in their clinical studies.

References

1. Everitt BS & Palmer CR. (2011). *Encyclopaedic Companion to Medical Statistics, Second Edition.* West Sussex, UK: John Wiley & Sons Ltd.
2. Armitage P. (1960). *Sequential Medical Trials, First Edition.* Blackwell: Oxford.
3. Armitage P, McPherson CK & Rowe BC. (1969). Repeated significance tests on accumulating data. *Journal of the Royal Statistical Society*, 132 (2): 235-244.
4. Kittelson JM & Emerson SS. (1999). A unifying family of group sequential test designs. *Biometrics*, 55 (3):874-882.
5. Pocock SJ. (1977). Group sequential methods in the design and analysis of clinical trials. *Biometrika*, 64 (2) 191-199.
6. O'Brien PC & Fleming TR. (1979). A multiple testing procedure for clinical trials. *Biometrics*, 35 (3): 549-556.
7. Haybittle JL. (1971). Repeated assessment of results in clinical trials of cancer treatment. *The British Journal of Radiology* 44: 793-797.
8. Peto R, Pike MC, Armitage P, Breslow NE, Cox DR, Howard SV, Mantel N, McPherson K, Peto J & Smith PG. (1976). Design and analysis of randomized clinical trials requiring prolonged observation of each patient. I. Introduction and design. *British Journal of Cancer*, 34 (6): 585-612.

9. Whitehead, J. (1997), *The Design and Analysis of Sequential Clinical Trials, Second Edition*, Chichester, UK: John Wiley & Sons.

10. Lan KKG & DeMets DL. (1983). Discrete sequential boundaries for clinical trials. *Biometrika*, 70 (3): 659-663.

11. Jennison C & Turnbull BW. (2000). *Group Sequential Methods with Applications to Clinical Trials, First Edition*. Boca Raton, FL: Chapman & Hall/CRC.

12. Todd S. (2007). A 25-year review of sequential methodology in clinical trials. *Statistics in Medicine*, 26: 237-252.

13. Wiegman A, Hutten BA, de Groot E, Rodenburg J, Bakker HD, Büller HR, Sijbrands EJG & Kastelein JJ. (2004). Efficacy and safety of statin therapy in children with familial hypercholesterolemia. *Journal of American Medical Association*, 292 (3): 331-337.

14. Leonardi C, Langley RG, Papp K, Tyring SK, Wasel N, Vender R, Unnebrink K, Gupta SR, Valdecantos WC & Bagel J. (2011). Adalimumab for treatment of moderate to severe chronic plaque psoriasis of the hands and feet: Efficacy and safety results from REACH, a randomized placebo-controlled, double-blind trial. *Archives of Dermatology*, 147 (4): 429-436.

15. Marrow PK, Wulf GM, Ensor J, Booser DJ, Moore JA, Flores PR, Xiong Y, Zhang S, Krop IE, Winer EP, Kindelberger DW, Coviello J, Sahin AA, Nuñez R, Hortobagyi GN, Yu D & Esteva FJ. (2011). Phase I/II study of trastuzumab in combination with everolimus (RAD001) in patients with HER2-overexpressing metastatic breast cancer who progressed on trastuzumab-based therapy. *Journal of Clinical Oncology*, 29: 3126-3132.

16. André F, O'Regan R, Ozguroglu M, Toi M, Xu B, Jerusalem G, Masuda N, Wilks S, Arena F, Isaacs C, Yap YS, Papai Z, Lang I, Armstrong A, Lerzo G, White M, Shen K, Litton J, Chen D, Zhang Y, Ali S, Taran T & Gianni L. (2014). Everolimus for women with trastuzumab-resistant HER2-positive, advanced breast cancer (BOLERO-3): a randomised, double-blind, placebo-controlled phase 3 trial. *Lancet Oncology*, 15: 580-591.

17. U.S. Food and Drug Administration. (2008). Guidance to Industry: Diabetes Mellitus - Evaluating Cardiovascular Risk in New Antidiabetic Therapies to Treat Type 2 Dia- betes. Rockville, MD: US FDA. Available at: http://www.fda.gov/downloads/drugs/guidancecomplianceregulatoryinformation/guidances/ucm071627.pdf (http://www.fda.gov/downloads/drugs/guidancecomplianceregulatoryinformation/guidances/ucm071627.pdf).

18. Soukup M. (2014). A two-stage approach to ruling out an excess amount of risk: statistical implications. Available at: http://www.fda.gov/downloads/Drugs/NewsEvents/UCM410139.pdf (http://www.fda.gov/downloads/Drugs/NewsEvents/UCM410139.pdf).

19. Scharfstein DO, Tsiatis AA & Robins JM. (1997). Semiparametric efficiency and its implication on the design and analysis of group-sequential studies. *Journal of the American Statistical Association*, 92: 1342-1350.

20. Tsiatis AA. (1981). The asymptotic joint distribution of the efficient scores test for the proportional hazards model calculated over time. *Biometrika*, 68: 311-315.

21. SAS Institute Inc. (2014). *SAS/STAT® 13.2 User's Guide*. Cary, NC: SAS Institute, Inc.

22. Wang SK & Tsiatis AA. (1987). Approximately optimal one-parameter boundaries for group sequential trials. *Biometrics*, 43(1): 193-199.

23. Pampallona S & Tsiatis AA. (1994). Group sequential designs for one-sided and two-sided hypothesis testing with provision for early stopping in favour of the null hypothesis. *Journal of Statistical Planning and Inference*, 42: 19-35.

24. Hwang IK, Shih WJ & De-Cani JS. (1990). Group sequential designs using a family of type I error probability spending functions. *Statistics in Medicine*, 9(12): 1439-1445.

25. Kim K & DeMets DL. (1987). Design and analysis of group sequential tests based on the type I error spending rate function. *Biometrika*, 74(1): 149-154.

26. Geiger MJ, Mehta C, Turner JR, Arbet-Engels C, Hantel S, Hirshberg B, Koglin J, Mendzelevski B, Sager PT, Shapiro D, Stewart M, Todaro TG & Gaydos B. (2015). Clinical development approaches and statistical methodologies to prospectively assess the cardiovascular risk of new antidiabetic therapies for type 2 diabetes. *Therapeutic Innovation & Regulatory Science* 49: 50-64.

27. Marchenko O, Jiang Q, Chakravarty A, Ke C, Ma H, Maca J, Russek-Cohen E, Sanchez-Kam M, Zink RC & Chuang-Stein C. (2015). Evaluation and review of strategies to assess cardiovascular risk in clinical trials in patients with type 2 diabetes mellitus. *Statistics in Biopharmaceutical Research* (in press).

28. U.S. Food and Drug Administration. (2014). Confidentiality of Interim Results in Cardiovascular (CV) Outcomes Safety Trials. Rockville, MD: US FDA. Available at: http://www.fda.gov/Drugs/NewsEvents/ucm405023.htm (http://www.fda.gov/Drugs/NewsEvents/ucm405023.htm).

29. Lan KKG, Simon R & Halperin M. (1982). Stochastic curtailed tests in long-term clinical trials. *Sequential Analysis* 1: 207-219.

30. Spiegelhalter DJ, Freedman LS & Blackburn PR. (1986). Monitoring clinical trials: conditional or predictive power? *Controlled Clinical Trials* 7: 8-17.

31. U.S. Food and Drug Administration. (2010). Guidance for Industry: Adaptive Design Clinical Trials for Drugs and Biologics. Rockville, MD: US FDA. Available at: http://www.fda.gov/downloads/Drugs/Guidances/ucm201790.pdf (http://www.fda.gov/downloads/Drugs/Guidances/ucm201790.pdf).

Authors

Joseph Wu, Biostatistics Manager, Global Innovative Pharma Business Unit, Pfizer Inc., Groton, CT, USA.

Sandeep Menon, Vice President and Head of Statistical Research and Consulting Center, Pfizer Inc, Cambridge, MA, USA.

Richard C. Zink, Principal Research Statistician Developer, JMP Life Sciences, SAS Institute Inc, Cary, NC, USA.

Inna Perevozskaya, Senior Director, Biometrics Statistical Research and Consulting Center, Pfizer Inc., Collegeville, PA, USA.

Chapter 3
Sample Size Re-estimation

3.1 Introduction

3.1.1 Motivation. Why Sample Size Re-estimation?

Sample size re-estimation (SSR) has received a lot of attention in recent years as a result of exploding interest in adaptive clinical trial designs in general. In February 2010, the Food and Drug Administration (FDA) issued a draft guidance on Adaptive Design Clinical Trials for Drugs and Biologics, which defined an adaptive design trial as "*a study that includes a prospectively planned opportunity for modification of one or more specified aspects of the study design and hypotheses based on analysis of data (usually interim data) from subjects in the study. Analyses of the accumulating study data are performed at prospectively planned time points within the study, can be performed in a fully blinded manner or in an unblinded manner, and can occur with or without formal statistical hypothesis testing*" [1]. By definition, an adaptive design can have many different types of adaptations and rules [2]. Sample size re-estimation is a specific sub-class of adaptive designs focusing on modifying a trial's sample size based on interim analysis results. It can be performed in either a blinded or unblinded manner. A blinded SSR does not require the knowledge of treatment assignment at the individual patient level, while an unblinded SSR procedure uses treatment assignment knowledge.

When sample size is planned for clinical trials, it depends heavily on assumptions used in sample size calculations, such as the hypothesized treatment effect size and the values of nuisance parameters. There is usually a considerable degree of uncertainty about either or both of these parameters at the trial planning stage. This translates into a wide range of possibilities for the study sample size needed to achieve a desired power level (e.g. 80%). Often the best guesses for effect size and nuisance parameter are utilized in power calculations in order to narrow down the choices for sample size to a single number. Unfortunately, when these assumptions are violated, the power of the study is negatively affected, sometimes quite dramatically. If the trial does not have an interim analysis (i.e. a fixed trial design), it is impossible to detect the gap between our assumptions and reality until the study ends and all available resources are used. The SSR methodology attempts to address this problem by looking at the interim estimates of the nuisance parameter alone (blinded SSR) or the treatment effect and nuisance parameter (unblinded SSR), and adjusting the sample size to maintain the originally planned study power. For example, in case of a normal endpoint with an unknown variance, the blinded SSR procedure will estimate only the variance using interim data. The originally hypothesized mean treatment difference along with the updated variance estimate will be used to calculate the adjusted sample size. In contrast, unblinded SSR will look at the patient-level unblinded data at the time of the interim analysis and calculate both the treatment effect and variability estimates, using both in the adjusted sample size calculations.

It is worthwhile to note that the unblinded SSR methodology is closely related to that of group sequential designs (GSDs) discussed in Chapter 2. In fact, unblinded SSR was originally developed as an extension of GSDs. Because of this relationship, these two classes of adaptive design are often compared and contrasted.

Even though GSDs satisfy the definition of adaptive design from FDA guidance described earlier, many people prefer to refer to them as classical rather than adaptive because their methodological development preceded that of unblinded SSR. There are important similarities and differences between GSD and unblinded SSR: the methodology for the latter builds upon the same distribution theory that was developed for GSDs (Chapter 2), allowing sponsors to adjust sample size upwards as well as downwards. In contrast, GSD only allows sample size reduction through early stopping. For that reason, the unblinded SSR methods are particularly appealing to developers with limited initial budgets. In such cases, the study can be initially sized small and additional sample size invested only if the interim results look promising [3]. Even if a larger budget is available upfront, more and more sponsors are exploring SSR options (both blinded and unblinded) in order to use their drug development resources efficiently.

3.1.2 Overview of Considerations and Issues

When considering a trial design involving SSR, one has to be aware of potential issues (statistical, regulatory, and implementation) that are associated with such designs. The specifics of these issues differ quite a bit between blinded and unblinded SSR procedures; therefore, we will discuss them in detail within their respective sections. In general, the core statistical issue for all methods is type I error control arising from multiple looks (interim and final) at the same data. The unblinded SSR procedure is more prone to type I error inflation than blinded SSR. Regulatory issues revolve primarily around classification of adaptive designs by FDA guidance [1] into "well-understood" (blinded SSR) and "less well-understood" (unblinded SSR). This classification is based on the maturity of the methodology and consequent regulatory experience with submissions involving each type of SSR. This classification is also closely related to implementation challenges: with unblinded SSR, there is always the risk of an accidental interim results leak or treatment effect reverse-engineering that results in compromised study integrity. Reverse-engineering refers to the ability of someone familiar with the interim decision algorithm to make guesses about the observed treatment effect based on the interim decision that was made. The blinded SSR procedure is less affected by such concerns. Because unblinded SSR methods are still considered "less well-understood", additional planning time for regulatory consultation should always be factored-in when considering such studies.

Other than the budgetary considerations discussed in [3], Chuang-Stein et al. [4] describe several scientific reasons why SSR may be desirable. These include (1) lack of information on how a new product candidate may affect a long-term clinical endpoint in the target population; (2) a newly approved product has become part of a treatment regimen to which a product candidate under development will be added; (3) emerging new medical or diagnostic practice that renders information from historical trials out of date; (4) newly issued regulatory guidance that departs from previous thinking on endpoint selection and statistical approaches. In addition, confirmatory trials are increasingly designed to be global trials to support global product registration. Depending on where phase II trials were conducted, a sponsor may face a situation where data from some geographic regions will contribute substantially to the registration trials, but no prior information is available on how patients in these regions respond to the product candidate.

For the above reasons, it is often prudent to use interim data to check the validity of the assumptions made at the design stage. If the assumptions appear to be erroneous, one should consider making a midcourse sample size adjustment to improve the chance that the trial will reach a definitive conclusion.

The main focus of this chapter will be unblinded SSR methodology, though we will give a brief overview of blinded methods in "3.2 Blinded SSR Methods" on page 75, in order to compare and contrast with unblinded SSR methods in "3.3 Unblinded SSR Methods " on page 77 . We conclude with summary and discussion in Section 3.4.

3.2 Blinded SSR Methods

A blinded SSR does not require knowledge of the treatment assignment at the individual patient level. It is designed to modify sample size due to inaccurate assumptions of the variability associated with a continuous endpoint or an assumed background event rate in the control arm for trials with a binary endpoint. Even though the treatment assignment information is very helpful in assessing such parameters, methods have been developed to allow their estimation without using the actual treatment assignment information.

Because blinded SSR does not involve treatment unblinding and can be conducted without worrying about introducing bias into a trial, blinded SSR is classified as a "well-understood" adaptive feature in the FDA guidance. From a practical standpoint, it is also easier to implement than unblinded SSR. For example, there is no potential risk of trial integrity loss due to accidental interim results leak, and no independent data monitoring committee (DMC) required. However, this simplicity comes at a cost: most blinded SSR methodologies rely implicitly on initially assumed treatment effect value to hold. In case of the actual treatment effect being larger than planned, these methods can mistakenly infer that the variance is larger than expected and increase the sample size unnecessarily. Alternatively, if the treatment effect is smaller than expected, the sample size increase will be insufficient, resulting in an underpowered trial, unable to reach meaningful conclusions. In other words, when nuisance parameters are assessed at the time of interim analysis in a blinded manner, it is impossible to determine for sure whether increased/decreased variability in the pooled data results from changes in variability alone or if it is also a consequence of changes in the treatment effect. For this reason, blinded SSR methods are typically reserved for situations where there is reasonable confidence to believe that treatment effect assumptions will hold and only nuisance parameter assumptions need to be reassessed at the interim analysis.

For the case of a two-treatment comparison of a normal endpoint, there are a few methods available to estimate the variance (nuisance parameter) in a blinded manner. The most popular is the one-sample variance method [5]. This method computes the overall estimate of variability from two treatment groups (active and control) essentially ignoring the different treatment assignments. For simplicity we discuss the case of equal allocation to treatment groups. For two normal samples with (unknown) means μ_{trt} and μ_{ctrl}, the common variance σ^2 (nuisance parameter) can be estimated as follows:

$$\widehat{\sigma}^2 = S_{OS}^2 = \frac{1}{2n-1}\left[\sum_{i=1}^{2}\sum_{j=1}^{n}\left(X_{ij} - \overline{X}\right)^2\right],$$

where n is an interim per-group sample size and X_{ij} is the observed interim data with overall mean $\overline{X}$. The key idea here is that the overall variability is a sum of between- and within-group variability, and the former is substantially smaller in clinical trials than the latter. Even though the above estimator of variance S_{OS}^2 is ignoring the between-treatment variability component (and therefore is biased upward when treatment difference is non-zero), it is still a practically useful estimate because the impact of this bias is small for typical noise-to-signal ratios encountered in clinical trials.

A natural extension of this method correcting for the bias is given in an adjusted one-sample variance method [6]:

$$S_{adj}^2 = S_{OS}^2 - \frac{n}{2(2n-1)}\Delta^2.$$

The magnitude of correction depends on the interim sample size n and the value of $\Delta = \mu_{trt} - \mu_{ctrl}$, where Δ is the hypothesized treatment effect for which the study was powered. Following the interim analysis, the originally planned sample size $N = f\left(\alpha,\ 1-\beta,\ \widehat{\sigma}_0^2,\ \Delta\right)$ is replaced by $M = f\left(\alpha,\ 1-\beta,\ \widehat{\sigma}^2,\ \Delta\right)$, where $\widehat{\sigma}^2$ is calculated as either S_{adj}^2 or S_{OS}^2 and function $f(.)$ refers to standard sample size calculations for a two-sample t test. Procedures allowing $M < N$ are called unrestricted designs. Alternatively, a restriction can be placed on the sample size adjustment requiring that the new sample size is max(M, N), resulting in a restricted design. The operating characteristics (power and type I error) depend very much on which version (restricted or unrestricted) is specified. It has been shown by simulation that blinded SSR trials using unrestricted design can lead to slight power losses and negligible type I error inflation [5]. They suggest using the more conservative one-sample variance method or using a restricted design to prevent inflation. Kieser and Friede also explored sensitivity of the adjusted one-sample variance estimator S_{adj}^2 to different values of Δ (ranging from null to alternative hypotheses values) and found that the impact was very minimal [5]. Additionally, they have shown that differences in sample sizes and operating characteristics between one-sample and adjusted one-sample SSR procedures are minimal. This finding is likely to be attributed to treatment effect sizes they explored: in most clinical trials noise to signal ratio is fairly high, i.e. between–group variability is much smaller than within-group variability. This is particularly true for non-inferiority trials (i.e. trials where very small treatment effect is expected and the success of the trial really depends on how well the variability can be nailed down). Such an assumption would also hold for superiority trails powered for a minimal clinically significant effect size. With the landscape of clinical trials constantly changing, this assumption has to be evaluated carefully on a case-by-case basis; as budgets get tighter and competition increases, many sponsors are forced into powering their trials more aggressively for larger commercially viable effect sizes. In these situations, blinded SSR methods should be applied with caution, as the key assumptions driving their performance (i.e. low signal to noise ratio) may get violated and they are likely to increase sample size unnecessarily or fail to increase sample size when needed.

Additional methods for blinded SSR with normal endpoints include the EM (expectation minimization) algorithm, the block-sum estimation of variance, and the unequal treatment allocation within blocks method [7-9]. These methods are less commonly used due to various statistical issues. In general, we will not discuss these challenges here and instead refer the reader to published reviews. For example, several references have a back-and-forth debate over the EM method [10-12].

For trials with a binary endpoint, several methods are also available. Gould describes a procedure for updating a sample size using the observed overall response rate at the interim analysis [13,14]. A similar strategy in the context of a non-inferiority trial with binary endpoint is described in [15]. Variance estimation using blocks of unequal treatment allocation for binary data is proposed in [16].

3.3 Unblinded SSR Methods

3.3.1 Overview

Unlike blinded sample size re-estimation methods described in the previous section, the unblinded SSR procedures utilize both the nuisance parameter and explicit treatment effect estimates in order to calculate the new sample size for the remainder of the trial. The methods vary in how they perform such adaptation but they all share a common feature: the methodology is focused on rigorously controlling the type I error. Type I error is very important to regulators in confirmatory trials (the majority of unblinded SSR trials are performed in confirmatory setting). Type I error inflation can potentially arise from multiple looks at the data (interim and final analyses) and data-driven sample size changes.

There are two major issues concerning unblinded SSR: 1) controlling the type I error rate mentioned earlier and 2) operational issues arising from interim unblinding (the potential to compromise the integrity of the trial). The first issue is statistical in nature and can be addressed by implementing an appropriate methodology assuring type I error control. The second concern is operational, which is much harder to address because it is largely based on perception. While one can implement certain procedures to minimize the chances of accidental unblinding and loss of study integrity, the concerns can never be eliminated completely. Operational issues can very easily become an extensive discussion on their own; for that reason we will not discuss it here and refer the reader to [17-18] for discussion of best practices for adaptive designs (unblinded SSR included).

Blinded SSR methods do not cause concerns about unblinding and their impact on type I error is minimal, so they don't suffer from the key issues of unblinded SSR as much. For that reason, they were classified as "well-understood" by the FDA guidance [1]. It is important to understand the circumstances under which the "less-well understood" procedure of unblinded SSR became preferred over the "well-understood" blinded SSR procedure.

The first reason to consider for unblinded SSR is that blinded methods may confound increased variability with increased treatment effect. An increase in the actual (but unobserved) treatment difference at the time of the (blinded) interim analysis leads to an increase in estimated variance. As a result, sample size may be potentially increased (compared to the original planned size). Conversely, in an unrestricted blinded SSR, a decrease in the actual treatment difference leads to reduced variance estimate, and a potential decrease in the sample size compared to the original planned size. These changes are the opposite to those that are actually needed. This can happen because blinded estimate of variance essentially ignores the between-treatment difference in its calculation. They are efficient only when there is a reason to believe that actual treatment difference is not too far from what was assumed at the design stage. In situations where there is great uncertainty about the underlying treatment effect, the unblinded SSR procedure may be well worth the additional effort to implement.

A second reason to consider an unblinded SSR procedure is that a sample size modification may not be the only objective of an interim analysis. In other words, other types of adaptations may be of interest. More and more trials routinely implement early stopping for efficacy or futility (e.g. classical GSD), both of which would require unblinding. If unblinding is already considered in the study plan, then using an unblinded SSR is a lot more precise than a blinded SSR. In fact, many unblinded SSR methodologies evolved as an adaptation to increase sample size on top of GSD-like boundaries for early stopping, i.e., as a way to expand the list of adaptation options available at the time of interim analysis. In general, it is very hard to get an overall recommendation on when to use one adaptation versus another. Each trial should be evaluated on a case-by-case basis, preferably by simulation that includes a good variety of reasonable treatment effect/variance scenarios. Based on the resulting operating characteristics and the likelihood of underlying assumptions, a final choice between blinded vs unblinded SSR procedures should be made.

For the remainder of this section, we focus on the statistical issues (e.g. controlling type I error rate resulting from multiple looks at the data) surrounding unblinded SSR. There are three main statistical issues to address (and pre-specify) when considering a method for unblinded SSR:

1. How to determine the new sample size?
2. How to set the final decision rule to accept/reject the null hypothesis so that type I error is preserved?
3. How to estimate the treatment effect in the final analysis?

Among these three issues, type I error control is probably the most researched topic in the statistical literature. The issue of determining the new sample is closely related to controlling type I error (just like power and type I error are related when planning a fixed-size trial) but it has some "degree-of-freedom." Most type I error control methodologies focus on defining an end-of-study rule for accepting or rejecting the null hypothesis following the unblinded SSR, but they leave some freedom as to how the new sample size is actually selected. This is understandable since sample size decisions are often heavily influenced by non-statistical considerations such as budget, regulatory, and market requirements. Because of the close relationship between issues #1 and #2 for some methods, we will discuss SSR methods in conjunction with type I error control, on a method-by-method basis.

Concerns over the final study analysis (estimation and confidence intervals) are not discussed here because the related literature is generally less mature and is still an active area of research for some methods. Nonetheless, estimation deserves attention because computing classic-point estimates and associated confidence intervals (CIs) following a trial with unblinded SSR may lead to biased results. Even if the final study inference is well defined and preserves the type I error rate, the methodology to compute point estimates and associated confidence intervals still needs to be addressed. At a minimum, simulations should be performed to quantify the magnitude of bias (often very small). For some methods, the theoretical framework addressing estimation at the end of trial is available [19-20].

3.3.2 Classification of Methods Used to Control Type I Error Rate

Historically, most of the original methods were developed and published as a standalone work referencing only closely related methodology. As the number of adaptive designs with SSR grew, so did the confusion about them and the need for a systematic review emerged. Perhaps one of the most comprehensive approaches to provide a unified view of type I error control in adaptive designs is the work by Posch, Bauer and Brannath [21]. They argue that most of the type I error control methods in adaptive trials that involve SSR can be viewed as some form of combination test, making it the cornerstone of the methodology. This is the approach that we will follow. A less philosophical and more pragmatic view is to break all methods into two categories: either performing a non-standard analysis by modifying test statistic/rejection region or performing a standard analysis, but restricting conditions under which this analysis can be done. Some examples are given bellow; the list is by no means exhaustive:

1. Perform a non-standard analysis at the end of the trial:
    a. Adjust the test statistic ([22] down-weighs the 2nd stage data in case of a sample size increase)
    b. Adjust critical region [23]
    c. Preserve conditional error function [24]
    d. Combine p-values for the 2 stages (before and after the SSR) and re-define the critical region for the combined value [25]
    e. Dual test (elaborates on the p-value combination test addressing some of its potential pitfalls) [26]
2. Perform a standard analysis at the end but state conditions under which sample size can be increased [3, 27, 28].

3.3.3 Methods Based on Combination Tests

3.3.3.1 Overview

For the sake of simplicity, we focus on the framework of a two-stage design (i.e. one interim analysis) comparing two treatment arms with equal allocation for a normally-distributed endpoint. It should be kept in mind that many of these methods generalize to binomial or time-to-event (TTE) endpoints based on asymptotic properties. Extension of these methodologies to trials with multiple interim analyses is possible but seldom used in practice.

As mentioned earlier, the cornerstone methodology of a p-value combination test is captured in [25,29]. The basic idea is that data from a two-stage trial can be viewed as two separate pieces from the two stages, before and after the interim analysis. When testing the null hypothesis of no difference between treatment arms,

H_0: $\delta = 0$ versus

$H_1: \delta > 0$,

the trial decisions could be based on p-values p_1 and p_2 generated from data in Stage 1 and Stage 2, respectively. For example, at the end of Stage 2 the decision to reject H_0 may be based on combination function $C(p_1, p_2) \le c_\alpha$, for an appropriate c_α chosen to preserve the type I error rate. The only requirement for the combination function

$C(p_1, p_2)$ above is that it is monotone increasing for both p_1 and p_2, and strictly increasing in one of them. It is also crucial that there is no overlap in Stage 1 and Stage 2 data, assuring independence of p_1 and p_2 (which is the foundation of p-value combination methodology).

In a trial with an unblinded SSR, the critical value for the final test is calculated so that the probability to reject H_0 at the final test is α. In practice it is very rare for a trial to include a chance for SSR but not offer an opportunity for an early efficacy/futility stop at an interim analysis. Combination test methods can be applied to such trials. Suppose that the trial has pre-specified efficacy/futility boundaries for Stage 1, similar to those under a group sequential design. In that case, the critical value has to be calculated accounting for the possibility of early stopping. The decision tree for a combination method takes the following form:

End of Stage 1

- If $p_1 < \alpha_1$, the trial stops early for efficacy

- If $p_1 > \beta_1$, the trial stops early for futility

- If $p_1 < \alpha_1 < \beta_1$, the trial continues into Stage 2, possibly with sample size change

End of Stage 2

- Decision to reject H_0 is made based on $C(p_1, p_2) \le c_\alpha$.

When calculating c_α in the above case, the overall type I error rate is

$$\Pr(p_1 < \alpha_1) + \Pr((\alpha_1 < p_1 < \beta_1) \cap (C(p_1, p_2) \le c_\alpha)),$$

where probabilities are calculated under the null hypothesis of no treatment difference. For the sake of simplicity, we put aside the issue of early efficacy/futility stopping and focus on unblinded SSR as the only adaptation for the remainder of this chapter.

Th most widely used combination tests include Fisher's combination test and the inverse normal method discussed below. Both combine p-values. Because there is a one-to-one correspondence between p-values and test statistics, they also can be viewed as test statistic combination methods. In Fisher's combination test, $C(p_1, p_2) = p_1 p_2$. In the case of the inverse normal method [21],

$$C(p_1, p_2) = 1 - \Phi\left[w_1 \Phi^{-1}(1 - p_1) + w_2 \Phi^{-1}(1 - p_2)\right],\ 0 < w_i < 1,\ w_1^2 + w_2^2 = 1 \quad (3.1)$$

The method of Lehmacher and Wassmer can be viewed as a special case of combination function (3.1) with equal weights w_1 and w_2, based on the sum of standardized Wald statistics obtained at the end of the trial [30]. The method of Cui, Hung, and Wang (discussed in detail in the next section) is also a special case where the second half of the trial is down-weighted in situations when the sample size is increased [22].

The above p-value combination tests do not rely on any particular rule for sample size adaptation, as long as sample size increase is the only change. Bauer and Köhne [25] recommended Stage 2 sample size adjustment for Fisher's combination test using a conditional power argument

$$Pr_\delta(\text{reject } H_0 \text{ at the end} \mid \text{interim data}) = Pr_\delta(p_2 < (c_\alpha / p_1) \mid \text{interim data})$$

where the Stage 2 p-value p_2 is calculated using the Stage 2 data only (i.e from $2(M - n)$ subjects based on adjusted final sample size $2M$). The final sample size is selected by equating the conditional power above to some reasonable number (e.g. 80%) and solving for M.

3.3.3.2 CHW Procedure as a Special Case of the Combination Test

The method of Cui, Hung, and Wang (CHW) was originally presented in [22]; we reproduce a simplified description of it here. Suppose an interim analysis with a decision to possibly increase the sample size is conducted after $2n$ patients and the originally planned sample size is N per group. Let Z_n be the normalized test statistic comparing the means of the two treatment groups based on the interim data. Under the null hypothesis $\delta = 0$, the statistic Z_n follows a standard normal distribution. If the sample size does not increase, the test statistic at the final analysis, denoted by Z_N, can be written as the weighted sum of the test statistics from the two stages Z_n and Z_{N-n}:

$$Z_N = \sqrt{\frac{n}{N}}Z_n + \sqrt{\frac{N-n}{N}}Z_{N-n}.$$

If after the interim analysis, the sample size is increased to $M(M > N)$ per group, the same statistic becomes

$$Z_M = \sqrt{\frac{n}{M}}Z_n + \sqrt{\frac{M-n}{M}}Z_{M-n},$$

where Z_{M-n} is the test statistic based on the last $2(M-n)$ subjects. Z_M is sometimes called a naïve statistic because it is based on the standard calculation of the final test statistic following a two-stage design calculated as if data-driven sample size adjustment did not take place. The naïve test statistic Z_M could inflate the overall type I error rate, sometimes quite dramatically. To counter the effect on the type I error rate, CHW methods propose modifying the weights on Z_n and Z_{M-n} as shown below:

$$Z'_M = \sqrt{\frac{n}{N}}Z_n + \sqrt{\frac{N-n}{N}}Z_{M-n}. \quad (3.2)$$

A closer examination of rule (3.2) and comparison with (3.1) reveals that the CHW method is a special case of a p-value combination method with $w_1 = \sqrt{n/N}$ and $w_2 = \sqrt{(N-n)/N}$. The type I error rate preservation property of the CHW test statistic does not depend on what rule is used to determine the new sample size M per group and it does not require any cap on M. The original CHW paper suggests selecting sample size M based on the conditional power argument or setting $M = g(\Delta_0/\Delta_L)^2$, where Δ_L is the estimated treatment effect at the interim analysis and Δ_0 is the treatment effect used to determine the original sample size. Another way to select the sample size M is to plug–in an interim estimate of treatment effect Δ_L into a usual sample size calculation formula for a normally-distributed endpoint. Regardless of how the sample size is selected, the type I error rate will be preserved as long as the sample size adjustment is the only modification.

The only difference between the naïve statistic Z_M and the CHW statistic Z'_M is that the result from the second part of the trial (i.e. Z_{M-n}) is down-weighted when $N < M$. This has led to numerous criticisms of CHW statistics as violating the principle of "all patients being equal." The same argument expressed in mathematical terms states that the CHW statistic Z'_M is different from the sufficient statistics Z_M, therefore leading to a loss of efficiency. While the debate over the loss of efficiency has generated a lot of theoretical research and publications, in practice this loss is not huge, especially if the sample size re-estimation rule is implemented reasonably, e.g. without multiple fold increase from N to M because the estimated treatment effect at the interim analysis is much smaller than the planned Δ.

The CHW method can be extended to trials with a TTE endpoint. In this case, weights given to the test statistics pre- and post-SSR interim analysis are the square root of the proportions of events in the respective periods under the original sample size plan.

Sample size re-estimation on the number of events in TTE trials should not be confused with increasing the number of patients only to achieve the same number of events due to lower than projected pooled event rate. The latter will not impact type I error rate. By comparison, if after the interim results are observed, that the target event number is adjusted upward to increase the amount of information for end-of-study testing, then one enters into the domain of sample size re-estimation. In the latter case, appropriate statistical and operational adjustments should be planned and pre-specified as part of the study design.

3.3.3.3 Example of the CHW Method

Let us consider a hypothetical two-arm trial with equal allocation to be designed to test the efficacy of an experimental new treatment compared to a control, which is also the standard of care. The primary endpoint is a binary outcome with a higher rate indicating improvement of the disease state. We denote p_t as the rate of response in the treatment and p_c as the rate of response in the control arm. The control treatment is based on findings from previous studies and is expected to have a response rate of 9%, while it is hypothesized that the new experimental treatment is expected to increase the response by 40%. Though an improvement of 40% is very desirable, in practice, even an improvement of 32% has clinical value. Hence, the sponsor would like to have an insurance policy to cover for improvement in range of clinical relevance.

While designing this study, we consider a few design options including a classical design (fixed sample size), a group sequential design, and an adaptive design with sample size re-estimation. There are pros and cons for each of the design options; however, we will specifically explore scenarios under which adaptive design with sample size re-estimation would be beneficial.

Classical Design

For a classical design with a single look, a total sample size of 2,326 subjects are needed to achieve 80% power to detect a 40% improvement for a one-sided α=0.025. If the improvement is around 32% then this trial would be underpowered with the power drop as low as 62% if the true improvement is 32%, while if the total sample size is increased to 3,532 and if the true improvement is 40% the trial is overpowered with power around 93%. Table 3.1 on page 82 shows the sample size and the power in the range of scenarios from a clinically meaningful improvement of 32% to a desirable improvement of 40%.

Table 3.1 Power for Classical Design

True Percent Improvement	**Optimistic Improvement (Δ_0 = 40%)** *N*=2326	**Pessimistic Improvement (Δ_0 = 32%)** *N*=3532
32%	62%	80%
34%	67%	84%
36%	72%	88%
38%	76%	91%
40%	80%	93%

There are some ways to deal with this situation:

1. Power the trial conservatively at 32% with a classical design and protect the trial in case the true percent improvement is as 32%, or
2. Power the trial conservatively at 32% with a group sequential design giving the option to decrease the average sample size through realistic futility or efficacy stopping boundaries, or
3. Start with the optimistic scenario of 40% and increase the sample size if the futility or efficacy boundary is not crossed.

Group Sequential Design

While considering the flexible designs, group sequential is the first natural consideration for any pivotal trial due to regulatory comfort in these designs. We consider a GSD with one interim look to detect an improvement of 32% with a possibility of stopping early for efficacy or futility. Group sequential designs can be a very safe and attractive option. However, the study population, the time at which the endpoint is observed, and the enrollment rate should be taken into consideration. In other words, the saving in the potential duration for the study should be balanced with the saving in the sample size. In our hypothetical example, we perform an interim analysis when approximately 50% of the subjects have observed the primary endpoint. We now choose the error spending function to evaluate the interim look. In most cases, the type I error or type II error is spent very conservatively in the early look so that a decision of efficacy or futility is triggered only if the results are compelling towards or against the new treatment.

The stopping boundaries can be chosen in several different ways and should be aligned to the project objectives. In this example, we choose the interim futility boundary such that the study can be stopped at interim if there is no difference between control and the test treatment, i.e., no improvement in the condition while the interim efficacy boundary is chosen such that the trial can be stopped at the interim if there is overwhelming efficacy. To achieve this objective, Example Code 3.1 on page 83 uses an error spending function using the conservative O'Brien-Fleming-like boundary to control type I error and an error spending function using a gamma boundary with $\gamma = -4$ to control type II error. In the program, **`proc seqdesign`** uses the **`method(alpha)=errfuncobf`** option for the type I error and the **`method(beta)=errfuncgamma(gamma=-4)`** option for the type II error. Hwang, Shih, and DeCani have shown that $\gamma = -4$ error spending is similar to using the conservative O'Brien Fleming boundary [31,32]. The option **`stop=both(betaboundary=nonbinding)`** gives a non-binding futility boundary. The non-binding futility means that the trial may be continued even if the futility boundary is crossed. There is a slight penalty that needs to be paid at the final analysis if the futility rule is non-binding as compared to the binding rule. The penalty is usually very negligible ; for instance using the above boundaries, the final critical value for the non-binding futility would be 1.969 while it would be 1.962 for a binding futility.

Example Code 3.1 *Sequential Design with Efficacy and Futility Boundaries*

```
proc seqdesign altref=0.0288 errspend;
   OneSidedErrorSpending: design nstages=2
   method(alpha)=errfuncobf
   method(beta)=errfuncgamma(gamma=-4)
   alt=upper stop=both(betaboundary=nonbinding)
   alpha=0.025 beta=0.20;
   samplesize model=twosamplefreq(nullprop=0.09 test=prop);
   ods output Boundary=Bnd_Prop;
run;
```

Here, the sample size is presented based on completers who are available for the primary endpoint evaluation. However, sample size savings should also consider overruns, those patients who are enrolled between the time the last patient is enrolled in the first stage until the completion of the interim analysis. The group sequential design does save expected sample size; however, for populations and indications where the study enrolls very rapidly or if the endpoint is observed after a delay, then the potential benefit of the interim analysis is severely diminished. Table 3.2 on page 84 summarizes the operating characteristics for the GSD with an initial total sample size 3,532.

Table 3.2 *Group Sequential Design with Improvement of 32%*

True Percent Improvement	Probability of Early Efficacy Stopping		Probability of Early Futility Stopping		Average Sample Size		Overall Power
	Under H_0	Under H_1	Under H_0	Under H_1	Under H_0	Under H_1	
32%	0.0016	0.160	0.518	0.026	2614	3205	80.0%
34%	0.0015	0.190	0.519	0.019	2611	3162	83.9%
36%	0.0017	0.224	0.522	0.014	2607	3111	87.6%
38%	0.0017	0.261	0.521	0.012	2606	3051	90.6%
40%	0.0017	0.297	0.522	0.008	2605	2992	93.1%

Based on Table 3.2 on page 84, this group sequential design has decent properties in that it has a low probability of stopping the trial for efficacy under the null hypothesis, while there is more than a 50% probability of stopping for futility if there is no improvement. It is recommended that readers assess different stopping boundaries to ensure desirable operating characteristics in order to incorporate program needs.

Adaptive Design with Unblinded Sample Size Re-estimation

In this design there is an opportunity to start with the optimistic total sample size of 2,326 and invest adaptively if the trial is not stopped for futility or efficacy. In this specific example, neither of the classical designs give us any flexibility. For example, in the first case when the improvement is 40%, a trial with 2,326 would lead to an underpowered trial if the true improvement is 32%, while the trial with 3,532 subjects would be overpowered if the true improvement is 32%. As discussed earlier, the GSD suffers from a large initial commitment of cost, and not sufficient gain if the trial recruits rapidly with a delayed endpoint. Some of these drawbacks encountered by a GSD can be mitigated by an adaptive design with sample size re-estimation. It provides an opportunity to start with an initial sample size of 2,326 subjects as in the optimistic scenario (design delta of 40%) of the classical design and adapt at an interim analysis. The interim analysis will be conducted when about 50% of the subjects complete the induction period.

At the interim analysis, one of the following decisions would be made:

1. Trial would be stopped for futility ($Z_1 < b_1$).

2. Trial would be stopped for efficacy ($Z_1 > c_1$), or

3. Trial would continue with a sample size re-estimation if neither futility nor efficacy is met ($b_1 \le Z_1 \le c_1$).

In this example, as done in GSDs, we choose the interim futility boundary such that the study can be stopped at the interim if there is no observed difference between control and the test treatment. For example, no improvement in the condition while the interim efficacy boundary is chosen such that the trial can be stopped at the interim if the improvement (i.e. the interim estimate) is at least 40%. If the interim statistic Z_1 is between b_1 and c_1; then the sample size would be increased using the interim estimate up to a maximum total sample size of 5,000 subjects. The type I error control at the final analysis would be done using the weighted Z-statistic as outlined in Cui, Hung, and Wang [22]. Table 3.3 on page 85 summarizes the results for this design with an initial total sample size of 2,326 i.e. $\Delta_0 = 40\%$.

Table 3.3 *Sample Size Re-Estimation*

True Percent Improvement	Probability of Early Efficacy Stopping		Probability of Early Futility Stopping		Average Sample Size		Overall Power
	Under H_0	Under H_1	Under H_0	Under H_1	Under H_0	Under H_1	
32%	0.0017	0.087	0.523	0.059	2870	3377	80.0%
34%	0.0017	0.102	0.523	0.046	2869	3293	83.2%
36%	0.0023	0.119	0.526	0.038	2856	3196	86.5%
38%	0.0023	0.137	0.526	0.031	2856	3101	88.9%
40%	0.0023	0.158	0.526	0.0257	2855	2994	91.3%

Based on Table 3.2 on page 84 and Table 3.3 on page 85, the properties are similar in that the saving of sample size for the GSD is through the average sample size. However, there is an initial upfront commitment. The sample size re-estimation gives a little more flexibility with a smaller initial sample size commitment. The properties of the adaptive sample size re-estimation can be increased further through the use of promising zone approach, which is discussed in the subsequent sections. Table 3.2 on page 84 and Table 3.3 on page 85 are generated using SAS macro **%SSR_EFF** in Example Code 3.2 on page 86.

Below we briefly summarize the macro. The initial macro calls are the following:

1. **nSamp** = number of simulations
2. **alpha** =desired α level
3. **beta** = desired β level
4. **cont** = control response to be simulated
5. **trt** = treatment response to be simulated
6. **pc** = assumed control response
7. **ptrt** = assumed treatment response
8. **delta** = difference between treatment and control response
9. **Nmax** = maximum sample size to be committed
10. **r** = randomization ratio of treatment and control
11. **t** = timing of interim analysis

12. **c1** = efficacy boundary at interim analysis in the standardized Z scale
13. **c2** = efficacy boundary at the final analysis in the standardized Z scale
14. **b1** = futility boundary at the interim analysis in the standardized Z scale

In the **%SSR_EFF** macro, **Nmax** is set to initial total sample size of 3,532 for the group sequential design, while it is set to a total sample size of 5,000 for the sample size re-estimation. Download sample code from the companion site to see explicit macro calls to reproduce Table 3.2 on page 84 and Table 3.3 on page 85.

Example Code 3.2 *SAS Macro SSR_EFF*

```
%macro SSR_EFF(nSamp=,alpha=,beta=, cont=, trt=,pc=,ptrt=, delta=, Nmax=,
r=,t=, c1=, c2=,b1=,titl=);
   data SSR_EFF;
   /*** r= randomization allocation ***/
   /*** total sample size by n and total numbers of subjects in each
   group by n1 = (1 - r)n and n2 = rn so that the fraction of subjects
   the active arm is r and total sample size is **/
   eSize=abs((&delta.)/((&pc.*(1-&pc.)+&ptrt.*(1-&ptrt.))/2)**0.5);
   nFixed=2*ceil(2*((probit(1-&alpha.)+probit(1-&beta.))/eSize)**2);
   /** Total Sample Size at the Interim Analysis**/
   n1=ceil(&t.*nfixed);
   n2=nFixed-n1;
   c_seed1=1736; t_seed1=6214;
   c_seed2=7869; t_seed2=9189;

   do i=1 To &nSamp;
      n11=round((1-&r.)*n1);
      n12=round(&r.*n1);
      cont1=Ranbin(c_seed1,N11,&cont.)/n11;
      trt1=Ranbin(t_seed1,N12,&trt.)/n12;
      deltahat1=trt1-cont1;
      pbar1=(cont1*n11+trt1*n12)/(n11 + n12);
      se1=sqrt(pbar1*(1-pbar1)*(1/n11+1/n12));
      z1=deltahat1/se1;
      improve=((trt1-cont1)/cont1)*100;
      rejectho=0;estop=0;fstop=0;power=0;
      if Z1 > &c1. then do;
         rejectho=1;
         ESTOP=1;
         nfinal=n1;
      end;
      if Z1 < &b1. then do;
         rejectho=0;
         FSTOP=1;
         nfinal=n1;
      end;
      if &b1. =< Z1 < &c1. then do;
         eRatio=abs(&delta/(abs(deltahat1)+0.0000001));
         n_adj=(eRatio**2)*nfixed;
         nFinal=Min(&Nmax,Max(nfixed,n_adj));
         nFinal=Min(&Nmax,Max(nfixed,n_adj));
      end;
      w1=sqrt(n1/(n1+n2));
      w2=sqrt(n2/(n1+n2));
```

```
      /***** Simulate Data for Stage II *******/;
      cont2=.;
      trt2=.;
      z2=.;
      zchw=z1;
      if nfinal > n1 then do;
         n21=round((1-&r.)*(nfinal-n1));
         n22=round(&r.*(nfinal-n1));
         n2=n21+n22;
         cont2=Ranbin(c_seed1,N21,&cont.)/n21;
         trt2=Ranbin(t_seed1,N22,&trt.)/n22;
         deltahat2=trt2-cont2;
         pbar2=(cont2*n21+trt2*n22)/(n21 + n22);
         se2=sqrt(pbar2*(1-pbar2)*(1/n21+1/n22));
         z2=deltahat2/se2;
         ZCHW=w1*Z1+w2*Z2;
      end;
      if ZCHW > &c2. then rejectho=1;
      else rejectho=rejectho;
      output;
   end;
   run;

   title "&titl";
   proc means data=SSR_EFF;
      var rejectho nfinal estop  fstop nfixed;
   run;
%mend SSR_EFF;

%SSR_EFF(nSamp=100000,alpha=0.025,beta=0.2,cont=0.1188,
trt=0.1188,pc=0.09,ptrt=0.1188,delta=0.0288,Nmax=3532,
r=0.5,t=0.5, c1=2.963, c2=1.969,b1=0.011,
titl=GSD with 32% Improvement under H0);
```

3.3.4 Sample Size Re-estimation Based on Promising Zone

3.3.4.1 Overview

This method builds on a series of work by several authors [3, 27, 28]; we will base our description on [3]. The core idea of this method is to derive a sample size re-estimation rule based on the conditional power, and use a standard (i.e. non-modified) statistic to test the null hypothesis at the end of trial. In order to protect type I error, the authors of [3, 27, 28] restrict the set of conditions under which such procedures can be performed rather than modifying the final analysis.

The idea of using conditional power for interim decisions is not really new or unique to this method. For example, see the extensive discussion in [21] who, among other things, point out that when observed treatment effect is small, the resulting SSR procedure based completely on the fact that the conditional power argument has undesirable properties of the new sample size being too large. Also, the fact that most SSR methods have to use a non-standard test statistic at the end of the trial to control for type I error rate creates some room for potential inconsistency in the final study inference between classical methods (GSD) and most unblinded SSR designs.

The promising zone design of Mehta and Pocock attempts to alleviate these concerns by using a conventional (in a sense of a GSD) Wald test statistic Z_M for the final decision, arguing that even if the final sample size is increased in a data-dependent manner, the overall type I error rate will not be inflated, provided that the sample size modifications are not too extreme [3]. The sample size modification rule is based on the conditional power assuming the treatment effect CP_δ in future observations:

$$CP_\delta(Z_{n,}, N - n) = P_\delta(Z_N > z_\alpha \mid Z_n = z_n). \quad (3.3)$$

Chen, DeMets, and Lan have shown that if sample size is increased only when the conditional power is above 50%, then one can use conventional statistics for the final testing and the type I error rate will not be inflated [28]. Mehta and Pocock took this approach further by lowering the 50% CP threshold as described below [3].

The new sample size M per group is selected so that $CP_\delta(Z_{n,}, M - n) = 1 - \beta$. A not too extreme sample size increase is quantified as 1) implementing a conservative cap on the total sample size $M < N_{\max}$ and 2) increasing sample size only if $CP_{\min} \le CP < 1 - \beta$, where $1 - \beta$ is the targeted study power and $CP_{\min}$ is the minimally acceptable conditional power that would still assure type I error preservation while using the conventional Wald statistic at the end of trial. The precise value of $CP_{\min}$ is determined based on the ratios $N_{\max}/N$ and n/N and on the targeted power $1 - \beta$. For most commonly used trial designs, $CP_{\min}$ will be in a range of 30-40%. For example, for a two-fold maximum allowed sample size increase, $N_{\max}/N = 2$, and one interim look midway through the trial, the $CP_{\min}$ would be 36% for 90% overall power [3].

One important (and controversial) point is which value of treatment effect to use in calculating the conditional power in equation (3.3). Should it be the treatment effect Δ_0 used to determine the original sample size or its interim estimate $\widehat{\Delta}$? There is no consensus or uniformly agreed upon answer. Mehta and Pocock recommend using the observed treatment difference, which may be justifiable given somewhat restrictive requirements under which the SSR is carried out [3]. Under their method, sample size adjustment will occur only if the observed treatment effect is in the ballpark of what was hypothesized, so it is unlikely to cause problems. Posch, Bauer, and Brannath give pros and cons of both approaches, pointing out that neither estimate is perfect in practice [21]. Other authors generally advise against plugging–in an estimated treatment effect into equation (3.3) and prefer using the originally planned effect size, citing lack of stability of mid-trial estimates and undesirable expected sample size properties of the former [4].

As a good rule of thumb, neither option should be ruled out a priori, and simulations should be conducted to evaluate operating characteristics of both options. The result may very well depend on the meaningful range of possible underlying treatment effects. If that range is too wide (i.e. extends way beyond clinically meaningful differences and the range of therapeutic value) then it is probably impossible to settle on a SSR rule that would give a uniformly good performance.

3.3.4.2 Promising Zone Example

Let us consider a hypothetical two-arm trial with equal allocation to be designed to test the efficacy of an experimental new treatment compared to the control which is also the standard of care. The primary endpoint is a continuous endpoint with high scores indicating improvement from baseline. We denote μ_t as the difference between the mean change from baseline for the treatment and μ_c as the difference between the mean change from baseline for the control arm. The treatment effect, i.e., the gain in efficacy between treatments is denoted by $\delta = \mu_t - \mu_c$.

The null hypothesis H_0 of this trial is $\delta = 0$ which is tested against the one-sided alternative hypothesis that $\delta > 0$. Based on previous studies, the new treatment is expected to have a δ of at least 0.25 units with a between-subject standard deviation to be around 1. Though the treatment difference is expected to be 0.25 units, a difference of 0.19 units and above is considered clinically and commercially meaningful. Hence, the sponsor would like to have a back plan to cover for uncertainty around the actual treatment difference to ensure that the trial can be appropriately powered in case the alternative hypothesis is less than expected but still in the range of clinical and commercial relevance.

While designing this study, we will consider few design options, including a classical design, i.e., fixed sample size, GSD, and an adaptive design with SSR. There are pros and cons for each of the design options; however, we specifically explore scenarios under which adaptive design with SSR would be beneficial.

Classical Design

It is expected that the treatment difference δ of at least 0.25 units with a between-subject standard deviation (σ) around 1. For a classical design with only a single look, a total of 504 subjects (252 subjects per arm) are needed to achieve 80% power to detect a difference of 0.25 at a one-sided $\alpha = 0.025$. If the treatment difference is indeed as expected, then classical design with 252 subjects per arm will have at least 80% power to detect the true difference. But, if the treatment difference is lower than 0.25, then this trial would be underpowered with the power drop as low as 57% if the true treatment difference is 0.19. There are several ways to deal with this situation. For example, the sponsor could decide to increase the initial sample size to total of 870 subjects (435 per arm) so that the trial is adequately powered at all δ values with at least 0.19. Table 3.4 on page 90 shows the sample size and the power in that scenario. We can see that in this case, the trial is very overpowered if the actual treatment difference is 0.25. The option of powering with δ of 0.19 would be the preferred and default option if the finances and resources for this project are not a constraint. However, in this example we assume that the sponsor does not have the flexibility to make such a large (i.e. total sample size of 870) commitment upfront. However, if the results are in the clinically and commercial relevance region, then the sponsor would be willing to invest more resources. Given this set up, this scenario blends into exploring more flexible designs with more than one look.

Group Sequential Design

We will consider a GSD with one interim look to detect a treatment difference of 0.19 with a possibility of stopping early if the interim treatment difference is more than 0.25. As mentioned before, a GSD can be a very appealing option if the savings in the potential study duration is adequately balanced with the savings in the sample size. In our hypothetical example, we conduct an interim analysis when approximately 50% of the subjects have observed the primary endpoint. For this design, we would assume that the sponsor is interested in early stopping for efficacy only and does not want to stop the trial for futility. Based on this assumption, we will now choose the error spending function to evaluate at the interim look. In most cases, the type I error is spent very conservatively in the early look so that a decision of early efficacy stop is triggered only if the results are compelling towards the new treatment. Hence, we will use an error spending function that mimics the conservative O'Brien-Fleming boundary. Example Code 3.3 on page 89 shows how this can be done in SAS using **`method (alpha)=ERRFUNCOBF`** or using **`method (alpha)=ERRFUNCGAMMA(GAMMA-4)`** in **`proc seqdesign`** [32].

Example Code 3.3 *Sequential Design with Efficacy Boundaries*

```
proc seqdesign altref=0.19 errspend pss(cref=0 0.5 1)
   stopprob(cref=0 0.5 1)
   plots=(asn power errspend)
   boundaryscale=stdZ;
```

```
   OneSidedErrorSpending: design nstages=2
   method(alpha)=ERRFUNCGAMMA(GAMMA=-4)
   alt=upper  stop=reject
   alpha=0.025 beta=0.2 info=cum(1 2);
   samplesize model=twosamplemean(stddev=1 weight=1);
run;
```

Again we emphasize that because this is a hypothetical example, the sample size is presented based on completers. However, sample size savings should consider overruns. Here, we assume no overruns. The GSD saves expected sample size; however, for populations and indications where the study enrolls very rapidly or if the endpoint is observed after a delay, then the potential benefit is severely diminished.

Table 3.4 on page 90 below compares sample size and power for three designs:

1. Classical design with optimistic $\delta = 0.25$

2. Classical design with pessimistic $\delta = 0.19$

3. Group sequential design with pessimistic $\delta = 0.19$ and with an option of stopping early for overwhelming efficacy.

Table 3.4 *Operating Characteristics of Classical and Group Sequential Design*

	Classical Design with optimistic δ		**Classical Design with pessimistic δ**		**Group Sequential Design with pessimistic δ**		
Delta	**Power**	**Total Sample Size**	**Power**	**Total Sample Size**	**Probability of Early Efficacy Stopping**	**Power**	**Average Sample Size**
0.19	0.57	504	0.80	870	0.163	0.799	799
0.20	0.61	504	0.84	870	0.190	0.837	787
0.21	0.65	504	0.87	870	0.220	0.871	774
0.22	0.70	504	0.90	870	0.252	0.899	760
0.23	0.73	504	0.92	870	0.286	0.923	745
0.24	0.77	504	0.94	870	0.323	0.942	729
0.25	0.80	504	0.96	870	0.361	0.957	713

Based on Table 3.4 on page 90, we can see that if 0.19 is a clinically meaningful difference, then the classical design based on optimistic $\delta = 0.25$ can be a risky option and can fail to achieve statistical significance, while the classical design based on pessimistic $\delta = 0.19$ will need a total sample size of 870. The added flexibility with a GSD does help by decreasing the sample size marginally and ensuring a 36% probability of stopping the trial for efficacy if the true $\delta = 0.25$. However, the gain with a GSD is not much as compared to designing a classical design, especially if the true δ is around 0.19.

Adaptive Design with Unblinded SSR in the Promising Zone

In this design there is an opportunity to start small and invest adaptively if results trend towards the promising zone. In our specific example, both classical designs do not provide any flexibility while the GSD, as discussed earlier, suffers from a large initial financial commitment. Further, as seen in Table 3.4 on page 90, the GSD does not provide much additional benefit as compared to the classical design with the pessimistic δ. We now explore an unblinded SSR using the promising zone approach. The adaptive design gives us the opportunity to start with the initial total sample size of 504 subjects as in the optimistic scenario of the classical design and adapt at interim analysis.

We define the promising zone when the conditional power is between 30% and 80%. We take an interim look when 252 subjects reach the primary endpoint and stop the trial early if the results are very compelling or the sample size would be re-estimated if the interim results fall into the promising zone or continue the trial if the results are favorable (conditional power ≥ 80%) or unfavorable (conditional power < 30%) zone. This approach of data-dependent decision making based on conditional power follows the method that is outlined in [3]. With this approach, type I error control can be done with (1) using the regular Wald test statistics once we find the $CP_{\min}$ as outlined in [3] and the previous section and then adjusting the final critical value, or (2) using the weighted Z-statistic as outlined in [22]. In this example, we use the weighted Z-statistic. In this set-up, any additional investment of resources is only warranted after an interim evaluation of data from the current study, rather than speculating treatment effect from previous studies.

Below are the steps planned for sample size re-estimation using the promising zone approach:

1. The initial sample size of 504 subjects is computed as in the classical design with 80% power to detect $\delta = 0.25$ with a one-sided $\alpha = 0.025$ text.

2. An interim analysis is planned when 252 subjects reach the primary endpoint.

3. An O'Brien Fleming-like critical value (c_1) is computed using a gamma spending function with $\gamma = -4$.

4. The trial is stopped if the test statistic crosses c_1 at an interim analysis.

5. If test statistic does not cross c_1; then the conditional power is computed using the estimated value of treatment difference. If the conditional power is between 30% and 80%, then the sample size is re-estimated to achieve 80% conditional power at the estimated treatment difference. The sample size is increased to a maximum of 1008, twice the original sample size of 504. If the re-estimated sample size is more than 1008, the final sample size is capped to 1008. If the conditional power is less than 30% or greater than 80% the study continues with the original sample size of 504 subjects.

Table 3.5 on page 92 compares three scenarios for an optimistic $\delta = 0.25$:

1. Power and total sample size for the classical design (as seen in Table 3.4 on page 90)
2. Overall power and average total sample size for the adaptive design
3. Power and average total sample size for the adaptive design in the promising zone.

Scenario 2 and 3 are the same design with an assessment presented overall and in the promising zone separately.

Table 3.5 Operating Characteristics of Classical and Adaptive Design

	Classical Design		Adaptive Design				
			Overall		Promising Zone		
Delta	Power	Total Sample Size	Power	Average Sample Size	Probability of Early Efficacy Stopping	Power	Average Sample Size
0.19	0.57	504	0.63	563	0.27	0.80	794
0.20	0.61	504	0.67	559	0.27	0.83	791
0.21	0.65	504	0.71	554	0.26	0.86	788
0.22	0.70	504	0.75	548	0.26	0.88	785
0.23	0.73	504	0.78	542	0.25	0.89	782
0.24	0.77	504	0.81	534	0.25	0.91	779
0.25	0.80	504	0.84	527	0.24	0.93	777

The results in the table show that the overall power for adaptive design is about 4% to 6% greater than the classical design with the optimistic δ, however, the additional sample size increase in the promising zone ensures that the trial has the desirable power of 80% at the clinically meaningful difference of 0.19. On average, the trial will land in the promising zone around 25% of the time. The promising zone approach gives the added flexibility so that the sample size is increased only if the results are promising at an interim analysis. This example is just an illustration on how to evaluate the promising zone approach. In practice, extensive simulations aligned to the project needs should be conducted to ensure desirable properties. For example, the minimum and maximum conditional power for the promising zone can be altered or an additional futility boundary can be added.

The adaptive and group sequential designs in Table 3.4 on page 90 and Table 3.5 on page 92 are generated using the SAS macro **%SSR_CP** in Example Code 3.4 on page 93.

Below we briefly summarize the macro. The initial macro calls are the following:

1. **nSamp** = number of simulations
2. **alpha** =desired α level
3. **beta** = desired β level
4. **cont** = control response to be simulated
5. **trt** = treatment response to be simulated
6. **delta** = difference between treatment and control response
7. **Nmax** = maximum sample size to be committed
8. **r** = randomization ratio of treatment and control
9. **t** = timing of interim analysis
10. **c1** = efficacy boundary at interim analysis in the standardized Z scale
11. **c2** = efficacy boundary at the final analysis in the standardized Z scale

In the macro **%SSR_CP**, **Nmax** is set to initial total sample size of 870 for group sequential design, while it is set to a total sample size of 1,008 for the SSR design. After Stage 1, the conditional power (CP) is calculated and the trial is categorized into four zones:

1. UNFAVORABLE (if CP < 0.3)
2. PROMISING (0.3 ≤ CP ≤ 0.8)
3. FAVORABLE (CP > 0.8 and $Z_1 < c_1$)
4. EFFICACY (CP > 0.8 and $Z_1 \geq c_1$)

The sample size is set to 504 (**nfixed**) in the unfavorable and favorable zone; in the efficacy zone the trial is stopped with a sample size of 254 (n_1), while the sample size is re-estimated in the promising zone so that the conditional power is 80%. If the re-estimated sample size is greater than 1,008, the final sample size (**nfinal**) is set to 1,008. Download sample code from the companion site to see all explicit macro calls to reproduce Table 3.4 on page 90 and Table 3.5 on page 92.

Example Code 3.4 *SAS Macro SSR_CP*

```
%Macro SSR_CP(nSamp=,alpha=,beta=, sigma=, cont=, trt=, delta=,
          Nmax=, r=,t=, c1=, c2=,titl=);
  data SSR;
  /*** r= randomization allocation ***/
  /*** total sample size by n and total numbers of subjects in each group by
  n1 = (1 - r)n and n2 = rn so that the fraction of subjects in the active arm
  is r and total sample size is **/

  esize=(&delta.)/&sigma.;
  nFixed=2*ceil(2*((probit(1-&alpha.)+probit(1-&beta.))/eSize)**2);
  /** Total Sample Size at the Interim Analysis**/
  n1=ceil(&t.*nfixed);
  n2=nFixed-n1;

  c_seed1=1736; t_seed1=6214;
  c_seed2=7869; t_seed2=9189;

  do i=1 To &nSamp;
     n11=round((1-&r.)*n1);
     n12=round(&r.*n1);
     cont1 = Rannor(c_seed1)*&sigma./Sqrt(n11)+&cont.;
     trt1 = Rannor(t_seed1)*&sigma./Sqrt(n12)+&trt.;
     deltahat1=trt1-cont1;
     se1=&sigma.*sqrt(1/(n1*&r.*(1-&r.)));
     Z1=deltahat1/se1;
     /*** Calculate Conditional Power ***/
     cp=1-probnorm(&c2.*sqrt(1+(n1/(nfixed-n1)))-Z1*(n1/(nfixed-n1))-
     (deltahat1*sqrt(&r.*(1-&r.))*sqrt(nfixed-n1)/&sigma.));
     if cp < 0.3 then zone="UNFAVORABLE";
     else if 0.3 =< cp =< 0.8 then zone="PROMISING";
     else if (cp > 0.8) and Z1 < &c1  then zone="FAVORABLE";
     else if (cp > 0.8) and Z1 >= &c1  then zone="EFFICACY";
     n2tilda=nfixed;
     w1=sqrt(n1/(n1+n2));
     w2=sqrt(n2/(n1+n2));
     if zone in("PROMISING") then do;
        a=&c2. / w2;
```

```
        zbt=Probit(1-&beta.);
        k=w1/w2;
        n2tilda=(n1*(((a+zbt)/z1)-k)**2)+n1;
    end;
    n2tilda=n2tilda;rejectho=0;estop=0;
    if zone in("EFFICACY") then do;
        n2tilda=n1;
        rejectho=1;
        zchw=z1;
        estop=1;
    end;

    if n2tilda > &nmax. then nfinal=&nmax.;
    else nfinal=n2tilda;

    /***** Simulate Data for Stage II *******/;
    cont2=.;trt2=.;z2=.;zchw=z1;
    if nfinal > n1 then do;
        n21=round((1-&r.)*(nfinal-n1));
        n22=round(&r.*(nfinal-n1));
        cont2 = Rannor(c_seed2)*&sigma./Sqrt(n21)+&cont.;
        trt2 = Rannor(t_seed2)*&sigma./Sqrt(n22)+&trt.;
        deltahat2=trt2-cont2;
        se2=&sigma.*sqrt(1/((nfinal-n1)*&r.*(1-&r.)));
        Z2=deltahat2/se2;
        ZCHW=w1*Z1+w2*Z2;
    end;
    if ZCHW > &c2. then rejectho=1;
    else rejectho=rejectho;
    output;
end;
run;

/** Calculating the power and average sample size **/
ods listing close;
PROC MEANS DATA=SSR;
    CLASS Zone;
    VAR nfinal rejectho estop;
    OUTPUT OUT=Results MEAN=AveSS Power ESTOP ;
RUN;

data results;
    set results;
    if _type_="0" then zone="Overall";
    else Zone=Zone;
    drop _type_ _freq_ ;
run;

ods listing;
title "&titl";
Proc Print data=Results noobs;
run;

/** Calculating the number of times in the promising zone **/
title " Zone Frequency - &titl";
Proc freq data=ssr;
```

```
      tables zone;
   run;
%mend SSR_CP;

***  GSD Design with 0.25 treatment difference **/
%SSR_CP(nSamp=1000000,alpha=0.025,beta=0.2, sigma=1, cont=0, trt=0.25,
delta=0.19, Nmax=870, r=0.5,t=0.5, c1=2.963, c2=1.969,titl=GSD
Design with 0.25 treatment difference);
```

There are potentially several rules for sample size increases that can be used. Extensive simulations should be used to see which rule best suits the project needs, as well as which one gives the best balance between overall power, power in the promising zone, and the average sample size. One simple way is the flat increase, where the sample size is increased to N_{max} or a percentage of N_{max} throughout the promising zone. For example, if the conditional power is between 30% to 80% the sample size can be increased to N_{max} or a percentage of N_{max}. The **%SSR_CP** macro can be modified easily to fit this sample size calculation rule. We further explore two scenarios where we increased the sample size: 1) 2 times the initial sample size, i.e., N_{max} = 1008 in the promising zone and 2) 1.5 times the initial sample size by setting the maximum sample size to 756 (i.e. 75% of N_{max} = 1008). Table 3.6 on page 95 and Table 3.7 on page 96 present three SSR rules used in the promising zone:

1. Sample size increased to achieve a conditional power of 80%
2. Sample size increased to N_{max}, i.e., 2 times the initial sample size
3. Sample size increased to 75% of N_{max}, equivalent to 1.5 times the initial sample size

The **%SSR_CP** macro can be updated easily to fit this flat increase rule. The only modification needed in the macro is the following: **if zone in ("PROMISING") then do; n2tilda=&Nmax; end;**.

The actual value of **&Nmax** could be any value, such as a percentage of the initial planned sample size.

Table 3.6 *Flat Increase SSR Rules in the Promising Zone – Overall Power*

	Achieve CP of 80%		**Flat Increase: 2 x initial sample size**		**Flat Increase: 1.5 x the initial sample size**	
δ	**Power**	**Average Sample Size**	**Power**	**Average Sample Size**	**Power**	**Average Sample Size**
0.19	0.63	563	0.65	620	0.62	553
0.20	0.67	559	0.69	616	0.67	550
0.21	0.71	554	0.73	611	0.71	545
0.22	0.75	548	0.76	606	0.75	541
0.23	0.78	542	0.80	598	0.78	535
0.24	0.81	534	0.83	590	0.81	529
0.25	0.84	527	0.85	581	0.84	522

Table 3.7 Flat Increase SSR Rules in the Promising Zone –Power in the Promising Zone

		Achieve CP of 80%		Flat Increase: 2 x initial sample size		Flat Increase: 1.5 x the initial sample size	
δ	Percent in Promsing Zone	Power	Average Sample Size	Power	Average Sample Size	Power	Average Sample Size
0.19	0.27	0.80	794	0.89	1008	0.80	756
0.20	0.27	0.83	791	0.92	1008	0.82	756
0.21	0.26	0.86	788	0.94	1008	0.85	756
0.22	0.26	0.88	785	0.95	1008	0.88	756
0.23	0.25	0.89	782	0.96	1008	0.90	756
0.24	0.25	0.91	779	0.97	1008	0.91	756
0.25	0.24	0.93	777	0.97	1008	0.93	756

From Table 3.6 on page 95 and Table 3.7 on page 96 we can see that the SSR rule with a flat increase of 1.5 times the initial sample size is better that the other two rules because the overall power and the power in the promising zone is comparable to the conditional power rule of achieving 80% but with a smaller average sample size. The SSR rule with a flat increase of 2 times the initial sample size may lead to an over-powered trial and an increased average sample size. In general, the flat increase rule can be attractive not only because it yields better operating characteristics, but because it can minimize reverse engineering of interim estimates based on the sample size increase since the increase is the same in the whole region of the promising zone.

The flat increase used in the example above can be further improved by using the method proposed by [33]. They propose a stepwise two-stage sample size adaptation using a step function with an inverted U-shaped observed treatment difference. This has the advantage of blinding the treatment effect, which can be potentially revealed at the interim. They use algorithms used for group sequential designs to further minimize expected sample size in the class of adaptive design, namely full optimized two-stage design, optimal two-stage group sequential design and designs based on promising zone.

3.3.5 Methods Based on the Conditional Type I Error Principle

This group of methods computes the probability of rejecting the null hypothesis at the end of the trial to the interim data and uses it to guide interim decisions. One of the most well-known methods from this category is the conditional error probability method by Proschan and Hunsberger [23]. The conditional rejection probability is defined as

$$CP_\delta\left(N-n,\ z_\alpha \middle| z_n\right) = \Pr\left(Z_N > z_\alpha \middle| Z_n = z_n,\ \delta\right)$$

where n and $N-n$ are the Stage 1 and Stage 2 sample sizes per group, respectively, Z_N is a standardized normal test statistic under the original design and δ is a standardized hypothesized effect size. When the above conditional probability is calculated under a non-zero δ (either hypothesized effect size or observed), it becomes a conditional power. If it is calculated under $\delta = 0$, then it becomes a conditional error probability. Integrated over all possible realizations of Z_n, the conditional error probability becomes the overall type I error rate. One could reduce the type I error rate inflation resulting from data-driven sample size adjustment by selecting a larger critical value z_α at the final stage and agreeing to continue the trial only if the first stage p-value $p_1 < p^*,\ p^* \in (0,\ 0.5]$ (e.g. if p^* is set to 0.15, which would translate into accepting the possibility of futility stop in case the p-value from the first stage $p_1 \geq p^* = 0.15$). However, these measures would only keep overall type I error rate below α, but not give an exact α-level procedure.

The key idea of the Proschan and Hunsberger method is to create an exact α-level test at the end. They rewrite type I error rate as

$$\int_{-\infty}^{\infty} A(z_n)\phi(z_n) = \alpha, \quad (3.4)$$

where $A(z_n)$ could be any increasing function with range [0,1], with the integration in (3.4) over all possible realizations of Z_n under the null hypothesis. Proschan and Hunsberger suggest using the following circular function:

$$A(z_n) = \begin{cases} 0 & z_n < z_{p^*} \\ 1 - \Phi\left(\sqrt{k^2 - z_n^2}\right) & z_{p^*} \leq z_n < k. \\ 1 & z_n \geq k \end{cases}$$

In the above equation, p^* is the cut-off for the Stage 1 futility stop and the critical value k for the Stage 1 test statistic z_n is selected (given p^*) so that condition (3.4) holds. The function $A(z_n)$ dictates how much conditional type I error rate to allow at the end of the study given the observed interim results $Z_n = z_n$.

When the design includes an unblinded SSR in addition to early stopping (efficacy and/or futility), the critical value c for the final testing and new sample size per group for second stage $n_2 = M - n$ are selected so that $CP_0(n_2,\ c|z_n) = A(z_n)$ and $CP_\delta(n_2,\ c|z_n) = 1 - \beta$.

It is important to note that the rule lets users decide on how to select n_2 (e.g. how high the conditional power should be or whether to use empirical vs hypothesized effect size). Once the rule is set, the type I error rate is guaranteed at level α. This method can also be viewed as a special case of the p-value combination principle.

Another method in the same category is by Müller and Schäfer [24]. The Müller and Schäfer method is a lot more general than the method by Proschan and Hunsberger and can be extended to multistage trials with adaptations other than sample size (e.g. hypotheses/endpoint changes). The latter also allows an unplanned interim analysis to be inserted into a sequence of pre-planned interim analyses in a group-sequential trial. Even though such extensions are beyond the scope of this chapter, the Müller and Schäfer principle is worth mentioning because even in case of a simple 2-stage procedure for SSR, it highlights a fundamental role of the conditional error function shared by the Proschan and Hunsberger method. That is, after the Stage 1 data have been observed, the conditional error probability (or conditional rejection probabilities, CRP, in their terminology) given $Z_n = z_n$ is all the information from Stage 1 that needs to be carried into Stage 2 of the study. As long as the Stage 2 in the new design has conditional type I error rate equal to the CRP calculated from Stage 1, the overall type I error will be preserved. Müller and Schäfer also recommend selecting Stage 2 sample size based on the conditional power argument [24]. When it comes to type I error rate control, the core idea of both methods is that the stronger evidence is contained in Z_n, the less the burden of showing significance in the final test statistic.

Because of the extensive computations required of the conditional type I error approach, this approach is seldom used in practice. However, with software development for SSR on the rise, this statement is likely to change in the future. Another reason why these methods are seldom used in practice is probably due to the fact that they are too flexible. For example, the Müller and Schäfer principle allows not just SSR change at interim but other more extensive changes such as hypothesis/endpoint changes and recursive insertion of interim analyses. While such flexibility is valuable in theory, it is rarely preferred by regulatory reviewers, especially for registration trials. Limited practical experience with such designs exist. One area where they may be of value is vaccine efficacy trial designs (see [34] for example). Because such trials typically rely on exact binomial distributions rather than a normal approximation for testing the null hypothesis, the flexibility of the Müller and Schäfer method could allow harnessing more precision in α-spending when using discrete (binomial) boundaries for stopping and sample size calculations.

3.4 Information-Based Design

Traditional sample size calculation takes into account both the magnitude of the treatment effect (δ) and values of the nuisance parameter (e.g., the variance for continuous endpoints or the placebo response for binary endpoints), with the best guesses of the nuisance parameter used for the initial sample size calculation. However, if initial estimates of the nuisance parameters are incorrect, this can adversely impact the statistical power to detect a clinically meaningful difference, if indeed a treatment difference exists. One way of addressing this uncertainty around nuisance parameters is to utilize an information-based design. Information-based design and analysis is based on the statistical information (defined below) that is available. In other words, the study continues until the required statistical information is achieved. Here, design and analysis is based on the statistical information or precision scale instead of the sample size scale. Information-based designs are based on the work of several authors, which is itself based on the fundamental concept that statistical information is obtained in the same manner irrespective of the parameter δ [35-37].

For the classical design, information is defined as $I_1 = \left(\frac{z_{\alpha/2} + z_{\beta}}{\delta}\right)^2$. Here, the statistical information depends on both the sample size and the magnitude of the nuisance parameter. For binary endpoints, information depends on the magnitude of the placebo response. For time-to-event (survival) endpoints, information is based on numerous factors, including accrual rate, event rate, length of follow up, and rate of drop outs. In longitudinal studies, information also depends on the number of time points observed per subject. In general, statistical information (I) is inversely related to the standard error of the estimator $\hat{\delta}$ of the parameter δ; that is, $I \approx \frac{1}{(SE^2)}$. Hence, the greater the information that is available, the higher the precision and the smaller the standard error. In a multistage design, the maximum information available is $I_{max} = I_1 {*} IF$, where IF is the inflation factor, a multiplicative constant which is a function of K (number of stages), the form of the error spending boundary (e.g. O'Brien Fleming or Pocock) , and the type I (α) and type II (β) errors. Tsiatis provides a table of inflation factors for different combinations of K, error spending boundaries, α and β [37]. The maximum sample size ($N_{\max}$) for a multistage design is a function of the maximum information ($I_{\max}$) and a nuisance parameter. For example, a test for the difference between two normally distributed means has $N_{\max} = 4\sigma^2 I_{\max}$; a test for the difference between two binomial proportions has $N_{\max} = 2[(p_T)(1 - p_T) + (p_C)(1 - p_C)]I_{\max}$, for treatments T and C.

We replicate an example for a binary endpoint described in Tsiatis [37]. Consider a hypothetical two-arm trial with equal allocation designed to test the efficacy of an experimental new treatment compared to the standard of care (control). We denote p_T as the rate of response in the treatment and p_C as the rate of response in the control arm.

The best guess for the response on the control arm is 0.15. In order to detect a meaningful difference of 0.15 with $p_T = 0.30$, 316 subjects are required for 90% power for a one-sided α=0.025 classical design. The information required is approximately 468. Partial output from **proc seqdesign** from Example Code 3.5 on page 99 is presented in Figure 3.1 on page 99.

Example Code 3.5 *Information Based Design - Fixed Sample Size*

```
proc seqdesign altref=0.15;
   OneSidedFixedSample: design nstages=1
   alt=upper alpha=0.025 beta=0.10;
   samplesize model=twosamplefreq(nullprop=0.15 test=prop);
run;
```

Figure 3.1 *Output for Example Code 3.5*

Sample Sizes (N) Two-Sample Z Test for Proportion Difference								
	Fractional N				Ceiling N			
Stage	N	N(Grp 1)	N(Grp 2)	Information	N	N(Grp 1)	N(Grp 2)	Information
1	315.22	157.61	157.61	467.0	316	158	158	468.1

Alternatively, suppose we design the study with 4 equally-spaced stages using an O 'Brien Fleming-like boundary using the Lan-DeMets error spending function. To obtain 90% power for a one-sided $\alpha = 0.025$ alternative, the total information needed is approximately 477, with a maximum sample size of 322. Partial output from **proc seqdesign** in Example Code 3.6 on page 99 is shown in Figure 3.2 on page 99 and Figure 3.3 on page 100.

Example Code 3.6 *Information Based Design – 4-Stage Design*

```
proc seqdesign altref=0.15;
   OneSidedErrorSpending: design nstages=4
   method(alpha)=errfuncobf
   alt=upper  stop=reject
   alpha=0.025 beta=0.10;
   samplesize model=twosamplefreq(nullprop=0.15 test=prop);
   ods output Boundary=Bnd_Count;
run;
```

Figure 3.2 *Sample Size and Maximum Information for 4-Stage Design*

Sample Sizes (N) Two-Sample Z Test for Proportion Difference								
	Fractional N				Ceiling N			
Stage	N	N(Grp 1)	N(Grp 2)	Information	N	N(Grp 1)	N(Grp 2)	Information
1	80.25	40.12	40.12	118.9	82	41	41	121.5
2	160.49	80.25	80.25	237.8	162	81	81	240.0
3	240.74	120.37	120.37	356.7	242	121	121	358.5
4	320.99	160.49	160.49	475.5	322	161	161	477.0

Figure 3.3 *Boundary Information for 4-Stage Design*

Boundary Information (Standardized Z Scale) Null Reference = 0					
				Alternative	Boundary Values
	Information Level			Reference	Upper
Stage	Proportion	Actual	N	Upper	Alpha
1	0.2500	118.8835	80.24637	1.63551	4.33263
2	0.5000	237.767	160.4927	2.31295	2.96318
3	0.7500	356.6505	240.7391	2.83278	2.35904
4	1.0000	475.534	320.9855	3.27101	2.01409

Suppose that the first interim analysis of 120 subjects (60 subjects per arm) provides an estimated treatment difference of 0. 0167 (15 responses out of 60 subjects in treatment while 14 responses out of 60 subjects in control) with a standard error of 0.0781. The information at Stage 1 is 163.9 (Figure 3.4 on page 100). The actual information is 0.34, slightly less than the expected information of 0.37 (120/322). Since the actual information is not very different from the expected information and the efficacy boundary is not crossed, the trial continues without any change.

Figure 3.4 *Information at First Interim Analysis for 4-Stage Design*

Test Information (Standardized Z Scale) Null Reference = 0						
			Alternative	Boundary Values	Test	
	Information Level		Reference	Upper	Trt	
Stage	Proportion	Actual	Upper	Alpha	Estimate	Action
1	0.3448	163.9449	1.92061	3.09023	0.21472	Continue
2	0.5632	267.8079	2.45473	2.70684	.	
3	0.7816	371.671	2.89182	2.31811	.	
4	1.0000	475.534	3.27101	2.03588	.	

Suppose the second interim analysis of 240 patients (120 patients per arm) provides an estimated treatment difference of 0.10 (41 responses out of 120 subjects in treatment while 29 responses out of 120 subjects in control) with a standard error of 0.0583. The cumulative information at Stage 2 is 292 (Figure 3.5 on page 101). The actual information is 0.61, far less than the expected information of 0.75 (240/322). Since the actual information is much lower than the expected information and the efficacy boundary is not crossed, we re-estimate the total sample size based on the currently available information in order to achieve an $I_{max} = 477$. Using the formula for N_{max} for two binomial proportions, an updated total sample size of 390 subjects is required. The trial continues to Stage 3 with an updated sample size of 390 subjects, instead of the originally planned sample size of 322 subjects.

Figure 3.5 *Information at Second Interim Analysis for 4-Stage Design*

Test Information (Standardized Z Scale) Null Reference = 0						
			Alternative	Boundary Values	Test	
	Information Level		Reference	Upper	Trt	
Stage	Proportion	Actual	Upper	Alpha	Estimate	Action
1	0.3448	163.9449	1.92061	3.09023	0.21472	Continue
2	0.6145	292.2054	2.56410	2.55757	1.76581	Continue
3	0.8072	383.8697	2.93889	2.28706	.	
4	1.0000	475.534	3.27101	2.04963	.	

Suppose the third interim analysis of 360 subjects (180 subjects per arm) provides an estimated treatment difference of 0. 11 (61 responses out of 180 subjects in treatment while 41 responses out of 180 subjects in control) with a standard error of 0.0471. Cumulative information at Stage 3 is 449 (Figure 3.6 on page 101). The actual information is 0.94, compared to the expected information of 0.92 (360/390). At Stage 3, the efficacy boundary is crossed (Figure 3.6 on page 101 and Figure 3.7 on page 102); the study is stopped early for efficacy. The results presented in Figures 3.4 through 3.7 were generated using the `%monitor` macro in Example Code 3.7 on page 102.

Figure 3.6 *Information at Third Interim Analysis for 4-Stage Design*

Test Information (Standardized Z Scale) Null Reference = 0						
			Alternative	Boundary Values	Test	
	Information Level		Reference	Upper	Trt	
Stage	Proportion	Actual	Upper	Alpha	Estimate	Action
1	0.3448	163.9449	1.92061	3.09023	0.21472	Continue
2	0.6145	292.2054	2.56410	2.55757	1.76581	Continue
3	0.9439	448.8653	3.17797	2.06657	2.33051	Reject Null
4	1.0000	475.534	3.27101	2.10100	.	

Figure 3.7 *Efficacy Boundary and Test Statistics at Stage 3 of 4-Stage Design*

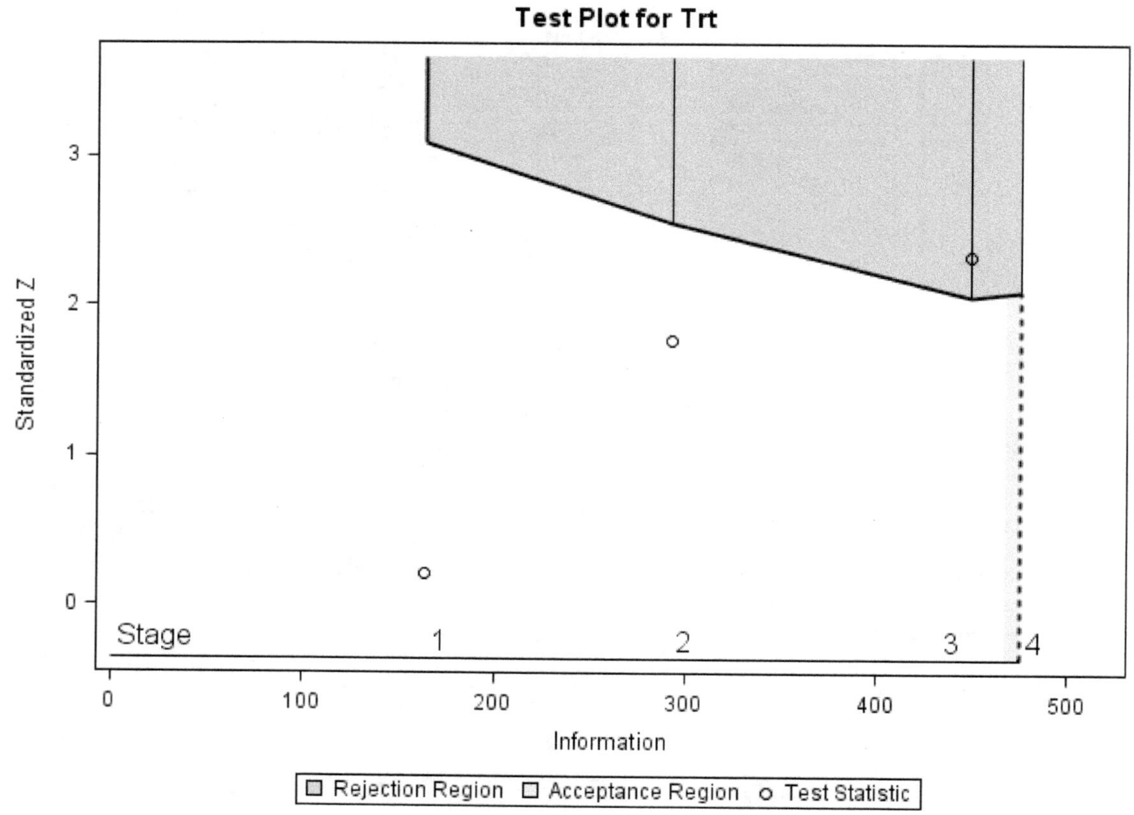

Example Code 3.7 *Information Based Monitoring – 4-Stage Design*

```
%macro monitor(dat=,estimate=,stderr=,Stage=,tit=, Boundary=, Parms=,test= );
   data parms_&dat;
      Parameter="Trt";
      Estimate=&estimate.;
      Stderr=&stderr.;
      _Scale_="mle";
      _Stage_=&stage;
   Run;

   title;
   proc seqtest Boundary=&boundary
      Parms(Testvar=Trt)=&parms
      infoadj=prop errspendmin=0.001
      boundaryscale=stdz errspend
      plots=errspend pss;
      ods output Test=&test;
   run;
%mend monitor;

%monitor(dat=count1,estimate=0.01677,stderr=0.0781,Stage=1,
Boundary=Bnd_Count,parms=Parms_Count1,test=Test_Count1);
%monitor(dat=count2,estimate=0.10330,stderr=0.0585,Stage=2,
Boundary=Test_Count1,parms=Parms_Count2,test=Test_Count2);
%monitor(dat=count3,estimate=0.11000,stderr=0.0472,Stage=3,
```

```
Boundary=Test_Count2,parms=Parms_Count3,test=Test_Count3);
```

3.5 Summary and Conclusions

Several different methods for blinded and unblinded sample size re-estimations were presented in this chapter for normally distributed data. Blinded methods reviewed included the one-sample variance method and the adjusted one-sample variance method. Unblinded SSR methods included Fisher's combination test, the inverse normal method, the CHW procedure, the promising zone design and conditional type I error preserving procedures (Proschan and Hunsberger, Müller and Schäfer). With the exception of the promising zone and the Müller and Schäfer procedure, all the other unblinded methods can be viewed as a special form of a combination test.

These procedures can be extended to the case of a binary endpoint based on the asymptotic normal approximation of binomial distribution in situations where such approximation is appropriate. In cases where exact binomial distribution has to be used, the problem of SSR becomes more complicated and was not investigated within this chapter.

Except for the promising zone and the Proschan and Hunsberger methods, unblinded SSR approaches reviewed were presented under the assumption that sample size adjustment is the only decision to be made at the interim analysis. This was chosen for the sake of simplicity (i.e. to focus on the concept of SSR under each method). In practice, other decisions such as early stop for futility or efficacy often accompany SSR. For these more real-life situations, the approaches presented in this section remain generally applicable, but the type I and type II error rate calculation needs to be adjusted to reflect opportunities for early stopping.

When a design includes the opportunity for an early efficacy stop, the need to preserve the overall type I error rate is well accepted. Early stopping due to futility is more subtle. It is common knowledge that stopping early for futility can, in fact, reduce the false positive rate, making it possible to use a higher significance level at the final analysis while maintaining the overall type I error rate at the desired level [38]. While the latter is theoretically justified, regulators have been unwilling to accept a higher significance level at the final analysis due to a planned interim futility analysis because futility rules are not binding and may not be rigorously enforced by a sponsor.

Many original manuscripts describing the unblinded SSR methodology focus solely on type I error control, because it is the most important topic to regulators (at least in a confirmatory trial setting) . When considering SSR, one has to address not only type I error control but also the rules to select the new sample size and how to estimate the treatment effect at the end of the trial. We did not get the opportunity to address these issues in detail within this chapter. Some general considerations are outlined below.

Sample size. With the exception of the promising zone design, a user is free to choose the method to re-estimate the sample size. It is commonly accepted to revise the sample size based on the desired conditional power (similar to how promising zone design does it). Even though in theory the sample size M does not have to be restricted, in practice most trials with unblinded SSR employ a cap on the maximum allowable sample size increase. The competing forces in selecting a maximum allowable sample size (MASS) are obvious. To maximize the chance of success in a trial (purely in terms of statistical power) we would select a value for the MASS that is as large as possible. This could potentially lead to increased trial costs and duration and carry a regulatory risk of achieving statistical significance for a treatment difference that is not clinically relevant. On the other hand, selecting too small a value for MASS could make the SSR effort useless, because power would not be maintained in situations of even mild departures from the assumptions used in the original sample size planning. As statisticians, we need to ensure that the selected value of the MASS is large enough to ensure the usefulness of a proposed SSR plan, while keeping in mind the implications of a large sample size increase to trial operations and interpretation.

Estimation. In a two-stage design, naive estimates from Stage 1 and Stage 2 are unbiased. But because the Stage 2 sample size is determined by using Stage 1 data, the naïve estimation approach based on data from both stages yields a biased estimate [39]. Final study inference (treatment difference estimate and associated confidence intervals) following a study with unblinded SSR remains an active area of research. For some methods analytical solutions exist and for others simulation remains the only way of quantifying the bias in estimation. For these reasons the authors did not attempt to give a comprehensive review of estimation methods here. With exception of the promising zone design, for most methods with a normal endpoint the final treatment effect estimation is usually accomplished by relying on the duality between CIs and a hypothesis test. Brannath and coauthors [19] extended the repeated confidence interval approach of [20] to flexible designs.

The promising zone design stands out from the other methods because it specifies the condition under which it can be used and does not require users to modify the test statistic or rejection region in the final analysis. The latter has an appealing property of simplicity. For example, one can use the standard Wald test statistic for final inference. All associated decisions that one has to make are "organically built into the promising-zone design," including the new sample size selection rule and early futility/efficacy stop boundaries [3]. We would generally recommend the promising zone design, but with one word of caution. Because of the very feature of simplicity mentioned above, the duality property between hypothesis testing and confidence intervals is lost and treatment effect estimation at the end of such trials remains an open problem. For trials implementing the promising zone design, we suggest using simulation to carefully assess the amount of bias in treatment effect estimates at the end of trial on a case-by-case basis.

Finally, we want to point out that in the unblinded SSR methodology literature, n, N and M often represent the total number of patients at the interim analysis, the original planned total sample size, and the revised total sample size, respectively. To be consistent with the notations used in this chapter, we used these symbols to note their counterparts per group in this section. Because we assume two treatment groups with equal allocation in this chapter, the unblinded SSR methods reported in the literature apply equally with the use of our notations even though the two sets of numbers differ by a factor of two.

References

1. U.S. Food and Drug Administration (2010). Draft Guidance for Industry: Adaptive Design Clinical Trials for Drugs and Biologics. Available at http://www.fda.gov/downloads/Drugs/GuidanceComplianceRegulatoryInformation/Guidances/UCM201790.pdf (http://www.fda.gov/downloads/Drugs/GuidanceComplianceRegulatoryInformation/Guidances/UCM201790.pdf).
2. Dragalin V. (2006). Adaptive designs: Terminology and classification. *Drug Information Journal* 40: 425–35.
3. Mehta CR & Pocock SJ. (2011). Adaptive increase in sample size when interim results are promising: A practical guide with examples. *Statistics in Medicine* 30: 3267-3284.

4. Chuang-Stein C, Anderson K, Gallo P & Collins S. (2006). Sample size re-estimation: A review and recommendations. *Drug Information Journal* 40: 475–484.

5. Kieser M & Friede T. (2003). Simple procedures for blinded sample size adjustment that do not affect the type I error rate. *Statistics in Medicine* 22: 3571–3581.

6. Zucker DM, Wittes JT, Schabenberger O & Brittain E. (1999). Internal pilot studies II: comparison of various procedures. *Statistics in Medicine* 18: 3493–3509.

7. Gould AL & Shih WJ. (1992). Sample size re-estimation without unblinding for normally distributed outcomes with unknown variance. *Communications in Statistics - Theory and Methods*: 21: 2833-2853.

8. Xing B & Ganju J. (2005). A method to estimate the variance of an endpoint from an ongoing blinded trial. *Statistics in Medicine* 24: 1807-1814.

9. Chen M & Kianifard F. (2003). Estimation of treatment difference and standard deviation with blinded data in clinical trials. *Biometrical Journal* 2003 2: 135-142.

10. Friede T & Kieser M. (2002). On the inappropriateness of an EM algorithm based procedure for the blinded sample size re-estimation. *Statistics in Medicine* 21: 165-176.

11. Gould AL & Shih WJ. (2005). On the inappropriateness of an EM algorithm based procedure for blinded sample size re-estimation by T Friede & M Kieser M. *Statistics in Medicine* 24: 147–154.

12. Friede T & Kieser M. (2005). Authors' reply. *Statistics in Medicine* 24: 154–156.

13. Gould AL. (1992). Interim analyses for monitoring clinical trials that do not materially affect the type I error rate. *Statistics in Medicine* 11: 55-66.

14. Gould AL. (1995). Planning and revisiting the sample size for a trial. *Statistics in Medicine* 14: 1039-1051.

15. Friede T, Mitchell C & Müller-Velten G. (2007). Blinded sample size reestimation in non-inferiority trials with binary endpoints. *Biometrical Journal* 49: 903-916.

16. Shih WJ & Zhao PL. (1997). Design for sample size re-estimation with interim data for double-blind clinical trials with binary outcomes. *Statistics in Medicine* 16: 1913-1923.

17. Gaydos B, Anderson KM, Berry D, Burnham N, Chuang-Stein C, Dudinak J, Fardipour P, Gallo P, Givens S, Lewis R, Maca J, Pinheiro J, Pritchett Y & Krams M. (2009). Good practices for adaptive clinical trials in pharmaceutical product development. *Drug Information Journal* 43: 539–556.

18. Antonijevic Z, Gallo P, Chuang-Stein C, Dragalin V, Loewy J, Menon S, Miller ER, Morgan CC & Sanchez M. (2013). Views on emerging issues pertaining to data monitoring committees for adaptive trials. *Therapeutic Innovation & Regulatory Science* 47: 495-502.

19. Brannath W, Konig F & Bauer P. (2006). Estimation in flexible two stage designs. *Statistics in Medicine* 25: 3366–3381.

20. Jennison C & Turnbull BW. (1984). Repeated confidence intervals for group sequential clinical trials. *Controlled Clinical Trials* 5: 33–45.

21. Posch M, Bauer P & Brannath P. (2003). Issues in designing flexible trials. *Statistics in Medicine* 22: 953–969.

22. Cui L, Hung HM & Wang SJ. (1999). Modification of sample size in group sequential clinical trials. *Biometrics* 55: 853– 857.

23. Proschan MA & Hunsberger SA. (1995). Designed extension of studies based on conditional power. *Biometrics* 51: 1315–1324.

24. Müller HH & Schäfer H. (2004). A general statistical principle for changing a design any time during the course of a trial. *Statistics in Medicine* 23: 2497–2508.

25. Bauer P & Kohne K. (1994). Evaluation of experiments with adaptive interim analyses. *Biometrics* 50: 1029-1041.

26. Burman CF & Lisovskaja V. (2010). The dual test: Safeguarding p-value combination tests for adaptive designs. *Statistics in Medicine* 29: 797-807.

27. Gao P, Ware JH & Mehta C. (2008). Sample size re-estimation for adaptive sequential design in clinical trials. *Journal of Biopharmaceutical Statistics* 18: 1184-1196.

28. Chen YH, DeMets DL & Lan KK. (2004). Increasing the sample size when the unblinded interim results is promising. *Statistics in Medicine* 23: 1023–1038.

29. Bauer P. (1989). Multistage testing with adaptive designs. *Biometrie und Informatik in Medizin und Biologie* 20: 130–148.

30. Lehmacher W & Wassmer G. (1999). Adaptive sample size calculations in group sequential trials. *Biometrics* 55: 1286–1290.

31. Hwang IK, Shih WJ & De-Cani JS.(1990). Group sequential designs using a family of type I error probability spending functions. *Statistics in Medicine* 9: 1439-1445.

32. O'Brien PC & Fleming TR. (1979). A multiple testing procedure for clinical trials. *Biometrics* 35: 549-556.

33. Hong W, Ellenberg S & Anderson K. (2015). Stepwise two-stage sample size adaptation. *Statistics in Medicine* 34: 27-38.

34. Anderson KM, Chan ISF & Li X. (2012). An adaptive design for case-driven vaccine efficacy study when incidence rate is unknown. *Statistics and Its Interface* 5: 391-399.

35. Lan KKG & Zucker D. (1993). Sequential monitoring of clinical trials: The role of information and brownian motion. *Statistics in Medicine* 12: 753–65.

36. Mehta CR & Tsiatis AA. (2001). Flexible sample size considerations using information based interim monitoring. *Drug Information Journal* 35: 1095–1112.

37. Tsiatis AA. (2006). Information based monitoring of clinical trials. *Statistics in Medicine* 25: 3236–3244.

38. Chang W & Chuang-Stein C. (2004). Type I error and power in trials with one interim futility analysis. *Pharmaceutical Statistics* 3:51-59.

39. Liu Q, Proschan AA & Pledger GW. (2002). A unified theory of two-stage adaptive designs. *Journal of the American Association* 97: 1034–1041.

Authors

Inna Perevozskaya, Senior Director, Biometrics Statistical Research and Consulting Center, Pfizer Inc., Collegeville, PA, USA.

Sandeep Menon, Vice President and Head of Statistical Research and Consulting Center, Pfizer Inc, Cambridge, MA, USA.

Chapter 4

Bayesian Survival Meta-Experimental Design Using Historical Data

4.1 Introduction

A typical drug development program may consist of multiple clinical studies with different study objectives, endpoints, and possibly different patient populations. There is rich literature for single trial Bayesian sample size determination [1-8]. Sutton et al. proposed a hybrid frequentist-Bayesian approach for sample size determination for a future randomized clinical trial (RCT) using the results of meta-analyses reported in the literature and suggested that the power can be highly dependent on the statistical model used for meta-analysis, and even very large studies may have little impact on a meta-analysis when there is considerable between study heterogeneity [9]. This raises a critical issue regarding how to appropriately account for between-study heterogeneity in a statistical model for meta-analysis. Recently, a Bayesian meta-analysis approach using survival models was developed for planning a phase II/III antidiabetes drug development program [10-12]. Their approach focuses on sample size determination and power at a drug development program level by taking into account between-study heterogeneity within a meta-analysis framework. The authors considered the fitting and sampling priors of Wang & Gelfand for designing a Bayesian meta-analysis clinical trial with a focus on controlling the type I error and power [1]. Their approach allows the incorporation of historical meta-survival data via the power priors of Ibrahim and Chen [13].

Built upon the work of [10-12], the goal of this chapter is the general and novel implementation of their proposed methodology into a user-friendly SAS macro, called **BSMED**, for Bayesian Survival Meta-Experimental Design using historical meta-survival data. In the development of the SAS macro, we extend the model and methodology of [10-12] for incorporating historical data. We note that in [10-12], it is assumed that the historical data are available only for the control arm from previous studies. As elaborated in Sections 4.2, 4.3, and 4.5 and illustrated in Section 4.7, the SAS macro **BSMED** allows for the incorporation of various types of historical meta-survival data, including those for the control arm only, those for the experimental arm only, those historical meta-survival data for both the control and experimental arms, or mixed historical meta-survival data of these three types from previous studies. In addition, the SAS macro **BSMED** allows users to input various randomization ratios between control and experimental arms, various accrual times and follow-up times, as well as different annualized event rates across studies. Furthermore, the SAS macro **BSMED** allows a single trial for the current data along with the historical data from one or more previous trials. Therefore, the macro can be used for the design of a Bayesian time-to-event clinical trial in the non-meta setting. Finally, we extend the computational algorithm discussed in [6, 10] to generate the prior predictive survival data by incorporating the trial duration, accrual time, and minimal follow-up time.

The rest of the chapter is organized as follows. "4.2 Meta Design Setting" on page 108 presents the general meta-experimental design setting. "4.3 Meta-Regression Survival Models" on page 111 discusses meta-regression survival models. "4.4 Bayesian Meta-Experimental Design" on page 113 outlines the general methodology of Bayesian meta-experimental design. "4.5 Specification of Prior Distributions" on page 114 gives a detailed discussion of the specification of prior distributions. "4.6 Computational Algorithms" on page 115 presents the computational algorithms. "4.7 SAS MACRO BSMED" on page 117 gives a detailed description and several illustrations of the SAS macro **BSMED**. We conclude this chapter with some discussion in "4.8 Summary" on page 127.

4.2 Meta Design Setting

4.2.1 Notation

We consider K randomized trials where each trial has two treatment arms denoted by control and experimental and $K \geq 1$. The control arm may be a placebo or an active control, and the experimental arm may be an investigational drug in the clinical trial setting. However, in the medical device application, the control arm may be an old generation medical device and the experimental arm may refer to a new generation medical device. For ease of presentation, we generically call these two arms as control and experimental.

Let n_{jk} denote the sample size for the jth treatment arm in the kth randomized trial, where $j = 1$ and $j = 2$ denotes control and experimental, respectively, for $k = 1, \ldots, K$. We write $n_k = n_{1k} + n_{2k}$, which denotes the total sample size for kth randomized trial. We also let p_k and r_k denote the proportion of subjects in the control arm and the annualized event rate, respectively, for $k = 1, \ldots, K$. The proportion of subjects in the control arm, which is also called the randomization ratio, plays a role to allocate the sample size to the control and experimental arms. Using this quantity, we have $n_{1k} = \lfloor p_k n_k \rfloor$ and $n_{2k} = n_k - n_{1k}$ where $\lfloor p_k n_k \rfloor$ is the largest integer less than or equal to $p_k n_k$. The annualized event rate is a prespecified probability that an event will occur in less than a year. It is also used to specify the design value of the mean survival time in the sampling prior discussed in "4.6 Computational Algorithms" on page 115. Finally, we let τ_k^A and τ_k^F denote accrual time and minimal follow-up time, respectively, for $k = 1, \ldots, K$.

4.2.2 Input Data for a Meta-Trial Design Variable

Table 4.1 on page 109 shows a general survival meta-experimental design setting for K randomized trials with two arms introduced in the previous section. From Table 4.1, we see that the input data contain trial ID (TID), the total sample size (n), proportion in control arm (p), annualized event rate (r) in the control arm, trial duration (TD, τ_k^D), and accrual time (TA, τ_k^A) for each trial. Using the relationship between trial duration and accrual time, we calculate the minimum follow-up time (TF, τ_k^F) for each trial; that is, $\tau_k^F = \tau_k^D - \tau_k^A$. We note that these input data are used to generate the predictive data discussed in "4.6 Computational Algorithms" on page 115. From the prior predictive data generation algorithm presented in "4.6 Computational Algorithms" on page 115, we impose the constraints on τ_k^D, τ_k^A, and τ_k^F, that is,

$$\tau_k^A \geq 0,\ \tau_k^F \geq 0,\ \tau_k^D \geq \tau_k^F, \text{ and } \tau_k^D > \tau_k^A. \quad (4.1)$$

In (4.1), if $\tau_k^A = 0$, all subjects enroll the trial at the trial entry time; if $\tau_k^F = 0$, there is no minimum follow-up requirement; and if $\tau_k^D \leq \tau_k^F + \tau_k^A$ subjects are followed-up during the entire trial after the subject enrolls in the trial. In addition, the number of studies (K), the number of MCMC samples ($NMCS$), the number of burn-in samples (nbi), the number of simulated data sets (REP), design margin (δ), and user-defined Bayesian credible level (η_0) are required as input variables to run the SAS macro, **BSMED**, discussed in Section 4.7.

Table 4.1 *A General Design of Meta-Trials with Two Arms*

Trial ID (TID)	Sample Size (n)	Proportion in Control Arm (p)	Annualized Event Rate (r)	Trial Duration (TD)	Accrual Time (TA)
1	n_1	p_1	r_1	τ_1^D	τ_1^A

Trial ID (TID)	Sample Size (n)	Proportion in Control Arm (p)	Annualized Event Rate (r)	Trial Duration (TD)	Accrual Time (TA)
2	n_2	p_2	r_2	τ_2^D	τ_2^A
…	…	…	…	…	…
K	n_k	p_k	r_k	τ_k^D	τ_k^A

4.2.3 Input Historical Data

Suppose that the historical data are available for the control and experimental arms from K_0 previous studies, where $K_0 \geq 1$. For the historical data, we define

$$x_{0k} = \begin{cases} x_{01k}, & x_{01k} = x_{02k} \\ (x_{01k}, x_{02k})', & x_{01k} < x_{02k} \end{cases},$$

where $x_{0jk} = 0$ for control or 1 for experimental for $j = 1{,}2$ and $x_{01k} \leq x_{02k}$. If x_{0k} is a scalar x_{01k} for $k = 1, \ldots, K_0$, then the historical data are available only for the control arm or experimental arm. On the other hand, if x_{0k} is the vector $(x_{01k}, x_{02k})'$ for all $k = 1, \ldots, K_0$, then the historical data are available for both arms. For example, if $x_{0k} = 0$ for $k = 1, \ldots, K_0$, this indicates that the historical data are available only for the control arm. If x_{0k} is the vector $(0{,}1)'$, then the historical data are available for both arms. Under this setting, we let $y_{0k} = \{y_{0jk}: x_{01k} \leq j - 1 \leq x_{02k}\}$ denote the total subject year duration and denote $\nu_{0k} = \{\nu_{0jk}: x_{01k} \leq j - 1 \leq x_{02k}\}$ to be the total number of events for $k = 1, \ldots, K_0$. Suppose that the trial-level aggregate data $D_0 = \{(y_{0k}, \nu_{0k}, x_{0k}), k = 1, \ldots, K_0\}$ are available for the K_0 historical studies. Table 4.2 on page 110 and Table 4.3 on page 111 show the four types of historical data D_0.

Table 4.2 Types of Single-Arm Historical Data

Type I (Control arm only)				Type II (Experimental arm only)			
TID	y_{0k}	ν_{0k}	x_{0k}	TID	y_{0k}	ν_{0k}	x_{0k}
1	y_{011}	ν_{011}	0	1	y_{021}	ν_{021}	1
2	y_{012}	ν_{012}	0	2	y_{022}	ν_{022}	1
…	…	…	…	…	…	…	…
K_0	y_{01K_0}	ν_{01K_0}	0	K_0	y_{012}	ν_{012}	1

Table 4.3 Types of Multi-Arm Historical Data

Type III (Both arms)				Type IV (Both arms mixed)			
TID	y_{0k}	ν_{0k}	x_{0k}	TID	y_{0k}	ν_{0k}	x_{0k}
1	y_{011}	ν_{011}	0	1	y_{011}	ν_{011}	0
1	y_{021}	ν_{021}	1	1	y_{021}	ν_{021}	1
2	y_{012}	ν_{012}	0	2	y_{022}	ν_{022}	1
2	y_{022}	ν_{022}	1	3	y_{013}	ν_{013}	0
…	…	…	…	…	…	…	…
K_0	y_{01K_0}	ν_{01K_0}	0	K_0	y_{01K_0}	ν_{01K_0}	0
K_0	y_{02K_0}	ν_{02K_0}	1	K_0	y_{02K_0}	ν_{02K_0}	1

From Table 4.2 on page 110 and Table 4.3 on page 111, we see that for the Type IV, the historical data are available for both arms for some studies and for either the control arm or the experimental arm for some other studies in a mixed fashion. For instance, the historical data are available only for the control arm in TID 3 ($x_{03} = 0$, scalar), only for the experimental arm in TID 2 ($x_{02} = 1$, scalar), and for both arms in TID 1, the vector $x_{01} = (x_{011}, x_{021})' = (0,1)'$ from historical studies. We note that historical data contain y_{0k}, ν_{0k} and x_{0k}. Moreover, the number of studies (K_0) and the discounting parameter (a_0) are also two input variables for the historical data in the SAS macro **BSMED**.

4.3 Meta-Regression Survival Models

4.3.1 Model for Future Survival Data

In this section, we discuss the meta-regression survival model under the general survival meta-experimental design setting discussed in "4.2 Meta Design Setting" on page 108. Let y_{ijk} denote the subject-level time-to-event (failure time) and also let ν_{ijk} denote the right censoring indicator such that $\nu_{ijk} = 1$ if y_{ijk} is a failure time and $\nu_{ijk} = 0$ if y_{ijk} is right censored for the ith subject in the jth arm and the kth trial for $i = 1, \dots, n_{jk}$, $j = 1,2$, $k = 1, \dots, K$. We write $y_{jk} = \sum_{i=1}^{n_{jk}} y_{ijk}$ and $\nu_{jk} = \sum_{i=1}^{n_{jk}} \nu_{ijk}$ which denote the total subject year duration and the total number of events, respectively, for $j = 1,2$, $k = 1, \dots, K$. We let $x_{jk} = 0$ for $j = 1$ (control) or 1 for $j = 2$ (experimental). Then, we have the observed aggregate meta-survival data denoted by $D_K = \left\{\left(y_{jk}, \nu_{jk}, n_{jk}, x_{jk}\right), j = 1,2,\ k = 1, \dots, K\right\}$.

We further assume that the individual-level failure time follows an exponential distribution with mean $1/\lambda_{jk}$, i.e., $y_{ijk} \sim Exp(\lambda_{jk})$, where $\lambda_{jk} > 0$ is the hazard rate. The density function of (y_{jk}, ν_{jk}) is given by

$$f(y_{jk}, \nu_{jk} | \lambda_{jk}) = \lambda_{jk}^{\nu_{jk}} e^{-\lambda_{jk} y_{jk}}. \quad (4.2)$$

The log-linear model for λ_{jk} assumes

$$\log(\lambda_{jk}) = \gamma_0 + \gamma_1 x_{jk} + \theta_k, \quad (4.3)$$

where $x_{jk} = 0$ for $j = 1$ (control) or 1 for $j = 2$ (experimental) for $k = 1, \ldots, K$. To ensure model identifiability in (4.2), we impose the constraint $\sum_{k=1}^{K} \theta_k = 0$. For simplicity, we take $\theta_K = -\sum_{k=1}^{K-1} \theta_k$. In (4.2), θ_k captures the differences among the trials. Note that under the exponential model, the design parameter γ_1 is the log hazard ratio of the treatment in the experimental arm. Let $\theta = (\theta_1, \ldots, \theta_K)'$ and $\gamma = (\gamma_0, \gamma_1)'$. Then, the likelihood function based on the meta-survival data D_K is given by

$$L(\gamma, \theta | D_K) = \prod_{k=1}^{K} \prod_{j=1}^{2} \exp\{\nu_{jk}(\gamma_0 + \gamma_1 x_{jk} + \theta_k)\}$$

$$\times \exp\{-\exp(\gamma_0 + \gamma_1 x_{jk} + \theta_k) y_{jk}\}. \quad (4.4)$$

In (4.4), we see that the likelihood function does not depend on the sample size n_{jk}. It implies that under the exponential model, the likelihood function based on the individual level meta-experimental survival data reduces to the likelihood function based on the treatment level meta-experimental survival data.

4.3.2 Model for Historical Survival Data

In this section, we consider meta-regression survival models for the different types of the historical data discussed in "4.2.3 Input Historical Data" on page 110. Suppose y_{0jk} is the total subject year duration and ν_{0jk} is the censoring indicator such that $\nu_{0jk} = 1$ if y_{0jk} is a failure time and $\nu_{0jk} = 0$ if y_{0jk} is right censored for the jth arm and the kth trial for $j = 1,2,\ k = 1, \ldots, K_0$. In addition, x_{0k} represents only one arm (control or experimental) if it is a scalar and both arms if it is a vector, as discussed in Section 4.2.3. Suppose that the trial-level aggregate data $D_0 = \{(y_{0k}, \nu_{0k}, x_{0k}), k = 1, \ldots, K_0\}$ are available from the K_0 historical studies. Assume that the individual-level failure time follows an exponential distribution, $Exp(\lambda_{0jk})$, where the hazard rate $\lambda_{0jk} > 0$. Then the model assumes

$$\log(\lambda_{0jk}) = \gamma_0 + \gamma_1(j-1) + \theta_{0k}, \quad (4.5)$$

for $x_{01k} \le j - 1 \le x_{02k}$, $k = 1, \ldots, K_0$. Suppose that the historical data are available only for the control arm. This is the first type of historical data discussed in Section 4.2.3 and it is easy to see that $x_{0k} = 0$ for this case. Then the models for the historical and current data share only one common parameter, namely, γ_0. However, if the historical data are available only for the experimental arm, which is the second type of historical data, then $x_{0k} = 1$ and the models for the historical and current data share one common composite parameter $\gamma_0 + \gamma_1$. Now, we consider the third type of historical data, in which the historical data are available for both arms. In this case, the models for the historical and current data share two common parameters γ_0 and γ_1. The likelihood function for the general form of the historical data is given by

$$L(\gamma, \theta_0 | D_K) = \prod_{k=1}^{K_0} \prod_{j=x_{01k}}^{x_{02k}} \exp\{\nu_{0,j+1,k}(\gamma_0 + \gamma_1 j + \theta_{0k})\}$$

$$\times \exp\{-\exp(\gamma_0 + \gamma_1 j + \theta_{0k}) y_{0,j+1,k}\}, (4.6)$$

where $\theta_0 = \left(\theta_{01}, \ldots, \theta_{0K_0}\right)'$. From (4.6), we see that if both x_{01k} and x_{02k} are 0, then it is the likelihood function based on the historical data only from the control arm. On the other hand, if both values are 1, then the likelihood function is based on the historical data only from the experimental arm. Also, if both values are 0 in some trials and 1 in other trials, then (4.6) represents the likelihood function that is based on the mixed historical data discussed in "4.2.3 Input Historical Data" on page 110.

4.4 Bayesian Meta-Experimental Design

In this section, we present a general methodology for Bayesian meta-experimental design for the log-linear regression models. We first define the hypotheses for non-inferiority testing, which can be formulated as follows:

$$H_0 : e^{\gamma_1} \geq \delta \text{ versus } H_1 : e^{\gamma_1} < \delta \ (4.7)$$

where e^{γ_1} is the hazard ratio of experimental versus control and δ is a prespecified non-inferiority margin. The meta-trials are successful if H_0 is rejected. The non-inferiority margin δ is a user's input value in the SAS macro **BSMED**. For example, for the meta-analysis design in evaluating cardiovascular risk, we may choose $\delta = 1.3$ according to [14].

Let (γ, θ) denote the collection of parameters for the regression model. Following [1], let $\pi^{(s)}(\gamma, \theta)$ and $\pi^{(f)}(\gamma, \theta)$ denote the sampling prior and the fitting prior under the meta-regression survival model, respectively. The sampling prior plays a role to capture a certain specified portion of the parameter space in achieving a certain level of performance in the Bayesian meta-experimental design. As discussed in [1, 6], the sampling prior, $\pi^{(s)}(\gamma, \theta)$, is used to generate the meta-experimental survival data D_K and the fitting prior, $\pi^{(f)}(\gamma, \theta)$, is used to fit the regression models once the meta-experimental survival data are generated.

Using the data D_K, the posterior distribution of (γ, θ) under the meta-regression survival model is given by

$$\pi(\gamma, \theta | D_K) \propto \prod_{k=1}^{K} \prod_{j=1}^{2} \exp\{\nu_{jk}(\gamma_0 + \gamma_1 x_{jk} + \theta_k)\} \exp\{-\exp(\gamma_0 + \gamma_1 x_{jk} + \theta_k) y_{jk}\}$$

$$\times \ \pi^{(f)}(\gamma, \theta). \ (4.8)$$

In (4.8), we note that the fitting prior, $\pi^{(f)}(\gamma, \theta)$, may be improper as long as the resulting fitting posterior $\pi(\gamma, \theta | D_K)$ is proper.

To complete the Bayesian meta-experimental design, we need to specify two proper sampling priors, $\pi_0^{(s)}(\gamma, \theta)$ and $\pi_1^{(s)}(\gamma, \theta)$, which are defined on the subsets of the parameter spaces induced by hypotheses H_0 and H_1. We define the key quantity as discussed in [6] as

$$\beta_{sl}^{(n)} = E_{sl}\left[1\left\{P\left(e^{\gamma_1} < \delta \middle| D_K, \pi^{(f)}\right) \geq \eta_0\right\}\right], \quad (4.9)$$

where the indicator function $1\{A\}$ is 1 if A is true and 0 otherwise, $0 < \eta_0 < 1$ is a prespecified Bayesian credible level, the posterior probability $P\left(e^{\gamma_1} < \delta \middle| D_K, \pi^{(f)}\right)$ is computed with respect to the posterior distribution of γ_1 given the data D_K under the fitting prior $\pi^{(f)}(\gamma, \theta)$, and the expectation E_{sl} is taken with respect to the predictive marginal distribution of D_K under the sampling prior $\pi_l^{(s)}(\gamma, \theta)$ for $l = 0,1$. From (4.9), we note that the quantities $\beta_{s0}^{(n)}$ and $\beta_{s1}^{(n)}$ correspond to the Bayesian type I error and power, respectively.

4.5 Specification of Prior Distributions

4.5.1 Fitting Priors

We extend the fitting prior in (4.8) to the partial borrowing power prior approach formally proposed in [6] and [10]. The partial borrowing power prior is that the historical data are borrowed only through the common parameters shared in the model for the historical data and the current data. Thus, the strength of the historical data is borrowed only through the common parameters. The fitting prior for (γ, θ) under the meta-regression survival model in (4.3) is given by

$$\pi^{(f)}(\gamma, \theta | D_0, a_0) \propto \left\{ \int \prod_{k=1}^{K_0} \prod_{j=x_{01k}}^{x_{02k}} \left(\exp\left\{ \nu_{0,j+1,k}(\gamma_0 + \gamma_1 j + \theta_{0k}) \right\} \right.\right.$$

$$\left.\left. \times \exp\left\{ -\exp(\gamma_0 + \gamma_1 j + \theta_{0k}) y_{0,j+1,k} \right\} \right)^{a_0} \pi_0^{(f)}(\theta_0) d\theta_0 \right\} \pi_0^{(f)}(\gamma, \theta), \quad (4.10)$$

where $0 \leq a_0 \leq 1$, $\pi_0^{(f)}(\theta_0)$ and $\pi_0^{(f)}(\gamma, \theta)$ are the initial priors. In (4.10), independent initial normal priors, $N\left(0, \sigma_0^2\right)$, $N\left(0, \sigma_1^2\right)$, $N\left(0, \tau_0^2\right)$, and $N\left(0, \tau^2\right)$ are assumed for γ_0, γ_1, θ_{0k}, and θ_k.

In (4.10), the parameter a_0 controls the influence of the historical meta-survival data D_0 on the current data D_K. The parameter a_0 can be interpreted as a discounting parameter for the historical meta-survival data. It is reasonable to restrict the range of a_0 between 0 and 1, and thus we take $0 \leq a_0 \leq 1$. One of the main roles of a_0 is that it controls the heaviness of the tails of the prior for γ_0 and γ_1 in the model. As a_0 becomes smaller, the tails of (4.10) become heavier. If $a_0 = 0$, then the prior does not depend on historical meta-survival data. That is, $a_0 = 0$ is equivalent to a prior specification with no incorporation of historical meta-survival data for the current study. Thus, the parameter a_0 controls the influence of the historical meta-survival data on the current study. Such control is important in the case where there is heterogeneity between the historical and current meta-survival data, or when the sample sizes of the historical and current meta-survival data are quite different.

In (4.10), we prefer to consider a fixed a_0. When a_0 is fixed, we know exactly how much historical meta-data are incorporated in the new meta-experimental trial, and also how the type I error and power are related to a_0. As shown in the simulation study in "4.7

SAS MACRO BSMED" on page 117, a fixed a_0 provides us additional flexibility in controlling the type I error. In addition, our informative prior specification only allows us to borrow historical meta-experimental data for the common parameters shared by the models for the historical and current data. Thus, the historical meta-experimental data has the most influence on γ_0 and γ_1. For this reason, [6] and [10] call the power priors given in (4.10) "partial borrowing power priors."

4.5.2 Sampling Priors

Now, we turn to our attention to specify the sampling priors. Under the proposed model in (4.3), we take the sampling priors $\pi_l^{(s)}(\gamma, \theta) \propto \pi^{(s)}(\gamma_0)\, \pi^{(s)}(\theta)\, \pi_l^{(s)}(\gamma_1)$ for $l = 0{,}1$. In the sampling prior, we first specify a point mass prior for γ_1 as $\pi_l^{(s)}(\gamma_1) = \Delta_{\{\gamma_1 = \log(\delta)\}}$ for $l = 0$ and $\pi_l^{(s)}(\gamma_1) = \Delta_{\{\gamma_1 = 0\}}$ for $l = 1$, where $\Delta_{\{\gamma_1 = \gamma_1^*\}}$ denotes a degenerate distribution at $\gamma_1 = \gamma_1^*$, i.e., $P(\gamma_1 = \gamma_1^*) = 1$. We then specify a point mass prior for each of $\pi^{(s)}(\gamma_0)$ and $\pi^{(s)}(\theta)$ as well. Note that the choices of design values, (γ_0, θ) are obtained by solving the following simultaneous equations:

$1 - \exp\{-\exp(\gamma_0 + \theta_k)\} = r_k$ and $\sum_{k=1}^{K} \theta_k = 0,$

where r_k is a pre-determined annualized event rate for $k = 1, \ldots, K$. As in the example discussed in "4.7 SAS MACRO BSMED" on page 117, we assume that the number of studies is $K = 9$ and the annualized event rates are $r_k = 0.012$ for $k = 1, \ldots, 8$ and $r_9 = 0.015$. Then, by solving the above equations, we obtain $\gamma_0 = -4.392$, $\theta_k = -0.025$ for $k = 1, \ldots 8$, and $\theta_9 = 0.2$. Therefore, we can specify the point mass priors based on those design values.

4.6 Computational Algorithms

4.6.1 Predictive Data Generation

In this section, we extend the computational algorithm discussed in [6] and [10] to generate the prior predictive survival data by incorporating the trial duration (τ_k^D) and accrual time (τ_k^A) discussed in "4.2 Meta Design Setting" on page 108. Specifically, we use τ_k^D and τ_k^A to construct the censoring time in the generation of the predictive survival data D_K in addition to the sampling prior $\pi^{(s)}(\gamma, \theta)$. Our new prior predictive data generation algorithm is given as follows:

1. Generate $(\gamma, \theta) \sim \pi^{(s)}(\gamma, \theta)$.
2. Generate $y_{ijk}^* \sim f(y_{ijk} | \gamma, \theta, x_{jk})$ independently for $i = 1, \ldots, n_{jk}$, $j = 1{,}2$, $k = 1, \ldots, K$.
3. Set $\tau_{ijk}^{*A} = 0$ if $\tau_k^A = 0$ and generate the accrual time $\tau_{ijk}^{*A} \sim U(0, \tau_k^A)$ independently if $\tau_k^A > 0$ for $i = 1, \ldots, n_{jk}$, $j = 1{,}2$, $k = 1, \ldots, K$.
4. Set $C_{ijk}^* = \tau_k^D - \tau_{ijk}^{*A}$ for $i = 1, \ldots, n_{jk}$, $j = 1{,}2$, $k = 1, \ldots, K$.

5. Compute $y_{jk} = \sum_{i=1}^{n_{jk}} \min\left(y^*_{ijk}, C^*_{ijk}\right)$ and $\nu_{jk} = \sum_{i=1}^{n_{jk}} 1\left(y^*_{ijk} \le C^*_{ijk}\right)$, where the indicator function $1\left(y^*_{ijk} \le C^*_{ijk}\right) = 1$ if $y^*_{ijk} \le C^*_{ijk}$ and 0 otherwise for $i = 1, \ldots, n_{jk}$, $j = 1,2$, $k = 1, \ldots, K$.
6. Set $D_K = \left\{\left(y_{jk}, \nu_{jk}, n_{jk}, x_{jk}\right), j = 1,2,\ k = 1, \ldots, K\right\}$.

4.6.2 Sampling from the Posterior Distributions

Under the model in (4.3), using (4.4) and (4.10), the posterior distribution of $\left(\gamma, \theta, \theta_0\right)$ is given by

$$\pi\left(\gamma, \theta, \theta_0 \middle| D_K, D_0, a_0\right) \propto \left\{\prod_{k=1}^{K} \prod_{j=1}^{2} \exp\left\{\nu_{jk}\left(\gamma_0 + \gamma_1 x_{jk} + \theta_k\right)\right\}\right.$$
$$\times \exp\left\{-\exp\left(\gamma_0 + \gamma_1 x_{jk} + \theta_k\right) y_{jk}\right\}\Big\}$$
$$\times \left\{\prod_{k=1}^{K_0} \prod_{j=x_{01k}}^{x_{02k}} \left(\exp\left\{\nu_{0,j+1,k}\left(\gamma_0 + \gamma_1 j + \theta_{0k}\right)\right\}\right.\right.$$
$$\left.\left.\times \exp\left\{-\exp\left(\gamma_0 + \gamma_1 j + \theta_{0k}\right) y_{0,j+1,k}\right\}\right)^{a_0}\right\} \pi_0^{(f)}\left(\theta_0\right) \pi_0^{(f)}\left(\gamma, \theta\right). \quad (4.11)$$

We use the Gibbs sampling algorithm to sample from the posterior distribution in (4.11) given D_K and D_0. The Gibbs sampling algorithm requires sampling from the full conditional distribution of each parameter given the other parameters. First, the full conditional density for $\left[\gamma \middle| \theta, \theta_0, D_K, D_0, a_0\right]$ is given by

$$\pi\left(\gamma \middle| \theta, \theta_0, D_K, D_0, a_0\right) \propto \left\{\prod_{k=1}^{K} \prod_{j=1}^{2} \exp\left\{\nu_{jk}\left(\gamma_0 + \gamma_1 x_{jk} + \theta_k\right)\right\}\right.$$
$$\times \exp\left\{-\exp\left(\gamma_0 + \gamma_1 x_{jk} + \theta_k\right) y_{jk}\right\}\Big\}$$
$$\times \left\{\prod_{k=1}^{K_0} \prod_{j=x_{01k}}^{x_{02k}} \left(\exp\left\{\nu_{0,j+1,k}\left(\gamma_0 + \gamma_1 j + \theta_{0k}\right)\right\}\right.\right.$$
$$\left.\left.\times \exp\left\{-\exp\left(\gamma_0 + \gamma_1 j + \theta_{0k}\right) y_{0,j+1,k}\right\}\right)^{a_0}\right\} \exp\left\{-\tfrac{1}{2}\gamma' \Sigma_\gamma^{-1} \gamma\right\}, \quad (4.12)$$

where $\Sigma_\gamma = \operatorname{diag}\left(\sigma_0^2, \sigma_1^2\right)$ denotes a 2×2 covariance matrix of γ.

The full conditional density for $\left[\theta_0 \middle| \gamma_0, D_0, a_0\right]$ is given by

$$\pi\left(\theta_0 \middle| \gamma_0, D_0, a_0\right) \propto \left\{\prod_{k=1}^{K_0} \prod_{j=x_{01k}}^{x_{02k}} \left(\exp\left\{\nu_{0,j+1,k}\left(\gamma_0 + \gamma_1 j + \theta_{0k}\right)\right\}\right.\right.$$
$$\left.\left.\times \exp\left\{-\exp\left(\gamma_0 + \gamma_1 j + \theta_{0k}\right) y_{0,j+1,k}\right\}\right)^{a_0}\right\} \exp\left\{-\tfrac{1}{2}\theta_0' \Sigma_{\theta_0}^{-1} \theta_0\right\}, \quad (4.13)$$

where $\Sigma_{\theta_0} = \tau_0^2 I_{K_0}$ denotes a $K_0 \times K_0$ covariance matrix of θ_0.

It is easy to show that the full conditional distributions in (4.11) to (4.13) are log-concave in each parameter. Then, we can implement the adaptive rejection algorithm of [15] to sample from the posterior distribution of $\left(\gamma, \theta, \theta_0\right)$. `PROC MCMC` in SAS also provides a Metropolis-Hastings algorithm [16] to sample from the posterior distribution of $\left(\gamma, \theta, \theta_0\right)$.

4.6.3 Power Calculation

We discuss how to calculate the type I error and power discussed in [6]. Let η_0 and a_0 denote prespecified Bayesian credible level and discounting parameter for the historical meta-experimental survival data, respectively. We also let $\left\{\gamma_1^{(m)},\ m = 1, \ldots, NMCS\right\}$ denote a Gibbs sample of γ_1 from the posterior distribution $\pi(\gamma, \theta | D_K, D_0, a_0)$, where $NMCS$ is the Gibbs sample size. Using this Gibbs sample, we obtain a Monte Carlo estimate of $P\left(e^{\gamma_1} < \delta \middle| D_K, \pi^{(f)}\right)$ given by

$$\widehat{P}_f = \frac{1}{NMCS} \sum_{m=1}^{NMCS} 1\left\{e^{\gamma_1^{(m)}} < \delta\right\}, \quad (4.14)$$

where $\pi^{(f)}$ is the fitting prior. To simultaneously compute the Bayesian type I error and power, $\beta_{sl}^{(n)}$ in (4.9), we use the following computational algorithm:

1. Set $l = 0$ and input D, D_0, η_0, δ, a_0, $NMCS$, nbi, and REP.
2. Generate $(\gamma, \theta) \sim \pi_l^{(s)}(\gamma, \theta)$ for $s = 0,1$.
3. Generate D_K via the predictive data generation algorithm in Section 4.6.1.
4. Run the Gibbs sampler to generate a Gibbs sample $\left\{\gamma_1^{(m)},\ m = 1, \ldots, NMCS\right\}$ of size $NMCS$ from the posterior distribution $\pi(\gamma, \theta | D_K, D_0, a_0)$.
5. Compute $\widehat{P}_f$ and repeat Steps 2 through 5. REP times.
6. Compute the proportions of $\left\{\widehat{P}_f \geq 0.90\right\}$, $\left\{\widehat{P}_f \geq 0.95\right\}$ and $\left\{\widehat{P}_f \geq 0.975\right\}$ (the default option) and the proportion of $\left\{\widehat{P}_f \geq \eta_0\right\}$ (the user's choice) in these REP runs, which give the estimates of $\beta_{sl}^{(n)}$.
7. $l = l + 1$ and go back to Step 2.

4.7 SAS MACRO BSMED

4.7.1 Implementation of BSMED

4.7.1.1 Detailed Macro Options

In this section, we present the details of SAS macro, **BSMED**, for Bayesian survival meta-experimental design. As discussed in "4.2 Meta Design Setting" on page 108, the macro **BSMED** requires two input data sets, namely, the current data and the historical data (optional), 11 input variables, and one output file (optional). Table 4.4 on page 118 shows the names and descriptions of the input variables and the design values in the SAS macro.

Table 4.4 Names and Descriptions of Input Variables and Design Values

Data	Names in macro	Description
Historical	`a0`	Discounting parameter (a_0)
	`sigma0`	Initial variance of γ_0 (σ_0^2)
	`sigma1`	Initial variance of γ_1 (σ_1^2)
Current	`tau0`	Initial variance of θ_{0k} (τ_0^2)
	`tau`	Initial variance of θ_k (τ^2)
Design	`delta`	Design non-inferiority margin (δ)
	`eta0`	User-defined Bayesian credible level (η_0)

The input variables, including the number of MCMC runs (**NMCS**), the number of simulation data sets (**REP**), and the number of burn-in samples (**nbi**), are required to run MCMC and generate predictive survival data in the macro. We also include an initial seed number (**SEEDGEN**) as the input variable. The input historical data should use SAS variable names **K**, **y**, **v** and **x** for the TID, the total subject year duration, the total number of events, and the treatment arm indicator, where 0 denotes control and 1 corresponds to experimental. The input current data requires the SAS variable names **K**, **n**, **p**, **r**, **TA** and **TD** for the trial ID, the total sample size, the proportion of subjects in the control arm, the annualized event rate, the accrual time, and the trial duration. The structure of the macro **BSMED** is given as follows:

```
%macro
BSMED(hist,curr,delta,eta0,NMCS,nbi,a0,REP,sigma0,sigma1,tau0,
tau,SEEDGEN,output);
```

1. Generate predictive survival data
2. Sample from the posterior distribution
3. Calculate type I error and power
4. Produce the desired output

```
%mend BSMED;
```

The **BSMED** macro does not require an input file for the historical data. If historical data are available, we call

```
%BSMED(HIST=hist,CURR=curr,delta=1.3,a0=0.10,eta0=0.96,NMCS=20
000,nbi=5000,REP=5000,sigma0=10,sigma1=10,tau0=10,tau=10,SEEDG
EN=123456789,OUTPUT=C:\...\BSMED);
```

and if no historical data are available, we simply use

```
%BSMED(CURR=curr,delta=1.3,a0=0.10,eta0=0.96,NMCS=20000,nbi=50
00,REP=5000,sigma0=10,sigma1=10,tau0=10,tau=10,SEEDGEN=1234567
89,OUTPUT=C:\...\BSMED);
```

As seen in the above macro, **BSMED** consists of the four main parts: generating predictive survival data, running **PROC MCMC** to sample from posterior distribution, calculating the type I error and power using posterior estimates, and producing the desired output. In the subsequent subsections, we provide a detailed development for each of these main components of the macro except for the desired output step using **PROC REPORT**.

4.7.7.2 Predictive Survival Data Generation

Following the algorithm described in "4.6.1 Predictive Data Generation" on page 115, we briefly present the prior predictive data generation in the macro. The SAS code to generate γ_0 and γ_1 from the sampling priors is shown in the first part of the Example Code 4.1 on page 119. For $s = 0$ and $s = 1$, we generate γ_1 from the sampling prior under the null hypothesis and the alternative hypothesis in (4.7). In the second part of Example Code 4.1 on page 119, we generate failure times $\left(y^*_{ijk}\right)$ and accrual times $\left(\tau^{*A}_{ijk}\right)$ as well as calculating censoring times $\left(C^*_{ijk}\right)$ using the information in the current data for $i = 1, \ldots, n_{jk}$, $j = 1,2$, $k = 1, \ldots, K$. Then, we compute the total subject duration $\left(y_{jk}\right)$ and the total number of events $\left(\nu_{jk}\right)$ for $j = 1,2$, $k = 1, \ldots, K$. These quantities are the key components in constructing the likelihood function for the current data for each simulated data set. In addition, we use the seed value generated from the initial seed (e.g. **SEEDGEN=123456789**) in the data generation to allow for reproducing the same simulation result.

Example Code 4.1 *Generation of the Prior Predictive Survival Data*

```
%do s=0 %to 1;
   data current&s;
      set current_new;
      gamma0=g0mean;
      if &s=0 then do;
         gamma1=log(&delta);
         end;
      else do;
         gamma1=0;
      end;
      theta_k=tk;
      lambda=exp(gamma0+gamma1*x+theta_k);
   run;
%end;

%do s=0 %to 1;
  %do m=1 %to &REP;

  ...(Use sets of seed numbers as macro variables)

   data current_sim;
      set current&s;
         y=0;
         v=0;
         call streaminit(&seedg);
         do i=1 to n;
            yi= -log(RAND('UNIFORM'))/lambda;
            if TA=0 then do;
               TAi=0;
            end;
```

```
            else do;
               TAi=RAND('UNIFORM')*TA;
            end;
            ci=TD-TAi;
            if yi<=ci then do;
               vi=1;
               timei=yi;
            end;
            else do;
               vi=0;
               timei=ci;
            end;
            y=y+timei;
            v=v+vi;
         end;
      output;
      keep K x y v group;
   run;

   ...(continue)
   %end;
%end;
```

4.7.1.3 Running MCMC to Sample from the Posterior Distribution

Example Code 4.2 on page 120 shows how to sample from the posterior distribution using the partial borrowing power prior. We allow the user to choose initial values of variances for the parameters γ_0, γ_1, θ_{0k}, and θ_k. Since we do not need to print out posterior estimates for each simulated data set, we use an option to suppress the posterior estimates in the SAS log window. The option, **ods exclude all**, also allows us to save storage space and reduce the computation time. To reproduce the simulation results, we use the seed values generated using the initial seed (e.g. **SEEDGEN** = 123456789) in **PROC MCMC**.

Example Code 4.2 *Running Markov Chain Monte Carlo (MCMC)*

```
ods graphics on;
ods exclude all;
proc mcmc data=sort_newdata outpost=postout nmc=&NMCS nbi=&nbi seed=&seedmc MAXTUNE=
            plots=none statistics=none diagnostics=none;
   %if (&hist ^= and &a0>0.00 and &a0<=1.00) %then %do;
      %if &N_hist > 1 %then %do;
         array theta_h[%eval(&N_hist-1)];
      %end;
      %if &N_curr > 1 %then %do;
         array theta_c[%eval(&N_curr-1)];
      %end;
   %end;
   %if (&hist= or &a0=0.00) %then %do;
      %if &N_curr > 1 %then %do;
         array theta_c[%eval(&N_curr-1)];
      %end;
   %end;

   ...(continue)

   %if (&hist= or &a0=0.00) %then %do;
```

```
   %if &N_curr > 1 %then %do;
      parms theta_c: 0;
   %end;
   %else %do;
      parms theta_c 0;
   %end;
%end;

parms gamma0 gamma1;
prior gamma0 ~ n(0,var=&sigma0);
prior gamma1 ~ n(0,var=&sigma1);

...(continue)

begincnst;
   discounta0=&a0;
endcnst;

tk=0;
%if (&hist ^= and &a0>0.00 and &a0<=1.00) %then %do;
   %if (&N_hist > 1 and &N_curr > 1) %then %do;
      if group eq "hist" then do;
         if K < &N_hist then tk=theta_h[K];
         else do;
            tk=0;
            do j=1 to %eval(&N_hist-1);
               tk=tk-theta_h[j];
            end;
         end;
      end;
      else do;
         if K < &N_curr then tk=theta_c[K];
         else do;
            tk=0;
            do j = 1 to %eval(&N_curr-1);
               tk=tk-theta_c[j];
            end;
         end;
      end;
   %end;

   ...(continue)

%end;
%if (&hist= or &a0=0.00) %then %do;
   discounta0=0;
   %if &N_curr > 1 %then %do;
      if K < &N_curr then tk=theta_c[K];
      else do;
         tk=0;
         do j = 1 to %eval(&N_curr-1);
            tk=tk-theta_c[j];
         end;
      end;
   %end;
   %else %do;
```

```
            tk=theta_c;
         %end;
      %end;
      regmean=gamma0+gamma1*x+tk;
      loglik=v*regmean-exp(regmean)*y;
      if (group eq "hist") then do;
         loglik=discounta0*loglik;
      end;
      model general(loglik);
   run;
   ods graphics off;
```

4.7.1.4 Calculation of the Type I Error and Power

To compute the type I error and power in (4.7), we use the algorithm discussed in "4.6.3 Power Calculation" on page 117. From the code (Example Code 4.3 on page 122) in the macro, we see that the macro allows the user to choose the Bayesian credible level (η_0). The macro also automatically produces the results using Bayesian credible levels, 0.90, 0.95, and 0.975 as a default option. This partial code shows the approach that is used to calculate the type I error and power, which are the proportions in (4.14) under various Bayesian credible levels based on the posterior sample of γ_1. In the code, the posterior estimates are saved in the data set **postout** and **pfhat** is the proportion satisfying $\exp\left\{\gamma_1^{(m)} < \delta\right\}$ calculated from the posterior samples for each simulated data set. From the data set **outpower**, we can accumulate the value of **phat** across simulated data sets. The data set **Type1Error** is used for calculating the type I error in (4.7) using the algorithm discussed in "4.6.3 Power Calculation" on page 117. The data set **BayesianPower** in the macro is used to calculate the power.

Example Code 4.3 *Calculation of the Type I Error and Power*

```
data indicator(keep=proportion);
   set postout;
   proportion=(exp(gamma1)<&delta);
run;

proc means data=indicator n mean noprint;
   var proportion;
   output out=outpower mean=pfhat;
run;

data outpower;
   set outpower;
   simid=&m;
   keep simid pfhat;
run;

%if &m=1 %then %do;
   data proportion&s;
      set outpower;
   run;
%end;
%else %do;
   data proportion&s;
      set proportion&s outpower;
   run;
%end;
```

```
data Type1Error;
   set proportion0;
   keep pfhat BP1 BP2 BP3 BP4;
   BP1=0;BP2=0;BP3=0;BP4=0;
   if pfhat>=0.90  then BP1=1;
   if pfhat>=0.95  then BP2=1;
   if pfhat>=0.975 then BP3=1;
   if pfhat>=&eta0 then BP4=1;
run;
```

4.7.2 Illustrative Examples

4.7.2.1 Evaluating Cardiovascular Risk

In this section, we illustrate the **BSMED** macro discussed in the previous section. As an illustrative example, we use the motivating case study for designing a phase II/III development program of a new T2DM therapy. A more detailed setting of this illustrative example can be found in [10,11].

Several authors considered a hypothetical drug development program for treating type 2 diabetes mellitus [10 -12]. The program includes eight randomized control efficacy superiority trials and one large randomized control CV outcome non-inferiority trial. For those traditional diabetes HbA1c superiority trials, the target subjects are at low or moderate CV risk with an assumed annualized event rate of 1.2%. On the other hand, for the non-inferiority trial, the subjects are at high risk with an assumed annualized event rate of 1.5% as the FDA guidance advocates the inclusion of such a population. A detailed description of the data can be found in [10 -12].

In this study, the historical data are available only for the control arm. This is the first type of historical data (control arm only) discussed in "4.2.3 Input Historical Data" on page 110 and the original historical data in [10] are shown in Table 4.5 on page 123 and Table 4.6 on page 123 . Also, we output the historical data shown in Table 4.6.

Table 4.5 *Original Historical Data for the Cardiovascular Risk Study*

Reference	Number of Subjects	Number of CV Events	Total Patient Years	Annualized Event Rate (%)
ACCORD (2008)	5,123	371	16,000	2.29
ADVANCE (2008)	5,569	590	27,845	2.10
Saxagliptin (2009)	1,251	17	1,289	1.31
Liraglutide (2009)	907	4	449	0.89
Liraglutide (2009)	1,474	13	1,038	1.24

Table 4.6 *Historical Data Shown in RTF Output File for the Cardiovascular Risk Study*

Trial ID	Total Subject Year Duration	Total Number of Events	Trial Arm
1	16,000	371	0

Trial ID	Total Subject Year Duration	Total Number of Events	Trial Arm
2	27,845	590	0
3	1,289	17	0
4	449	4	0
5	1,038	13	0

For the predetermined design values, the non-inferiority design margin δ is specified as in (4.7), and to ensure that the type I error is controlled under 0.05, we choose $\eta_0 = 0.96$ as discussed in [6] and recommended in the FDA guidance [14]. We define in advance the proportion in the control arm, annualized event rates, and accrual times as well. Under these settings, we compile the current data shown in Table 4.7 on page 124.

Table 4.7 Current Data in the Cardiovascular Risk Study

Trial ID	Total Sample Size	Proportion in Control Arm	Annualized Event Rate	Accrual Time	Trial Duration	Minimum Follow-up Time
1	150	0.17	0.012	0	0.077	0.077
2	350	0.40	0.012	0	0.462	0.462
3	3,500	0.40	0.012	0	2	2
4	400	0.25	0.012	0	0.462	0.462
5	375	0.20	0.012	0	0.462	0.462
6	740	0.25	0.012	0	0.462	0.462
7	750	0.33	0.012	0	0.462	0.462
8	564	0.33	0.012	0	0.462	0.462
9	8,000	0.50	0.015	2	4	2

Using `PROC REPORT` in the macro, we reproduce the predetermined design values in the study. Table 4.8 on page 124 shows the predetermined design margin, the discounting parameter (a_0) for the historical data, and the initial variances of the parameters, $\gamma_0, \gamma_1, \theta_{0k}$ for $k = 1, \ldots, K_0$ and θ_k for $k = 1, \ldots, K$.

Table 4.8 Design Values in the Cardiovascular Risk Study

Design Margin	Discounting Parameter	User-Defined Credible Level	Initial Variance of `gamma0`	Initial Variance of `gamma1`	Initial Variance of `theta_0k`	Initial Variance of `theta_k`
1.3	0.10	0.96	10	10	10	10

The type I error and power can be obtained by running the **BSMED macro**, and are shown in Table 4.8 on page 124 and Table 4.9 on page 125. These quantities are calculated from 5,000 simulation data sets. As shown in Table 4.9 and Table 4.10 on page 125, the Bayesian type I error and power are 0.0506 and 0.8774, respectively. We note that the type I error was not controlled at 5%, but the power was above 0.80 when we borrowed 10% $(a_0 = 0.10)$ from the historical data.

Table 4.9 *Type I Error Provided from BSMED*

Type I with Credible Level 0.90	Type I with Credible Level 0.95	Type I with Credible Level 0.975	Type I with User Choice 0.96
0.1190	0.0614	0.0324	0.0506

Table 4.10 *Power Provided from BSMED*

Power with Credible Level 0.90	Power with Credible Level 0.95	Power with Credible Level 0.975	Power with User Choice 0.96
0.9454	0.8994	0.8310	0.8774

4.7.2.2 Evaluating Cardiovascular Risk Study with Artificial Experimental Arm Data

We consider a hypothetical study similar to the one discussed in the previous section but with historical data available only for the experimental arm. To do this, we artificially generated the total subject duration and the number of CV events using the annualized event rates in the historical study in Table 4.4 on page 118. From the relationship between the homogeneous Poisson process and the exponential distribution, we generated the total subject year duration of the experimental arm in the historical data, and the total number of events are easily obtained using those annualized event rates. Table 4.11 on page 125 shows the artificial historical data for the experimental arm and we see that this is the second type of historical data (experimental arm only) discussed in "4.2.3 Input Historical Data" on page 110.

Table 4.11 *Artificial Historical Data for the Experimental Arm*

Trial ID	Total Subject Year Duration	Total Number of Events	Trial Arm
1	301	4	1
2	438	4	1
3	318	4	1
4	152	4	1
5	164	3	1

By combining the two historical data sets (Table 4.6 on page 123 and Table 4.11 on page 125), we obtained the third type of historical data which are available for both the control and the experimental arms. To illustrate one possible case of the last type of historical data, we deleted the control arm in trial ID 2 and the experimental arm in trial ID 3 from the combined historical data. Then, we finally had the last type of historical data. Based on these four types of the historical data types, denoted by historical data types I, II, III, and IV, we calculated the Bayesian type I errors and powers for the different types of historical data, and the results are shown in Table 4.12 on page 126. We specified 0.96 as the user choice of Bayesian credible level and produced 20,000 posterior estimates with 5,000 burn-in samples in each simulation. Based on the constructions of these four historical data sets, the historical data type III is most informative and the historical data type IV is less informative than type III, but more informative than types I and II. From Table 4.12, we see that type III yielded the highest powers, while type IV had higher powers than types I and II for $a_0 = 0.10, 0.15, 0.20,$ and 0.30. However, the types of historical data that had higher powers also resulted in larger type I errors in general.

Table 4.12 *Type I Error and Power Using the Four Types of Historical Data*

		Type I error				**Power**			
a_0	**Historical Data Forms**	**0.90**	**0.95**	**0.975**	**User 0.96**	**0.90**	**0.95**	**0.975**	**User 0.96**
0.0	-	0.1046	0.0544	0.0308	0.0436	0.9342	0.8792	0.8118	0.8544
0.10	I	0.1190	0.0614	0.0324	0.0560	0.9454	0.8994	0.8310	0.8774
	II	0.1118	0.0574	0.0280	0.0458	0.9378	0.8792	0.8000	0.8574
	III	0.1226	0.0650	0.0344	0.0540	0.9452	0.8942	0.8324	0.8738
	IV	0.1170	0.0594	0.0314	0.0478	0.9520	0.9044	0.8270	0.8816
0.15	I	0.1250	0.0642	0.0342	0.0538	0.9504	0.9084	0.8438	0.8902
	II	0.1108	0.0558	0.0292	0.0448	0.9356	0.8790	0.8004	0.8558
	III	0.1292	0.0696	0.0374	0.0570	0.9492	0.9062	0.8426	0.8826
	IV	0.1222	0.0608	0.0320	0.0490	0.9542	0.9088	0.8382	0.8872
0.20	I	0.1294	0.0684	0.0366	0.0556	0.9530	0.9312	0.8502	0.8958
	II	0.1110	0.0558	0.0288	0.0452	0.9362	0.8780	0.7994	0.8572
	III	0.1392	0.0732	0.0400	0.0632	0.9536	0.9130	0.8508	0.8922
	IV	0.1278	0.0636	0.0348	0.0528	0.9578	0.9154	0.8462	0.8942
0.30	I	0.1376	0.0732	0.0388	0.0622	0.9568	0.9196	0.8672	0.9034
	II	0.1070	0.0538	0.0284	0.0432	0.9350	0.8768	0.7940	0.8510
	III	0.1542	0.0840	0.0456	0.0690	0.9614	0.9230	0.8654	0.9038
	IV	0.1372	0.0692	0.0392	0.0562	0.9618	0.9234	0.8602	0.9080

4.8 Summary

In this chapter, we presented a general Bayesian methodology and a detailed development of a SAS macro, **BSMED**, for meta-experimental design for survival data. Throughout this chapter, we only consider the exponential regression model, which is a potential limitation of the SAS macro **BSMED**. However, the exponential model is attractive in the sense that the individual patient-level survival data is not required. Another major motivation for using the exponential model in this chapter is that the historical data itself were often only available in aggregate form. Thus, the exponential model was most natural in this setting, even if we had individual patient-level data for the trials themselves.

We note that the assumed meta-regression survival model in the SAS macro **BSMED** is a log-linear fixed-effects model. There are several advantages of the fixed effects model over the random effects model. First, the fixed effects model is easier and more convenient to implement in **PROC MCMC**. Second, the fixed effects model does not require the specification of the design values for the variability of the random effects, which is a major task from a design perspective. Third, the fixed effects model is more flexible to accommodate different annualized event rates of historical meta-survival data across previous trials. In addition, as shown in [11, 12], the fixed effects model and the random effects model essentially yield a similar sample size. If individual patient-level meta-survival data are available, then the Bayesian methodology discussed in this chapter can be easily extended to other survival regression models discussed in [17].

As a future project, we will extend the SAS macro **BSMED** to allow different survival models, such as the Weibull regression model and other survival models discussed in [17] for the setting of the meta-design with individual patient level data.

Acknowledgements

The research of JGI and MHC was partially supported by NIH grants #GM 70335 and #P01 CA42538.

References

1. Wang F & Gelfand AE. (2002). A simulation-based approach to Bayesian sample size determination for performance under a given model and for separating models. *Statistical Science* 17: 193-208.
2. Spiegelhalter DJ, Abrams KR & Myles JP. (2004). *Bayesian Approaches to Clinical Trials and Health-Care Evaluation*. New York, NY: Wiley.
3. Inoue LYT, Berry DA & Parmigiani G. (2005). Relationship between Bayesian and frequentist sample size determination. *The American Statistician* 59: 79-87.
4. De Santis F. (2007). Using historical data for Bayesian sample size determination. *Journal of the Royal Statistical Society, Series A* 170: 95-113.
5. M'Lan CE, Joseph L & Wolfson DB. (2008). Bayesian sample size determination for binomial proportions. *Bayesian Analysis* 3: 269-296.
6. Chen MH, Ibrahim JG, Lam P, Yu A & Zhang Y. (2011). Bayesian design of noninferiority trials for medical devices using historical data. *Biometrics* 67: 1163-1170.

7. Chen MH, Ibrahim JG, Zeng D, Hu K & Jia C. (2014). Bayesian design of superiority clinical trials for recurrent events data with applications to bleeding and transfusion events in myelodyplastic syndrome. *Biometrics* 70: 1003-1013.

8. Li W, Chen MH, Tan H & Dey DK. (2015). Bayesian design of non-inferiority clinical trials with co-primary endpoints and multiple dose comparison. In: Chen A, Liu Y, Qu LT, Ting N & Song YT. Eds. *Applied Statistics in Biomedicine and Clinical Trials Design: Selected Papers from 2013 ICSA/ISBS Joint Statistical Meetings*. New York: Springer.

9. Sutton AJ, Cooper NJ, Jones DR, Lambert PC, Thompson JR & Abrams KR. (2007). Evidence-based sample size calculations based upon updated meta-analysis. *Statistics in Medicine* 26: 2479-2500.

10. Ibrahim JG, Chen MH, Xia HA & Liu T. (2012). Bayesian meta-experimental design: Evaluating cardiovascular risk in new antidiabetic therapies to treat type 2 diabetes. *Biometrics* 68: 578-586.

11. Chen MH, Ibrahim JG, Xia HA, Liu T & Hennessey V. (2014). Bayesian sequential meta-analysis design in evaluating cardiovascular risk in a new antidiabetic drug development program. *Statistics in Medicine* 33: 1600-1618.

12. Ibrahim JG, Chen MH, Xia HA, Liu T & Hennessey V. (2014). Bayesian meta-experimental design for evaluating cardiovascular risk. In: Jiang Q & Xia HA, eds. *Quantitative Evaluation of Safety in Drug Development: Design, Analysis and Reporting*. Boca Raton: Chapman Hall/CRC.

13. Ibrahim JG & Chen MH. (2000). Power prior distributions for regression models. *Statistical Sciences* 15: 46-60.

14. U.S. Food and Drug Administration. (2008). Guidance to Industry: Diabetes Mellitus - Evaluating Cardiovascular Risk in New Antidiabetic Therapies to Treat Type 2 Diabetes. Rockville, MD: US FDA. Available at: http://www.fda.gov/downloads/Drugs/GuidanceComplianceRegulatoryInformation/Guidances/ucm071627.pdf (http://www.fda.gov/downloads/Drugs/GuidanceComplianceRegulatoryInformation/Guidances/ucm071627.pdf)

15. Gilks WR & Wild P. (1992). Adaptive rejection sampling for Gibbs sampling. *Applied Statistics* 41: 337-348.

16. Hastings WK. (1970). Monte Carlo sampling methods using Markov chains and their applications. *Biometrika* 57: 97-109.

17. Ibrahim JG, Chen MH & Sinha D. (2001). *Bayesian Survival Analysis*. New York, NY: Springer.

Authors

Joseph G. Ibrahim, Alumni Distinguished Professor, Department of Biostatistics, University of North Carolina at Chapel Hill, Chapel Hill, NC, USA.

Yeongjin Gwon, Graduate Assistant, Department of Statistics, University of Connecticut, Storrs, CT, USA.

Ming-Hui Chen, Professor and Director of Statistical Consulting Services, Department of Statistics, University of Connecticut, Storrs, CT, USA.

Appendix

Macro Call

The SAS macro **BSMED** could be stored in a folder named **BSMED**. Then **%BSMED** can be accessed by including the following lines:

```
%include BSMED (macroBSMED.sas);

%BSMED (HIST=, CURR=, delta=, eta0=, NMCS=, nbi=, a0=, REP=,
sigma0=, sigma1=, tau0=, tau=, SEEDGEN=, OUTPUT=);
```

Inputs

Below are the requirements for **%BSMED**:

Required Inputs

1. **CURR**: data set with the seven columns, K (trial ID) in the same format as for the historical data, n (the total sample size), p (the proportion of subjects in the control arm), r (the annualized event rate), TD (the trial duration), and TA (the accrual time), where all variables should be arranged in columns. TF (the minimal follow-up time) is easily calculated using TA and TD.

2. **delta**: indicates a prespecified design margin of non-inferiority trial.

3. **eta0**: indicates the user's choice of a Bayesian credible level in calculating the Bayesian type I error and power.

4. **NMCS**: indicates the number of Markov chain Monte Carlo (MCMC) samples.

5. **nbi**: indicates the number of burn-in samples in each run of PROC MCMC.

6. **a0**: indicates a discounting parameter for the historical survival meta-experimental data.

7. **REP**: indicates the number of simulated data sets.

8. **sigma0**: indicates the initial prior variance of the parameter γ_0.

9. **sigma1**: indicates the initial prior variance of the parameter γ_1.

10. **tau0**: indicates the initial prior variance of the parameters, θ_{0k}, for the historical data sets.

11. **tau**: indicates the initial prior variance of the parameters, θ_k, for the current data sets.

12. **SEEDGEN**: indicates the initial seed to generate sets of seed numbers in generating predictive data and running MCMC.

Optional Inputs

1. **HIST**: data set with the first three columns, K (trial ID), y (total subject year duration), υ (total number of events), and an additional column for treatment indicator (x), where K, y, and υ should be arranged in the first, second, and third columns, and x should be placed after column 3. Note that x is an indicator variable of the treatment arm, which takes a value of 0 if it comes from the control arm and 1 if it comes from the

experimental arm. The values of K should be consecutive integers starting with 1. For example, if the total number of historical data sets is 5, the values of K should be enumerated as 1, 2, 3, 4, and 5.

2. **OUTPUT**: name of the output rich text file (RTF). One can also specify a directory/folder in which the file will be stored. For example, the output file named `output_a0` will be stored in `C:\...\BSMED` by `%BSMED (OUTPUT=C:\...\BSMED)`. If `OUTPUT` is not specified, the file will be indexed by the name `BSMED_Output_a0` as default. In the filename, `a0` indicates a discounting parameter for the historical survival meta-experimental data which the user specifies in the macro.

Notes

1. The name of the K (trial ID) variable in HIST should be the same as that of the K (trial ID) variable in CURR.
2. TD and TA should be in the same time unit such as years.
3. TD is always greater than TA, and TD is allowed to be greater than or equal to or less than or equal to the sum of TA and TF.
4. The indicator variable x must be coded as 0 and 1.
5. No missing values are allowed in both data sets. However, it is possible to leave a blank in historical data sets if historical data are not available.
6. Four different types of historical data sets are allowed:
    a. hist1: only the control arm
    b. hist2: only the experimental arm
    c. hist3: both the control and experimental arms
    d. hist4: mixed control and experimental arms.
7. The total number of trials in the current data is allowed to be 1 or greater and the total number of trials in the historical data is also allowed to be 1 or greater.

Output

The macro automatically produces an RTF file indexed by the user-specified name. If a user does not specify the filename, the macro uses the filename as `BSMED_Output_a0.rtf` by default. The RTF file includes five tables:

1. Historical Data if a filename is specified in `HIST=`
2. Current Data with the Input Variables
3. Design Values
4. Type I Error for the Bayesian Survival Meta-Experimental Design
5. Power for the Bayesian Survival Meta-Experimental Design.

Note: In the absence of historical data, the macro does not produce the table for historical data and thus, it produces only four tables instead. For historical data, the macro allows users to input four different types of data sets. In the construction of tables for the Bayesian type I error and power, the macro produces three default Bayesian credible levels 0.90, 0.95, and 0.975 and one user choice Bayesian credible level.

Running Time

It takes approximately 2 hours to run this macro for 5,000 simulated data sets.

Chapter 5

Continual Reassessment Methods

5.1 Dose Finding in Oncology

In cancer drug development, phase I clinical trials are mainly designed to determine the maximum tolerated dose (MTD), which is typically defined as the maximum dosage that can be administered to patients without exceeding the unacceptable level of toxicity. In practice, the investigators specify a target toxicity rate so that the toxicity probability of the identified MTD should be closest to the target among all the doses under investigation. Phase I trials, often known as dose-escalation studies, involve only a single arm. The collected data are typically binary, indicating whether patients have experienced the dose-limiting toxicity (DLT). The DLTs are predefined drug-related toxicities that would prohibit continuing the treatment.

In phase I trials, a common assumption is that toxicity monotonically increases with the dose, and so does efficacy. Once the MTD is determined, the treatment would exert the maximum effectiveness as long as patients can tolerate the dosage. For practicality, patients are typically grouped into cohorts according to their enrollment dates and each cohort is adaptively assigned to the most appropriate dose based on the cumulative data. The first cohort of patients may be treated at the lowest dose level or that specified by investigators.

5.2 Continual Reassessment Method

To incorporate the monotonic toxicity order, a dose-toxicity curve or a parametric model is often assumed. In contrast to algorithm-based designs, such as the 3+3 design, where dose escalation or de-escalation is solely based on the data collected at the current dose level, model-based designs can pool all the information across different doses for decision making. Among a variety of model-based dose-finding methods, the continual reassessment method (CRM) is a very popular approach which is often cast in the Bayesian framework [1]. The CRM may take a single-parameter power model, a two-parameter logistic regression model, or a probit model. Different parametric models represent different patterns of the dose-toxicity curve, while the underlying true curve is typically unknown.

With a focus on the one-parameter power model [2], let $p_1 < \cdots < p_J$ denote the prespecified toxicity probabilities of a set of J doses for the drug under consideration, which is often known as the skeleton of the CRM. Let ϕ denote the target toxicity probability specified by the investigator. We model the toxicity probability at dose level j, $j = 1, \ldots, J$, in the form of

$$P(\text{toxicity at dose level } j) = \pi_j(\alpha) = p_j^{\exp(\alpha)},$$

where α is an unknown parameter. Suppose that at a certain stage of the trial, we observe the data that y_j patients have experienced the DLT among the n_j patients treated at dose level j, for $j = 1, \ldots, J$. If we let D denote the observed data, the binomial likelihood function is given by

$$L(\alpha \mid D) \propto \prod_{j=1}^{J} \left(p_j^{\exp(\alpha)}\right)^{y_j} \left(1 - p_j^{\exp(\alpha)}\right)^{n_j - y_j}.$$

In the Bayesian paradigm, we often take a normal prior distribution for α, i.e. $\alpha \sim N(0, \sigma^2)$, with a prior mean of zero and a prior variance σ^2. Using Bayes' theorem, we can estimate the toxicity probability at dose level j by the corresponding posterior mean,

$$\hat{\pi}_j = \int p_j^{\exp(\alpha)} \frac{L(\alpha \mid D) f(\alpha)}{\int L(\alpha \mid D) f(\alpha) d\alpha} d\alpha.$$

Once a cohort of patients is treated, the toxicity data would be updated in light of the new information, and so would the likelihood function $L(\alpha \mid D)$ which includes all the patients enrolled in the trial thus far. As a result, we re-estimate the toxicity probabilities at all the dose levels using the posterior means $\hat{\pi}_1, \ldots, \hat{\pi}_J$.

In detail, the CRM dose-finding procedure is described as follows:

1. Treat the first cohort of patients at the lowest or the physician-specified dose level.
2. Denote the current dose level as j^{curr}. Based on the data observed thus far, we obtain the posterior means of the toxicity probabilities for all the doses under consideration, $\hat{\pi}_1, \ldots, \hat{\pi}_J$. We then find the dose level j^* that has a toxicity probability closest to ϕ, $j^* = \underset{j \in \{1, \ldots, J\}}{\operatorname{argmin}} \left|\hat{\pi}_j - \phi\right|$, and make decisions as follows:
   a. if $j^{curr} > j^*$, de-escalate to dose level j^{curr} - 1;
   b. if $j^{curr} < j^*$ escalate to dose level $j^{curr} + 1$;
   c. otherwise, the dose stays at the same level for the next cohort of patients.
3. Once the maximum sample size is reached, the dose with the toxicity probability closest to ϕ is selected as the MTD.

The sample size for the CRM trial is calibrated through simulation studies in order to achieve desirable operating characteristics. In addition, if the lowest dose is still too toxic, as noted by

$$P(\pi_1 > \phi \mid D) = \int_{-\infty}^{\log\{\log(\phi)/\log(p_1)\}} f(\alpha \mid D)d\alpha > 0.9,$$

the trial would be terminated for safety. The tuning parameter 0.9 can be adjusted to control how stringent the safety rule is.

As an example, we illustrate the CRM with a phase I clinical trial to find the MTD of a new drug. Six dose levels of the drug are considered, and the CRM skeleton is prespecified as $(p_1, p_2, p_3, p_4, p_5, p_6) = (0.05, 0.10, 0.25, 0.40, 0.55, 0.65)$. The MTD is defined as the dose that has a toxicity probability closest to the target toxicity ϕ = 30%. Suppose the trial has treated 5 cohorts with a cohort size of 3, and the toxicity outcomes and dose assignments are listed below in Table 5.1 on page 135.

Table 5.1 *Toxicity Outcomes and Dose Assignments for First Hypothetical Trial*

Cohort Sequence	Dose Level	Cohort Size	# of DLTs
1	1	3	0
2	2	3	1
3	2	3	0
4	3	3	2
5	2	3	0

The SAS macro **%CRM** in Example Code 5.1 on page 135 can be used to analyze the cumulative data and determine the next dose assignment under the CRM framework. The input parameters for the **%CRM** macro are **currentdata**, **skeleton**, **target**, and **toxstop**. The **currentdata** parameter stores the observed data set based on the treated patients, and each row corresponds to the accumulated information for each cohort, where the three entries in each row represent the number of DLTs observed for each cohort, dose level, and number of patients for that cohort, respectively. The user must also specify the **skeleton** parameter, which is the prespecified $(p_1, \ldots, p_J)$. The target toxicity rate is denoted as **target** in the **% CRM** macro, which is set to be 0.3 as the default. In addition, the user can adjust the toxicity tolerance by changing the value of **toxstop**. **%CRM** creates a plot that overlays the curves for the initial guess and the posterior estimate of toxicity probability for each dose level. The output variable of the **%CRM** macro is the suggested dose level for the next cohort of patients.

Example Code 5.1 *Continual Reassessment Method Macro*

```
%macro CRM(currentdata,skeleton,target=0.3,toxstop=0.9);
   proc iml;
      use &currentdata.;
      read all;
      use &skeleton.;
      read all;
      pihat={};
      ndose=nrow(p);
      dosecurr=doselevel[nrow(doselevel)];
      stop=0;
      /* posterior=likelihood * prior */
      start posterior(alpha) global(DLT,doselevel,p,cohortsize);
```

```
        sigma2=2;
        lik=1;
        nn=nrow(DLT);
        do k=1 to nn;
           pi=(p[doselevel[k]])##exp(alpha);
           lik=lik*(pi##(DLT[k]))*((1-pi)##(cohortsize[k]-DLT[k]));
        end;
        lik=lik*exp(-0.5*alpha*alpha/sigma2);
        return(lik);
     finish;

     /* used to calculate the posterior mean of pi */
     start posttoxf(alpha) global(j,DLT,doselevel,p,cohortsize);
        post=p[j]##exp(alpha)*posterior(alpha);
        return(post);
     finish;

     call quad(marginal, "posterior", {.M .P}) eps=1E-4 peak=0.1;

     pi={};
     do j=1 to ndose;
        call quad(pij,"posttoxf",{.M .P}) ;
        pij=pij/marginal;
        pi=pi//pij;
     end;

     lb=log(log(&target)/log(p[1]));
     call quad(povertox,"posterior",-35||lb) eps=1E-4 peak=0.1;
     povertox=povertox/marginal;

     if povertox>&toxstop then stop=1;

     diff=abs(pi-&target);
     dosebest=diff[>:<];
     dosenext=dosecurr;

     if dosebest>dosecurr then
        if dosecurr<ndose then do;
        dosenext=dosecurr+1;
     end;

     if dosebest<dosecurr then
        if dosecurr>1 then do;
        dosenext=dosecurr-1;
     end;

     if stop=1 then dosenext="The trial should be terminated early";
     print dosenext;
     doselevel=1:ndose;
     doselevel=doselevel`;
     create doselevel from doselevel[colname="doselevel"];
     append from doselevel;

     create pi from pi[colname="pi"];
     append from pi;
  quit;
```

```
   data &skeleton.;
      merge &skeleton. pi doselevel;
   run;

   *title "Skeleton Versus Estimated Toxicity Probability";
   proc sgplot data = skeleton;
      vline doselevel / response = p markers legendlabel='p'
 markerattrs=(symbol=circlefilled size=10pt) lineattrs=(pattern = solid);
      vline doselevel / response = pi markers legendlabel='pi'
 markerattrs=(symbol=trianglefilled size=10pt) lineattrs=(pattern = solid);
      yaxis min = 0 max = 1 label="Toxicity Probability";
      xaxis label="Dose Level";
      refline &target / axis=y label="Toxicity Target"
LABELLOC= INSIDE LABELPOS= min lineattrs=(pattern = shortdash);
      keylegend / location=inside noborder;
   run;
%mend CRM;

data currentdata;
   input DLT doselevel cohortsize;
   datalines;
   0 1 3
   1 2 3
   0 2 3
   2 3 3
   0 2 3
   ;
run;

data skeleton;
   input p;
   datalines;
   0.05
   0.1
   0.25
   0.40
   0.55
   0.65
   ;
run;

%CRM(currentdata,skeleton,target=0.3,toxstop=0.9);
```

As shown in Figure 5.1 on page 138, the estimated toxicity probability of dose level 3 is closest to the target, while the most recent cohort has been treated at dose level 2. Based on the dose-finding algorithm, dose escalation should be taken and thus the next cohort will be treated at dose level 3.

Figure 5.1 *Prespecified and Estimated Toxicity Probabilities in the CRM*

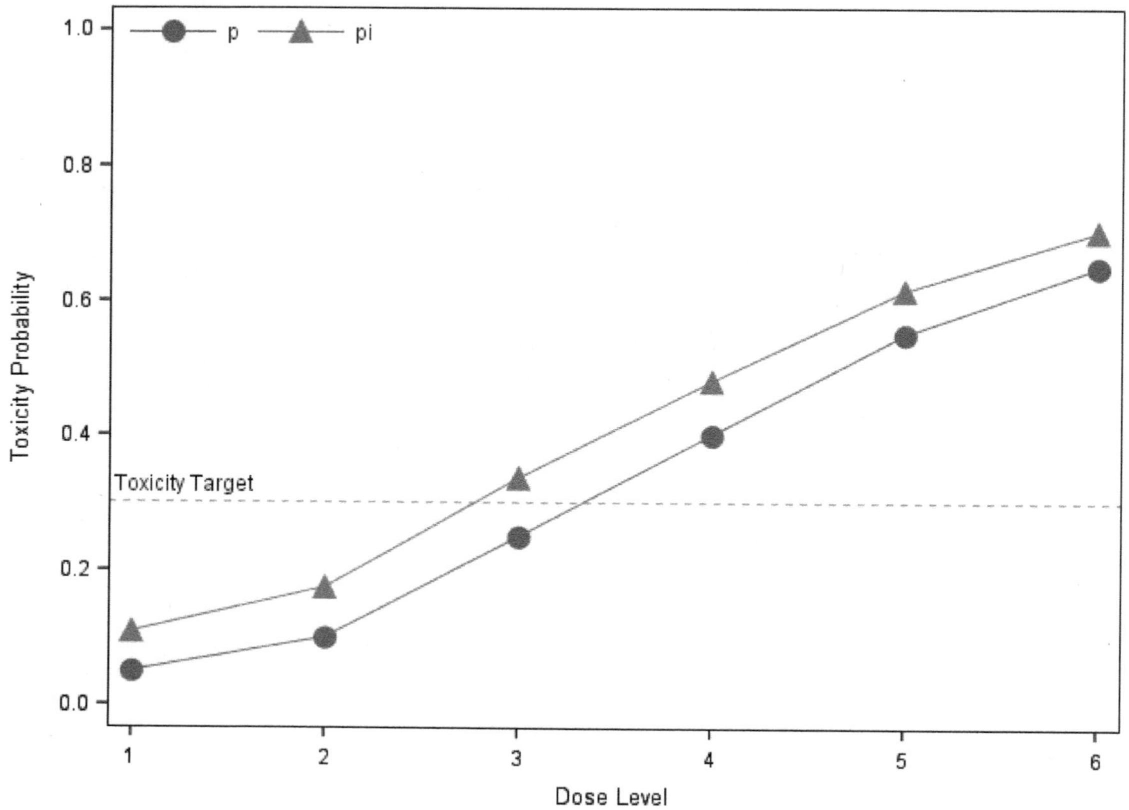

5.3 Bayesian Model Averaging Continual Reassessment Method

In the CRM, the prespecified skeleton $(p_1, \ldots, p_J)$ is usually arbitrary and subjective. As a result, the performance of the CRM may be compromised due to model misspecifications, which is a common drawback of parametric models. To enhance the robustness of the CRM, we can construct multiple CRM models in parallel, such that each model is equipped with a different skeleton representing uncertainty in the parametric modeling structure [3]. If there is no preference on different modeling structures, then we assign a discrete uniform prior probability to each CRM model. Through the Bayesian model averaging (BMA) procedure [4, 5], we let the data determine the weight of each model based on the posterior model probability. Automatically, the BMA-CRM assigns a larger weight to a model with a better fit, which ensures the robustness of the estimated toxicity probabilities even when some CRM models are misspecified.

To be more specific, let M_k denote the CRM model that is associated with the kth skeleton $(p_{k1}, \ldots, p_{kJ})$ for $k = 1, \ldots, K$. Under the working model M_k, the toxicity probability at dose level j is defined as

$$\pi_{kj}(\alpha_k) = p_{kj}^{\exp(\alpha_k)}, \quad j = 1, \ldots, J,$$

where α_k is the unknown parameter that is associated with model M_k. Suppose that at a certain stage of the trial, y_j patients have experienced the DLT among the n_j patients treated at dose level j. Based on the observed data D, the likelihood function under model M_k is

$$L(\alpha_k|D, M_k) \equiv P(D|\alpha_k, M_k) \propto \prod_{j=1}^{J} \left\{ p_{kj}^{\exp(\alpha_k)} \right\}^{y_j} \left\{ 1 - p_{kj}^{\exp(\alpha_k)} \right\}^{n_j - y_j}.$$

In the Bayesian hierarchical modeling framework, we specify $P(M_k)$ to be the prior probability that model M_k is the true model. If there is no preference *a priori* for any single CRM model, we simply take a discrete uniform distribution for the prior model probability; that is, $P(M_k) = 1/K$; otherwise, prior information can be incorporated by assigning a higher probability to a more preferred model. Under model M_k, we further specify $f(\alpha_k|M_k)$ to be the prior distribution of α_k. As in the single CRM model, we may take a zero-mean normal distribution as the prior for α_k. We apply Bayes' theorem to calculate the posterior model probability of M_k,

$$P(M_k|D) = \frac{P(D|M_k)P(M_k)}{\sum_{i=1}^{K} P(D|M_i)P(M_i)},$$

where $P(D|M_k)$ is the marginal likelihood of model M_k obtained by integrating out α_k with respect to the corresponding prior distribution,

$$P(D|M_k) = \int P(D|\alpha_k, M_k) f(\alpha_k|M_k) \mathrm{d}\alpha_k.$$

The BMA estimate of the toxicity probability at dose level j is then given by a weighted average,

$$\bar{\pi}_j = \sum_{k=1}^{K} \hat{\pi}_{kj} P(M_k|D), \quad j = 1, \ldots, J,$$

where $\hat{\pi}_{kj}$ is the posterior mean of the toxicity probability at dose level j under model M_k,

$$\hat{\pi}_{kj} = \int p_{kj}^{\exp(\alpha_k)} \frac{P(D|\alpha_k, M_k) f(\alpha_k|M_k)}{\int P(D|\alpha_k, M_k) f(\alpha_k|M_k) \mathrm{d}\alpha_k} \mathrm{d}\alpha_k.$$

The BMA estimator $\bar{\pi}_j$ assigns each $\hat{\pi}_{kj}$ a weight of $P(M_k|D)$, and the better the model fit the larger the weight. Under the BMA-CRM, the decision on dose escalation or de-escalation is based upon the BMA estimate $\bar{\pi}_j$ as opposed to $\hat{\pi}_{kj}$ from each single CRM model.

In contrast to averaging over multiple CRM models, one can also take a model selection approach by identifying the best fitting model at each step of dose assignment. Model selection can be based on certain criteria that penalizes a large model [6], for example, Akaike information criterion (AIC), Bayesian information criterion (BIC), and Deviance information criterion (DIC). Because all the candidate models in the multiple CRMs are of the same structure, except for different skeletons, for simplicity, we can take the posterior model probability as the basis for model selection: The higher the posterior model probability, the better the model fit. Therefore, we can select the CRM model that is associated with the highest posterior model probability to determine each dose assignment.

To illustrate the BMA-CRM, we consider six dose levels and the target toxicity probability is 30%. Four sets of initial guesses of the toxicity probabilities (skeletons 1-4) are specified as follows,

$$(p_{11}, \ldots, p_{16}) = (0.02,\ 0.08,\ 0.12,\ 0.20,\ 0.30,\ 0.50),$$

$$(p_{21}, \ldots, p_{26}) = (0.01,\ 0.05,\ 0.14,\ 0.22,\ 0.26,\ 0.30),$$

$$(p_{31}, \ldots, p_{36}) = (0.10,\ 0.20,\ 0.30,\ 0.40,\ 0.50,\ 0.60),$$

$$(p_{41}, \ldots, p_{46}) = (0.20,\ 0.30,\ 0.40,\ 0.50,\ 0.60,\ 0.65).$$

The prior model probabilities are set equally for the four skeletons, i.e., $P(M_k) = 1/4$, for $k = 1, \ldots, 4$. After seven cohorts of patients have been treated in the trial, their toxicity outcomes are presented in Table 5.2 on page 140.

Table 5.2 *Toxicity Outcomes and Dose Assignments for Second Hypothetical Trial*

Cohort Sequence	Dose Level	Cohort Size	# of DLTs
1	1	3	0
2	2	3	0
3	3	3	1
4	3	3	0
5	4	3	1
6	4	3	1
7	5	3	2

The SAS macro **%BMACRM** in Example Code 5.2 on page 140 can be used to analyze the cumulative data and recommend the most appropriate dose for the next cohort of patients. The input parameters in the **%BMACRM** macro are similar to those in the **%CRM** macro, but the **%BMACRM** macro requires users to specify several skeletons instead of a single skeleton. In addition, the prior probability of each skeleton is stored in the **priormodel** data set for which we use equal probabilities as a default. The **%BMACRM** macro has the same output as the **%CRM** macro. To illustrate the **%BMACRM** macro, we consider the above example with seven cohorts of patients treated in the trial and the goal is to determine the dose assignment for the next cohort.

Example Code 5.2 *Bayesian Model Averaging CRM Macro*

```
%macro BMACRM(currentdata,skeleton,priormodel,target=0.3,toxstop=0.9);
   proc iml;
      use &currentdata.;
      read all;
      use &skeleton.;
      read all into skeleton;
      use &priormodel.;
      read all;

      nmodel=nrow(priormodel);
```

```
ndose=nrow(skeleton);

dosecurr=doselevel[nrow(doselevel)];
stop=0;
/* posterior=likelihood * prior */
start posterior(alpha) global(DLT,doselevel,p,cohortsize);
   sigma2=2;
   lik=1;
   nn=nrow(DLT);
   do k=1 to nn;
      pi=(p[doselevel[k]])##exp(alpha);
      lik=lik*(pi##(DLT[k]))*((1-pi)##(cohortsize[k]-DLT[k]));
   end;
   lik=lik*exp(-0.5*alpha*alpha/sigma2);
   return(lik);
finish;

/* used to calculate the posterior mean of pi */
start posttoxf(alpha) global(j,DLT,doselevel,p,cohortsize);
   post=p[j]##exp(alpha)*posterior(alpha);
   return(post);
finish;

marginalm={};
povertoxm={};
pim=repeat(0,ndose,nmodel);
do md=1 to nmodel;
   p=skeleton[,md];
   lb=log(log(&target)/log(p[1]));
   call quad(marginal, "posterior", {.M .P}) eps=1E-4 peak=-3 scale=0.5;
   /* default: PEAK=1 */
   marginalm=marginalm//marginal;

   do j=1 to ndose;
      call quad(pij,"posttoxf",{.M .P}) eps=1E-4 peak=-3 scale=0.5;
      pij=pij/marginal;
      pim[j,md]=pij;
   end;

   call quad(povertox,"posterior",-35||lb) eps=1E-4 peak=-3 scale=0.5;
   povertox=povertox/marginal;
   povertoxm=povertoxm//povertox;
end;

posmodel=marginalm#priormodel/sum(marginalm#priormodel);
pi=pim*posmodel;
povertox=sum(povertoxm#posmodel);

if povertox>&toxstop then stop=1;

diff=abs(pi-&target);
dosebest=diff[>:<];
dosenext=dosecurr;

if dosebest>dosecurr then
   if dosecurr<ndose then do;
```

```
         dosenext=dosecurr+1;
      end;

      if dosebest<dosecurr then
         if dosecurr>1 then do;
         dosenext=dosecurr-1;
      end;

      if stop=1 then dosenext="The trial should be early terminated";
      print dosenext;
      doselevel=1:ndose;
      doselevel=doselevel`;
      create doselevel from doselevel[colname="doselevel"];
      append from doselevel;

      create pi from pi[colname="pi"];
      append from pi;
   quit;

   data &skeleton.;
      merge &skeleton. pi doselevel;
   run;

   *title "Skeleton versus Estimated Toxicity Probability";
   proc sgplot data = skeleton;
      vline doselevel / response = p1 markers legendlabel='p1'
markerattrs=(symbol=circlefilled size=10pt) lineattrs=(pattern = solid);
      vline doselevel / response = p2 markers legendlabel='p2'
markerattrs=(symbol=trianglefilled size=10pt) lineattrs=(pattern = solid);
      vline doselevel / response = p3 markers legendlabel='p3'
markerattrs=(symbol=diamondfilled size=10pt) lineattrs=(pattern = solid);
      vline doselevel / response = p4 markers legendlabel='p4'
markerattrs=(symbol=squarefilled size=10pt) lineattrs=(pattern = solid);
      vline doselevel / response = pi markers legendlabel='pi'
markerattrs=(symbol=starfilled size=10pt) lineattrs=(pattern = solid thickness = 3);
      yaxis min = 0 max = 1 label="Toxicity Probability";
      xaxis label="Dose Level";
      refline &target / axis=y label="Toxicity Target"
LABELLOC= INSIDE LABELPOS= min lineattrs=(pattern = shortdash);
      keylegend / location=inside noborder;
   run;

%mend BMACRM;

/* Observed data:
   1st col: # of DLTs for each cohort
   2nd col: Treated dose level
   3rd col: # of patients for each cohort
*/
data currentdata;
   input DLT doselevel cohortsize;
   datalines;
   0 1 3
   0 2 3
   1 3 3
   0 3 3
```

```
   1 4 3
   1 4 3
   2 5 3
   ;
run;

/* Prespecified skeleton:
   Four skeletons are used in this example,
   each column corresponds to a skeleton.
*/
data skeleton;
   input p1 p2 p3 p4;
   datalines;
   0.02 0.01 0.10 0.20
   0.08 0.05 0.20 0.30
   0.12 0.14 0.30 0.40
   0.20 0.22 0.40 0.50
   0.30 0.26 0.50 0.60
   0.50 0.30 0.60 0.65
   ;
run;

/* Prior probability for each skeleton */
data priormodel;
   input priormodel;
   datalines;
   0.25
   0.25
   0.25
   0.25
   ;
run;

%BMACRM(currentdata,skeleton,priormodel,target=0.3,toxstop=0.9);
```

As shown in Figure 5.2 on page 144, the four skeletons represent quite different prior opinions on the dose toxicity curve. The BMA-CRM naturally integrates the posterior estimates from the individual CRM under each skeleton. Based on the cumulative data of the first seven treated patients, the estimated toxicity curve is also presented in Figure 5.2, and clearly dose level 4 should be recommended for the next cohort of patients.

Figure 5.2 *Four Prespecified Skeletons and Estimated Toxicity Probabilities in the BMA-CRM*

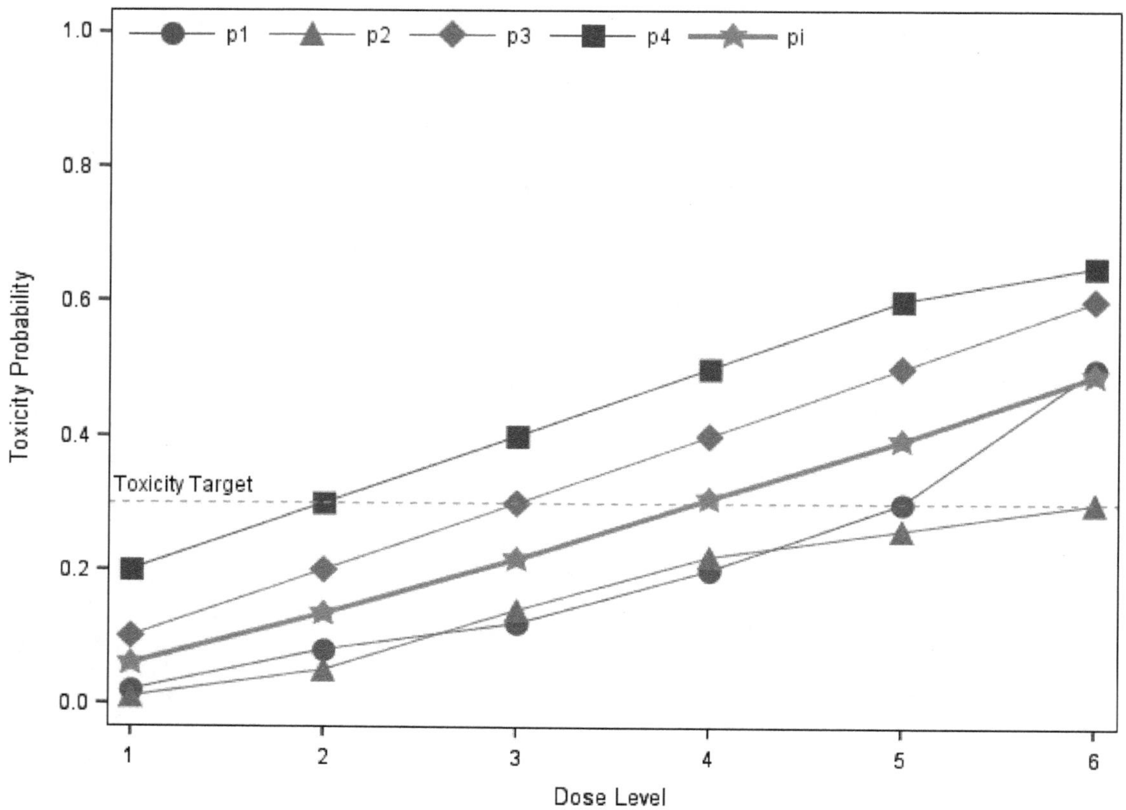

Prior to implementation of a phase I clinical trial, extensive simulation studies should be conducted to examine the operating characteristics of the design, so that the design parameters such as the skeletons and the prior distributions can be properly calibrated. A good design should have robust and acceptable behaviors under various toxicity scenarios. To investigate the practical performance of the CRM and BMA-CRM, we consider six dose levels with monotonically increasing toxicity. The target toxicity probability is $\phi = 30\%$. We use a non-informative prior distribution for α, with $\alpha \sim N(0, \sigma^2)$ and σ^2=2. The first cohort is treated at the lowest dose level, and the maximum sample size is 30. Table 5.3 on page 145, Table 5.4 on page 146, and Table 5.5 on page 146 summarize the true toxicity probability, the selection percentage, the number of patients treated at each level, the total number of observed DLTs, and the percentage of trial early stopping, where 1000 trials are replicated under each scenario. As expected, the BMA-CRM delivers more robust dose-finding performance in comparison to the four individual CRMs using a single skeleton. Macros **`%CRMSIM`** and **`%BMACRMSIM`** generate the results for Table 5.3 through Table 5.5 and are included in the supplemental material for the book available from the companion website.

The input parameters in the %CRMSIM macro are listed below.

1. **`skeleton`** stores the prespecified skeleton (first column) and the true toxicity probabilities (second column).
2. **`target`** is the target toxicity rate.
3. **`ncohort`** is the total number of cohorts.
4. **`cohortsize`** is the number of patients in each cohort.

5. **toxstop** is the threshold probability to early terminate the trial if the lowest dose level is too toxic.

6. **ntrial** is the number of replications in the simulation.

As an illustration, we consider the CRM with skeleton 1 under scenario 1 in Example Code 5.3 on page 145.

Example Code 5.3 *Simulation of CRM Design*

```
data skeleton1;
   input p ptrue;
   datalines;
   0.02 0.07
   0.08 0.12
   0.12 0.17
   0.20 0.30
   0.30 0.45
   0.50 0.60
   ;
run;
%CRMsim(skeleton,target=0.3,ncohort=10,cohortsize=3,toxstop=0.9,ntrial=1000);
```

The output table includes the following variables.

1. **doseselect** is the percentage of each dose level being selected as the MTD.

2. **ntox** is the average number of DLTs observed at each dose level.

3. **ntrted** is the average number of patients assigned to each dose level.

4. **nstop** is the percentage of early termination.

The **%BMACRMSIM** macro has similar input and the same output variables as those of **%CRMSIM**. **%BMACRMSIM** requires users to create the skeletons and true toxicity rates in different data sets (**skeleton** and **truerate**). In addition, users should specify the prior probability for each skeleton in the **priormodel** data set.

Table 5.3 *Scenario 1 of Simulation Study Comparing the BMA-CRM and CRM*

Dose Level	1	2	3	4	5	6	# DLTs	% Stop
P(Tox)	0.07	0.12	0.17	0.30	0.45	0.60		
BMA-CRM	0.0	3.0	24.0	51.1	20.6	1.3		
# of Pts	4.1	4.2	7.2	9.1	4.5	0.9	7.3	0
CRM 1	0.0	2.6	20.3	53.0	23.0	1.1		
# of Pts	4.0	4.2	6.7	9.2	5.4	0.7	7.5	0
CRM 2	0.0	3.5	33.4	45.0	14.3	3.8		
# of Pts	4.0	4.6	8.2	7.6	3.8	1.6	7.3	0
CRM 3	0.0	3.0	24.1	53.0	18.6	1.3		
# of Pts	4.1	4.2	7.6	9.1	4.2	0.8	7.2	0
CRM 4	0	2.6	24.1	54.2	17.6	1.5		

Dose Level	1	2	3	4	5	6	# DLTs	% Stop
# of Pts	4.1	4.3	7.4	9.4	4.0	0.9	7.2	0

Table 5.4 *Scenario 2 of Simulation Study Comparing the BMA-CRM and CRM*

Dose Level	1	2	3	4	5	6	# DLTs	% Stop
P(Tox)	0.10	0.20	0.30	0.40	0.50	0.60		
BMA-CRM	1.6	26.7	41.7	23.1	5.7	0.9		
# of Pts	5.4	7.9	9.2	4.4	1.7	0.3	8.0	0.3
CRM 1	2.2	25.0	38.4	26.6	6.9	0.6		
# of Pts	5.2	7.8	8.8	5.8	2.1	0.2	8.1	0.3
CRM 2	1.5	27.2	47.0	18.5	3.4	2.1		
# of Pts	5.1	8.6	9.8	4.3	1.4	0.7	8.0	0.3
CRM 3	1.7	26.6	43.6	21.4	5.7	0.7		
# of Pts	5.4	7.9	9.6	5.2	1.6	0.3	8.0	0.3
CRM 4	1.8	26.1	43.5	22.7	5.0	0.6		
# of Pts	5.4	8.0	9.4	5.4	1.5	0.3	8.0	0.3

Table 5.5 *Scenario 3 of Simulation Study Comparing the BMA-CRM and CRM*

Dose Level	1	2	3	4	5	6	# DLTs	% Stop
P(Tox)	0.05	0.14	0.18	0.20	0.23	0.30		
BMA-CRM	0.0	2.9	11.0	21.9	32.3	31.9		
# of Pts	3.8	4.4	5.7	6.5	5.5	4.2	5.7	0
CRM 1	0.0	2.6	8.9	21.6	43.0	23.9		
# of Pts	3.7	4.2	5.3	6.6	7.0	3.2	5.7	0
CRM 2	0.0	3.9	14.1	19.0	16.1	46.9		
# of Pts	3.7	4.7	6.5	5.2	3.5	6.4	5.9	0
CRM 3	0.0	2.8	12.0	24.0	31.4	29.8		
# of Pts	3.8	4.3	6.2	6.4	5.5	3.9	5.7	0
CRM 4	0.0	2.7	11.8	25.2	27.2	33.1		
# of Pts	3.8	4.3	6.0	6.6	5.1	4.2	5.7	0

5.4 Fractional Continual Reassessment Method

Most of the dose-finding methods, including the aforementioned CRM and BMA-CRM, require the DLT outcomes to be ascertainable shortly after treatment. In other words, the toxicity outcomes of all the previously treated patients must be available in order to determine the next dose assignment. However, it may take a long period of time to measure the DLT outcomes after treatment. In a more common scenario, if the patient accrual is fast and the toxicity measurements cannot keep pace with the enrollment, missing toxicity data arise as the outcomes of the patients under treatment may still be unavailable when that information is needed. For example, in radiotherapy trials, DLTs often occur long after the treatment is finished. In a phase I trial with pancreatic cancer, the goal was to determine the MTD of oxaliplatin for combination with gemcitabine and the concurrent radiation therapy [7]. The accrual rate was one patient every two weeks, whereas, it took on average nine weeks to assess the toxicity outcome of each patient after the treatment was initiated. Consequently, at the moment of dose assignment for a newly arrived patient, the patients under treatment might not have yet completed the full assessment period and, thus, the non-toxicity outcomes could be considered missing or censored at that time.

To accommodate late-onset toxicity, we can model the underlying times to toxicity through the well-known Kaplan-Meier estimator [8,9]. An alternative approach to handling censored data is to redistribute the mass of each censored observation to the right [10,11]. Typically, there is a prespecified toxicity evaluation window to determine the DLT outcome. Within the evaluation window $[0, \tau]$, if a patient experiences the DLT, we take the toxicity outcome Y=1; if a patient still has not experienced the DLT after time τ, we take Y=0. Due to continual decision making on dose assignment for each new cohort, patients currently under treatment may have not experienced the DLT when a new cohort of patients is ready for treatment. Under such circumstances, the toxicity event can be viewed as censored data, and we adopt the redistribution to the right approach by splitting the point mass of 1 between the censoring point and somewhere beyond τ (anywhere that is larger than τ). In the construction of the likelihood function, only the weight assigned to the censoring time point within $[0, \tau]$ makes the contribution, and the weight assigned beyond τ does not contribute to the likelihood. Thus, due to censoring, we can only count on fractional information of the censored data. In contrast, the naïve method may simply discard the missing data as if no toxicity would ever occur in the future, which inevitably loses useful information for decision making.

To fully utilize the follow-up time information, more data need to be collected during the trial conduct, for example, patients' enrollment dates, decision-making dates (censoring times), and the dates of toxicity occurrences (event times). For subject i, let t_i denote the time to toxicity occurrence, and let u_i $(u_i \le \tau)$ denote the actual follow-up time (up to the decision-making time on dose assignment for the next cohort) that may censor t_i. We assume u_i to be independent of t_i, because the arrival time of a new cohort is typically independent of the time to toxicity due to patients' staggered entry. Censoring times arise when patients have not experienced the DLT $(u_i < t_i)$ and have not completed the follow-up to τ $(u_i < \tau)$. If the toxicity event of subject i is censored, the corresponding fractional contribution of this subject is given by

$$\Pr(t_i < \tau \mid t_i > u_i) = \frac{\Pr(u_i < t_i < \tau)}{\Pr(t_i > u_i)},$$

which is the conditional probability of occurrence of the toxicity event in (u_i, τ) given that no toxicity has occurred yet by time u_i. As a result, the collected data in the trial include 0, 1, and some fraction between 0 and 1. The fractional contribution for a censored toxicity outcome can be easily estimated by

$$\hat{y}_i = \frac{\hat{S}(u_i) - \hat{S}(\tau)}{\hat{S}(u_i)}$$

where $\hat{S}(\cdot)$ is the usual Kaplan-Meier estimator. More specifically, for subject *i*, we define y_i=0 if the DLT has not occurred by time τ, y_i=1 if the DLT has occurred by time τ, or $y_i = \hat{y}_i$ if the DLT is censored before time τ. For notational clarity, denote $p_{j(i)} = p_j$ if subject *i* is treated at dose level *j*, let *n* be the total number of patients treated in the trial thus far, and let *D* denote the observed data. Based on the fractional scheme, the likelihood function under the CRM power model can be written as

$$L(\alpha \mid D) \propto \prod_{i=1}^{n} p_{j(i)}^{y_i \exp(\alpha)} \left\{1 - p_{j(i)}^{\exp(\alpha)}\right\}^{1 - y_i},$$

where y_i takes a value of 0 or 1 for complete data, or a fraction of 1 for a censored observation. Once the censored data are fractionized, the rest of implementation of the fractional CRM (fCRM) is straightforward as the usual CRM.

As an illustration, we consider a phase I dose-finding study to identify the MTD of a new drug with six doses. The skeleton of the trial is set as $(p_1, \ldots, p_6) = (0.1,\ 0.2,\ 0.3,\ 0.4,\ 0.5,\ 0.6)$. In the trial, each patient is followed for 90 days, i.e., τ =90. Suppose that twelve patients have been treated with three DLTs observed, and their detailed information is provided in Table 5.6 on page 148.

Table 5.6 *Cumulative Data of the First Twelve Patients in the fCRM Trial*

Patient	Dose Level	DLT	Follow-up	Date of Entry	Date of DLT	Imputed DLT
1	1	0	0	01-Jan-11		0
2	1	0	0	02-Jan-11		0
3	1	0	0	15-Jan-11		0
4	2	0	0	01-Feb-11		0
5	2	0	0	05-Feb-11		0
6	2	1	0	20-Feb-11	13-Apr-11	1
7	3	1	1	03-Mar-11	20-Apr-11	1
8	3	0	1	07-Mar-11		0
9	3	0	1	10-Mar-11		0
10	3	0	1	01-Apr-11		0.22
11	3	1	1	02-Apr-11	28-Apr-11	1
12	3	0	1	02-Apr-11		0.22

Suppose that a new patient enters the trial on 10-May-2011, then we can use the SAS macro **% fCRM** to determine the dose level for this participant. If the cohort size is three, each patient's information in the cohort must be recorded separately to compute each individual contribution to the likelihood. Towards this goal, one needs to input the information of the twelve patients, including their observed toxicity outcomes, indicators of whether they have been fully followed, their entering dates and the dates of DLT occurrences. If a patient has completed the follow-up period without experiencing toxicity, then we input the date as the last day of the follow-up period. If a patient has not experienced toxicity but is still in the follow-up period, his/her date of censoring is specified as the current decision-making date: 10-May-2011.

The **% fCRM** macro (Example Code 5.4 on page 149) requires the following input variables. The location of the **km.sas** file should be specified in the **%include** statement.

1. **currentdata** is the data set that stores the accumulated information. More specifically, users need to input the dose level (**doselevel**), DLT outcome (**DLT**, 1 if DLT is observed, 0 otherwise), the indicator variable (**followup**) that denotes whether the patient is still under the follow-up in the trial, the entry date (**entrydate**), and the event date (**timetoevent**) of the patient.

2. **skeleton** is the data set that stores the prespecified skeleton.

3. **currenttime** is the current date (entry date for the new patient).

4. **tau** is the length of the full follow-up period for toxicity evaluation.

5. **target** is the target toxicity rate.

6. **toxstop** is the threshold probability to early terminate the trial if the lowest dose level is too toxic.

Example Code 5.4 *Fractional CRM Macro*

```
data currentdata;
   input doselevel DLT followup entrydate timetoevent;
   informat entrydate timetoevent date7.;
   datalines;
   1 0 0 01Jan11 01Apr11
   1 0 0 02Jan11 02Apr11
   1 0 0 15Jan11 15Apr11
   2 0 0 01Feb11 02May11
   2 0 0 03Feb11 05May11
   2 1 0 20Feb11 13Apr11
   3 1 1 03Mar11 20Apr11
   3 0 1 07Mar11 10May11
   3 0 1 10Mar11 10May11
   3 0 1 01Apr11 10May11
   3 1 1 02Apr11 28Apr11
   3 0 1 02Apr11 10May11
   ;
run;

data skeleton;
   input p;
   datalines;
   0.1
   0.2
   0.3
   0.4
```

```
   0.5
   0.6
   ;
run;

%macro fCRM(currentdata,skeleton,currenttime,tau=90,target=0.3,toxstop=0.9);
   proc iml;
      use &skeleton.;
      read all;
      use &currentdata.;
      read all;

      start posterior(alpha) global(DLT,doselevel,p);
         sigma2=2;
         lik=1;
         nn=nrow(DLT);
         aa=sum(DLT);

         if aa=0 then do;
            do k=1 to nn;
               pi=(p[doselevel[k]])##exp(alpha);
               lik=lik*((1-pi)##(1-DLT[k]));
            end;
         end;
         else do;
            do k=1 to nn;
               pi=(p[doselevel[k]])##exp(alpha);
               lik=lik*(pi##(DLT[k]))*((1-pi)##(1-DLT[k]));
            end;
         end;

         lik=lik*exp(-0.5*alpha*alpha/sigma2);
         return(lik);
      finish;

      /* used to calculate the posterior mean of pi */
      start posttoxf(alpha) global(j,DLT,doselevel,p);
         post=p[j]##exp(alpha)*posterior(alpha);
         return(post);
      finish;

      currenttime=inputn(&currenttime.,'date7.');

      ndose=nrow(p);
      doseselect={};
      dosecurr=doselevel[nrow(doselevel)];

      stop=0;
      Time=DLT#(timetoevent-entrydate)+(1-DLT)#((1-followup)
      #&tau+followup#(timetoevent-entrydate));

      if sum(DLT)=0 then do;
         if dosecurr<ndose then dosenext=dosecurr+1;
      end;
      else do;
         create survivaldata var{Time DLT};
```

```
   append;
close survivaldata;

*** Need to specify directory of file ***;
%include "KM.sas";

use survivalcurve;
   read all;
close survivalcurve;
*compute S(&tau);
k = loc( Time<=&tau );
k=k[ncol(k)];
stau=SURVIVAL[k];
if missing(stau)=1 then stau=min(SURVIVAL);

print stau;
*compute S(t) for censored data;
do j=1 to nrow(DLT);
if (followup[j]=1) then
   if (DLT[j]=0) then do;
      k=loc( Time<=(timetoevent[j]-entrydate[j]) );
      k=k[ncol(k)];
      st=SURVIVAL[k];
      if missing(st)=1 then st=min(SURVIVAL);
      DLT[j]=(st-stau)/st;
   end;
end;

imputedDLT=DLT;

print imputedDLT;
/* posterior=likelihood * prior */

call quad(marginal, "posterior", {.M .P}) eps=1E-4 peak=-1 scale=0.5;
/* default: PEAK=1 */
pi={};
do j=1 to ndose;
   call quad(pij,"posttoxf",{.M .P}) eps=1E-4 peak=-1 scale=0.5;
   pij=pij/marginal;
   pi=pi//pij;
end;

lb=log(log(&target)/log(p[1]));

call quad(povertox,"posterior",-35||lb) eps=1E-4 peak=-1 scale=0.5;
povertox=povertox/marginal;

if povertox>&toxstop then do;
   stop=1;
end;

diff=abs(pi-&target);
dosebest=diff[>:<];

if dosebest>dosecurr then
   if dosecurr<ndose then do;
```

```
            dosenext=dosecurr+1;
         end;

         if dosebest<dosecurr then
            if dosecurr>1 then do;
            dosenext=dosecurr-1;
         end;
      end;

      if stop=1 then dosenext="The trial should be early terminated";

      print dosenext[colname='doselevel level for next cohort'];

      doselevel=1:ndose;
      doselevel=doselevel`;
      create doselevel from doselevel[colname="doselevel"];
      append from doselevel;

      create pi from pi[colname="pi"];
      append from pi;
   quit;

   data &skeleton.;
      merge &skeleton. pi doselevel;
   run;

   proc sgplot data = skeleton;
      vline doselevel / response = p markers legendlabel='p'
markerattrs=(symbol=circlefilled size=10pt) lineattrs=(pattern = solid);
      vline doselevel / response = pi markers legendlabel='pi'
markerattrs=(symbol=trianglefilled size=10pt) lineattrs=(pattern = solid);
      yaxis min = 0 max = 1 label="Toxicity Probability";
      xaxis label="Dose Level";
      refline &target / axis=y label="Toxicity Target"
LABELLOC= INSIDE LABELPOS= min lineattrs=(pattern = shortdash);
      keylegend / location=inside noborder;
   run;
%mend fCRM;

%fCRM(currentdata,skeleton,'10May11',tau=90,target=0.3,toxstop=0.9);
```

The **% fCRM** macro uses **proc lifetest** to generate a Kaplan-Meier estimator. Two plots are produced: one is for the Kaplan-Meier estimator of the survival function, and the other is the overlay of the curves for the initial guess and the posterior estimate of the toxicity probability for each dose level. The output variables include:

1. **stau** is the survival probability after the follow-up period.
2. **imputedDLT** denotes the imputed value for each censored observation.
3. **dosenext** is the suggested dose level for the next cohort of patients.

The Kaplan-Meier estimator of the survival function for the time to toxicity based on all the observed data (including censored observations) is presented in Figure 5.3 on page 153. The fractional contributions for the censored toxicity outcomes are given in the last column of Table 5.6 on page 148. As the current 12th patient is treated at dose level 3, while the optimal one is at dose level 2 from the estimated toxicity probability curve in

Figure 5.4 on page 154, this indicates that dose level 2 should be recommended for the next patient.

Figure 5.3 Kaplan-Meier Estimator of the Survival Curve Based on the First 12 Patients

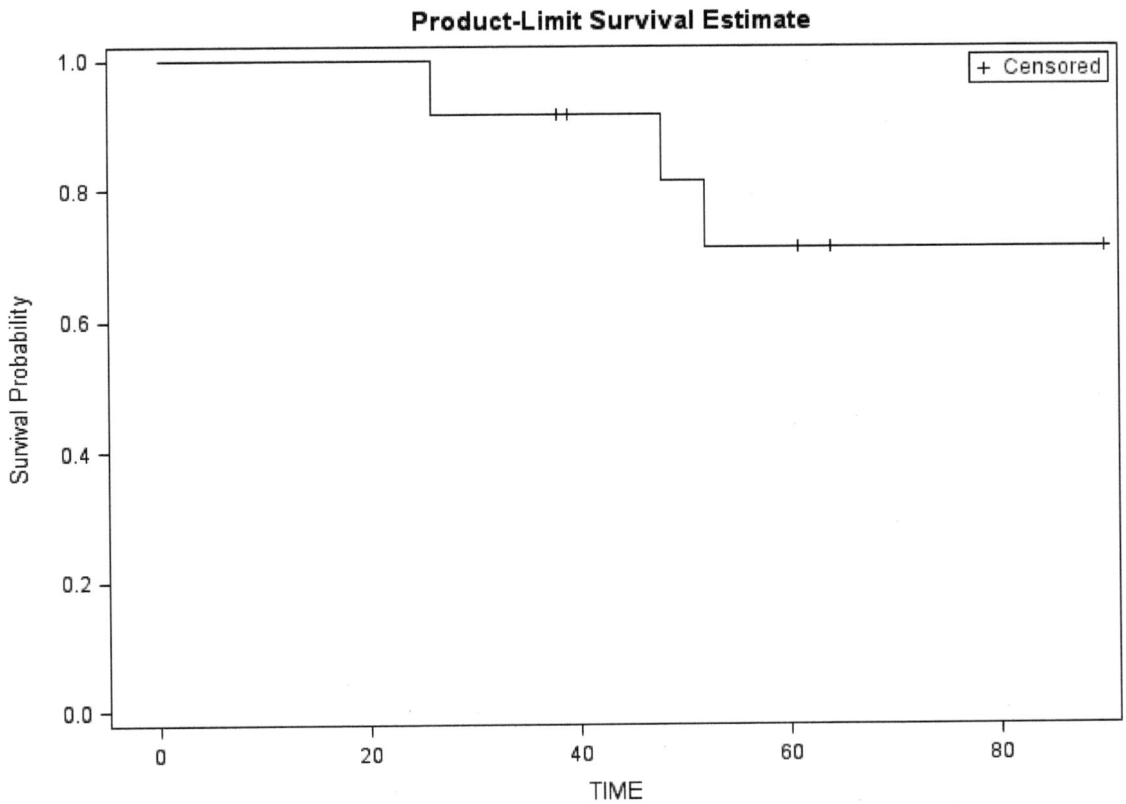

Figure 5.4 Prespecified and Estimated Toxicity Probabilities in the fCRM

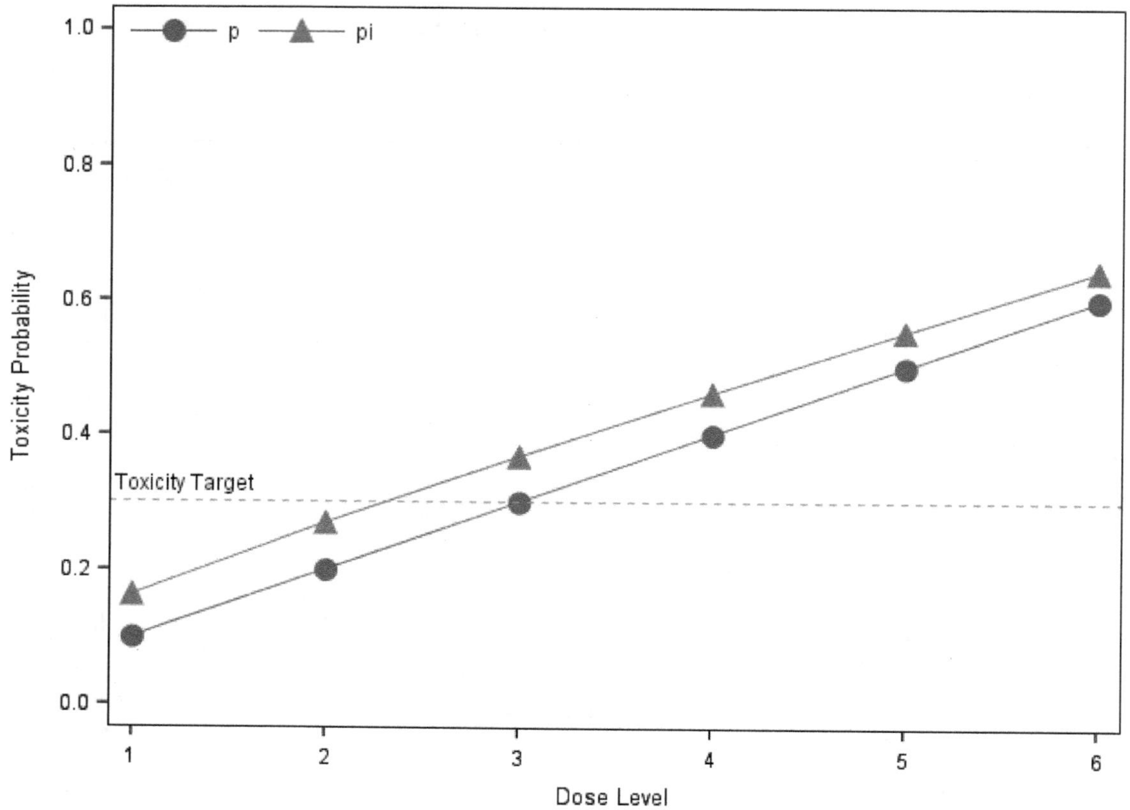

5.5 Time-to-Event Continual Reassessment Method

Using patients' exposure times as weights, Cheung and Chappell [12] proposed the time-to-event continual reassessment method (TITE-CRM) to incorporate information of follow-up times into toxicity evaluation. Let u_i be the actual follow-up time for subject i, and let y_i be the observed toxicity outcome at time u_i. If the ith patient has not experienced the DLT, y_i takes a value of 0, and otherwise y_i=1. Often a uniform weighting scheme is assumed in the form of $w_i = u_i/\tau$. The longer the follow-up, the higher the weight. The weight takes a value of 1, if the patient has experienced the DLT by time u_i. Under the CRM model, the pseudo-binomial likelihood function is given by

$$L(\alpha \mid D) \propto \prod_{i=1}^{n} \left\{ w_i p_{j(i)}^{\exp(\alpha)} \right\}^{y_i} \left\{ 1 - w_i p_{j(i)}^{\exp(\alpha)} \right\}^{1-y_i}.$$

Under this formulation, patients who have not experienced toxicity and have not been fully followed are treated as “no toxicity” with y_i=0, although their data are in fact missing.

To illustrate the TITE-CRM, we consider a hypothetical trial that includes six dose levels. The target toxicity rate is 0.3, and the skeleton is specified as

$(p_1, \ldots, p_6) = (0.1,\ 0.2,\ 0.3,\ 0.4,\ 0.5,\ 0.6)$. In the trial, each patient is followed for 90 days, i.e., $\tau = 90$. Suppose the entry date for the new patient is 20-April-2011. Before the entry of the new patient, nine patients have been treated, of whom the data are provided in Table 5.7 on page 155.

Table 5.7 *Cumulative Data for the First Nine Patients in the TITE-CRM Trial*

Patient	Dose Level	DLT	Follow-up	Date of Entry
1	1	0	0	01-Jan-11
2	1	0	0	02-Jan-11
3	1	0	0	15-Jan-11
4	2	0	1	01-Feb-11
5	2	0	1	05-Feb-11
6	2	1	1	20-Feb-11
7	3	1	1	03-Mar-11
8	3	0	1	07-Mar-11
9	3	0	1	10-Mar-11

The **%TITECRM** macro (Example Code 5.5 on page 155) implements the TITE-CRM to determine the dose level for the new patient. The input variables are similar to those in the **% fCRM**.

Example Code 5.5 *Time-to-Event CRM Macro*

```
data currentdata;
   input doselevel DLT followup entrydate date7.;
   datalines;
   1 0 0 01Jan11
   1 0 0 02Jan11
   1 0 0 15Jan11
   2 0 1 01Feb11
   2 0 1 05Feb11
   2 1 1 20Feb11
   3 1 1 03Mar11
   3 0 1 07Mar11
   3 0 1 10Mar11
   ;
run;

data skeleton;
   input p;
   datalines;
   0.1
   0.2
   0.3
   0.4
   0.5
   0.6
```

```
    ;
run;

%macro TITECRM(currentdata,skeleton,currenttime,tau=90,target=0.3,toxstop=0.9);
   proc iml;
      use &skeleton.;
      read all;
      use &currentdata.;
      read all;
      currenttime=inputn(&currenttime.,'date7.');
      ndose=nrow(p);
      doseselect={};
      dosecurr=doselevel[nrow(doselevel)];
      w=(followup=0)+(followup=1)#(currenttime-entrydate)/&tau;
      stop=0;

      start posterior(alpha) global(DLT,doselevel,p,w);
         sigma2=2;
         lik=1;
         nn=nrow(DLT);
         aa=sum(DLT);

         if aa=0 then do;
            do k=1 to nn;
               pi=(p[doselevel[k]])##exp(alpha);
               lik=lik*((1-w[k]*pi)##(1-DLT[k]));
            end;
         end;
         else do;
            do k=1 to nn;
               pi=(p[doselevel[k]])##exp(alpha);
               lik=lik*((w[k]*pi)##(DLT[k]))*((1-w[k]*pi)##(1-DLT[k]));
            end;
         end;

         lik=lik*exp(-0.5*alpha*alpha/sigma2);
         return(lik);
      finish;

      /* used to calculate the posterior mean of pi */
      start posttoxf(alpha) global(j,DLT,doselevel,p);
         post=p[j]##exp(alpha)*posterior(alpha);
         return(post);
      finish;

      call quad(marginal, "posterior", {.M .P}) eps=1E-4 peak=-1
      scale=0.5;  /* default: PEAK=1 */
      pi={};
      do j=1 to ndose;
         call quad(pij,"posttoxf",{.M .P}) eps=1E-4 peak=-1 scale=0.5;
         pij=pij/marginal;
         pi=pi//pij;
      end;

      lb=log(log(&target)/log(p[1]));
```

```
      call quad(povertox,"posterior",-35||lb) eps=1E-4 peak=-1 scale=0.5;
      povertox=povertox/marginal;
      if povertox>&toxstop then stop=1;
      diff=abs(pi-&target);
      dosebest=diff[>:<];
      if dosebest>dosecurr then
         if dosecurr<ndose then do;
         dosenext=dosecurr+1;
      end;
      if dosebest<dosecurr then
         if dosecurr>1 then do;
         dosenext=dosecurr-1;
      end;

      if stop=1 then dosenext="The trial should be early terminated";
      *title "dose for next patient";
      print dosenext;

      doselevel=1:ndose;
      doselevel=doselevel`;
      create doselevel from doselevel[colname="doselevel"];
      append from doselevel;

      create pi from pi[colname="pi"];
      append from pi;
   quit;

   data &skeleton.;
      merge &skeleton. pi doselevel;
   run;

   *title "Skeleton Versus Estimated Toxicity Probability";
   proc sgplot data = skeleton;
      vline doselevel / response = p markers legendlabel='p'
markerattrs=(symbol=circlefilled size=10pt) lineattrs=(pattern = solid);
      vline doselevel / response = pi markers legendlabel='pi'
markerattrs=(symbol=trianglefilled size=10pt) lineattrs=(pattern = solid);
      yaxis min = 0 max = 1 label="Toxicity Probability";
      xaxis label="Dose Level";
      refline &target / axis=y label="Toxicity Target"
LABELLOC= INSIDE LABELPOS= min lineattrs=(pattern = shortdash);
      keylegend / location=inside noborder;
   run;
%mend TITECRM;

%TITECRM(currentdata,skeleton,'20Apr11',tau=90,target=0.3,toxstop=0.9);
```

The posterior estimate of the toxicity rate is presented in Figure 5.5 on page 158, and the dose level to be assigned to the new patient is level 2.

Figure 5.5 *Prespecified and Estimated Toxicity Probabilities in the TITE-CRM*

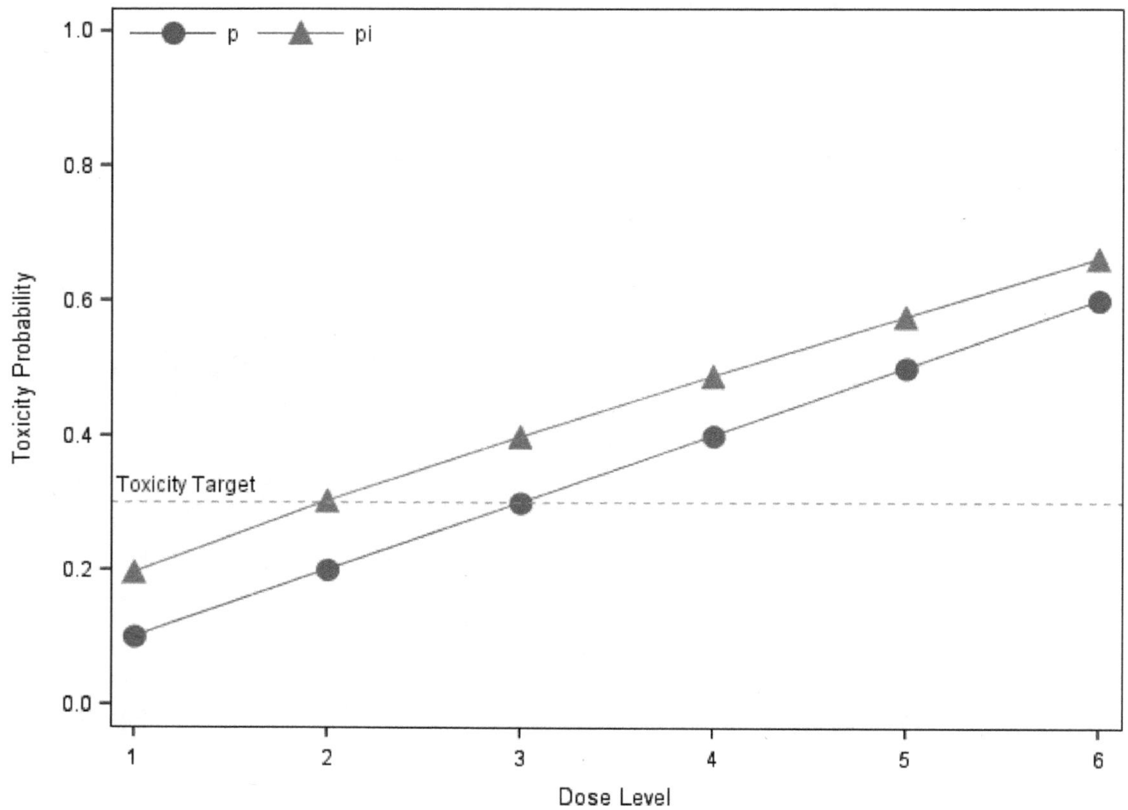

Based on an exposure-time weighting scheme, the weight function in the TITE-CRM may take various forms, among which the uniform weight is the most straightforward but needs justification. By contrast, the fractional CRM applies the Kaplan-Meier estimator to redistribute the censored data to the right [11]. As a result, the censored data can be fractionized to yield an outcome between 0 and 1, and thus, still make contributions to the likelihood. The **%TITECRM** macro is included in the supplemental material for the book from the companion website.

We conduct simulation studies to compare the performance of fCRM and TITE-CRM. The times to toxicity are simulated from Weibull distributions. The toxicity probability of each dose is set equal to the cumulative distribution function that is evaluated at the end of the follow-up time τ. Among all the DLTs that would occur in $(0, \tau)$, 70% of them are observed in $(\tau/2, \tau)$, the latter half of the assessment period. We take the sample size to be 36 patients and the skeleton as (0.1,0.2,0.3,0.4,0.5,0.6). Under each scenario, 1,000 trials are replicated. As shown in Table 5.8 on page 159 and Table 5.9 on page 160, the results from the fCRM and TITE-CRM are similar in terms of both the selection percentages of the MTDs and the number of patients treated at each dose. The fCRM pools all the data across different dose levels to estimate the Kaplan-Meier survival curve, because the data at each dose level are quite sparse. Similarly, the TITE-CRM uses the same weight function for different dose levels, which also does not take into account the dose information. Due to the sparsity of the data, it would be difficult to accommodate dose levels in the Kaplan-Meier estimator or the weight function via stratification. Macros **% fCRMSIM** and **%TITECRMSIM** generate the results for Table 5.8 and Table 5.9 and are included in the supplemental material for the book from the companion website. The location of the **kmsim.sas** file should be specified in the **%include** statement in the **% fCRMSIM** macro.

The simulation is performed with the **% fCRMsim** and **% TITECRMsim** macros. The input variables for the two macros are the same:

1. **skeleton** is the data set that includes the true toxicity rate and the skeleton.
2. **target** is the target toxicity rate.
3. **ncohort** is the total number of cohorts.
4. **cohortsize** is the cohort size.
5. **tau** is the length of the follow-up period for full evaluation of toxicity.
6. **a** is the length between the recruitment times of two adjacent cohorts.
7. **toxstop** is the threshold probability to early terminate the trial if the lowest dose level is too toxic.
8. **ntrial** is the number of trial replications.

As an example, Example Code 5.6 on page 159 generates the results for scenario 2 in Table 5.9; the output variables are the same as those in the **% CRMsim**.

Example Code 5.6 *Simulation of fCRM and TITE-CRM Designs*

```
data skeleton;
   input p ptrue;
   datalines;
   0.1 0.15
   0.2 0.30
   0.3 0.45
   0.4 0.55
   0.5 0.60
   0.6 0.70;
run;
%fCRMsim(skeleton,target=0.3,ncohort=12,tau=3,a=1,cohortsize=3,
toxstop=0.9,ntrial=1000);
%TITECRMsim(skeleton,target=0.3,ncohort=12,tau=3,a=1,cohortsize=3,
toxstop=0.9,ntrial=1000);
```

Table 5.8 *Scenario 1 of Simulation Study Comparing the fCRM and TITE-CRM*

Dose Level	**1**	**2**	**3**	**4**	**5**	**6**	**# DLT**	**% Stop**
P(Tox)	0.04	0.08	0.12	0.20	0.30	0.50		
fCRM	0	0.1	3.4	29.6	55.4	11.5		
# of Pts	3.3	3.7	5.1	8.7	9.5	5.7	8.5	0
TITE-CRM	0	0.1	3.5	30.9	53.9	11.6		
# of Pts	3.4	3.7	5.2	8.5	9.5	5.6	8.5	0

Table 5.9 Scenario 2 of Simulation Study Comparing the fCRM and TITE-CRM

Dose Level	1	2	3	4	5	6	# DLT	% Stop
P(Tox)	0.15	0.30	0.45	0.55	0.60	0.70		
fCRM	17.5	63.7	17.6	0.8	0.0	0.0		
# of Pts	10.4	14.5	7.9	2.7	0.4	0.0	11.3	0.4
TITE-CRM	18.6	62.9	16.4	0.8	0.0	0.0		
# of Pts	9.4	14.4	8.5	2.8	0.6	0.0	11.6	1.4

5.6 Summary

The continual reassessment method and its variations have been studied extensively and their performances are in general better than algorithm-based methods, such as the 3+3 design. All the cumulative data can be integrated and modeled for better decision making. In the Bayesian paradigm, more direct comparisons and early stopping rules can be implemented, which can help pin down the right dose faster.

References

1. O'Quigley J, Pepe M & Fisher L. (1990). Continual reassessment method: A practical design for phase 1 clinical trials in cancer. *Biometrics* 46: 33-48.
2. O'Quigley J & Shen LZ. (1996). Continual reassessment method: A likelihood approach. *Biometrics* 52: 673-684.
3. Yin G & Yuan Y. (2009). Bayesian model averaging continual reassessment method in phase I clinical trials. *Journal of the American Statistical Association* 104: 954-968.
4. Raftery AE, Madigan D & Hoeting JA. (1997). Bayesian model averaging for linear regression models. *Journal of the American Statistical Association* 92: 179-191.
5. Hoeting JA, Madigan D, Raftery AE & Volinsky CT. (1999). Bayesian model averaging: A tutorial. *Statistical Science* 14: 382-401.
6. Spiegelhalter DJ, Best NG, Carlin BP & Van Der Linde A. (2002). Bayesian measures of model complexity and fit. *Journal of the Royal Statistical Society: Series B (Statistical Methodology)* 64: 583-639.
7. Desai SP, Ben-Josef E, Normolle DP, Francis IR, Greenson JK, Simeone DM, Chang AE, Colletti LM, Lawrence TS & Zalupski MM. (2007). Phase I study of oxaliplatin, full-dose gemcitabine, and concurrent radiation therapy in pancreatic cancer. *Journal of Clinical Oncology* 25: 4587–4592.
8. Kaplan EL & Meier P. (1958). Nonparametric estimation from incomplete observations. *Journal of the American Statistical Association* 53: 457-481.

9. Yin G, Zheng S & Xu J. (2013). Fractional dose-finding methods with late-onset toxicity in phase I clinical trials. *Journal of Biopharmaceutical Statistics* 23: 856-870.

10. Efron B. (1967). The two-sample problem with censored data. In: Le Cam L & Neyman J, eds. *Proceedings, Fifth Berkeley Symposium in Mathematical Statistics, Volume IV*. New York: Prentice Hall, 831-853.

11. Portnoy S. (2003). Censored regression quantiles. *Journal of the American Statistical Association* 98:1001-1012.

12. Cheung YK & Chappell R. (2000). Sequential designs for phase I clinical trials with late-onset toxicities. *Biometrics* 56: 1177-1182.

Authors

Guosheng Yin, Professor, Department of Statistics and Actuarial Science, The University of Hong Kong, Hong Kong, China.

Ruitao Lin, Ph.D. Candidate, Department of Statistics and Actuarial Science, The University of Hong Kong, Hong Kong, China.

Chapter 6
Classical Dose-Response Study

6.1 Introduction

In the drug development process, a candidate compound needs to go through a stringent series of testing for toxicity, pharmacokinetics/pharmacodynamics, efficacy, and safety before it can be released to the market for patient use. The process involves different phases of nonclinical studies on animals and clinical studies in healthy volunteers and in the targeted patient population with the disease [1, 2]. Clinical studies can be categorized into 4 phases (phase I-IV), corresponding to four levels of stage-gate drug development: human pharmacology, therapeutic exploratory, therapeutic confirmatory, and therapeutic use studies [3]. Phases I and II are generally considered exploratory and learning phases. The goal of phase III studies is mainly for therapeutic confirmation. Phase IV trials are post marketing studies. Because phase III pivotal studies are typically large scale and so very high cost (the cost in some of phase III studies could be even more than the total cost spent from the very beginning of a compound to the end of phase II studies), phase II studies are one of the most critical components before entering into the phase III confirmatory stage. In addition, regulatory agencies generally recommend that a full dose range of the test therapy has been explored prior to initiating phase III and that identification of minimum effective dose (MinED) be encouraged [4]. Given the substantial resources invested in phase III and beyond, a well-designed phase II study could be very beneficial to both patients and sponsors and, consequently, reduce the time to market launch and/or increase the probability of success.

This chapter describes the general consideration in a classical dose response study, and demonstrates two simulated examples for the analysis of such data using the E_{max} model approach in SAS.

6.2 Statistical Design Considerations in a Classical Dose-Response Study

6.2.1 Dose-Response Relationship

In most cases, phase II features a learning period when the patient population may be first exposed to the test therapy for evidence of clinical benefit and risk; it is also a period to explore and recommend alternative doses to be tested in the later phase (e.g., phase III) confirmatory clinical trials. In the development of a first-in-class new chemical entity, the first phase IIa study is referred to as a proof-of-concept (PoC) study followed by phase IIb study called dose-ranging studies. A PoC study is often faster and cheaper because it only requires a well-tolerated dose of test therapy plus a control group (e.g., placebo), as appropriate. A dose-ranging study, however, needs multiple doses of the test therapy to characterize the dose-response relationship. Therefore, a classical phase II development program usually consists of a small-scale PoC trial followed by moderately sized dose-ranging studies.

Dose ranging studies are too often designed with a very small number of doses [5]. A dose ranging trial typically includes a placebo (representing zero dose), and several doses of the test product. One very common design is a four-group study with placebo, low dose, medium dose, and high dose groups of the drug candidate under development. When designing a dose ranging study, it is important to keep the following questions in mind to achieve the study objective:

1. What dose-range should be considered in the study?
2. Was the concept proven?
3. How do you space the test dosages from the placebo to the maximum tolerated dose (MTD)?
4. How many treatment arms or dosage levels should be included?
5. What are the total sample size and allocation schedule?

Conceptually, the efficacy of a drug increases as the dose increases (Figure 6.1). The left curve plotted in Figure 6.1 on page 165 can be viewed as an efficacy–response curve; that is, the response (y-axis) represents some measure of the drug efficacy. In addition to efficacy response, there are also toxicity dose–response curves. We will assume, as shown in Figure 6.1, when the dose increases, both efficacy and toxicity increase. Based on these curves, the maximum tolerated dose (MTD) can be defined. The MTD is the maximal dose acceptably tolerated by a particular patient population.

Figure 6.1 *Possible Efficacy and Toxicity Dose-Response Curves*

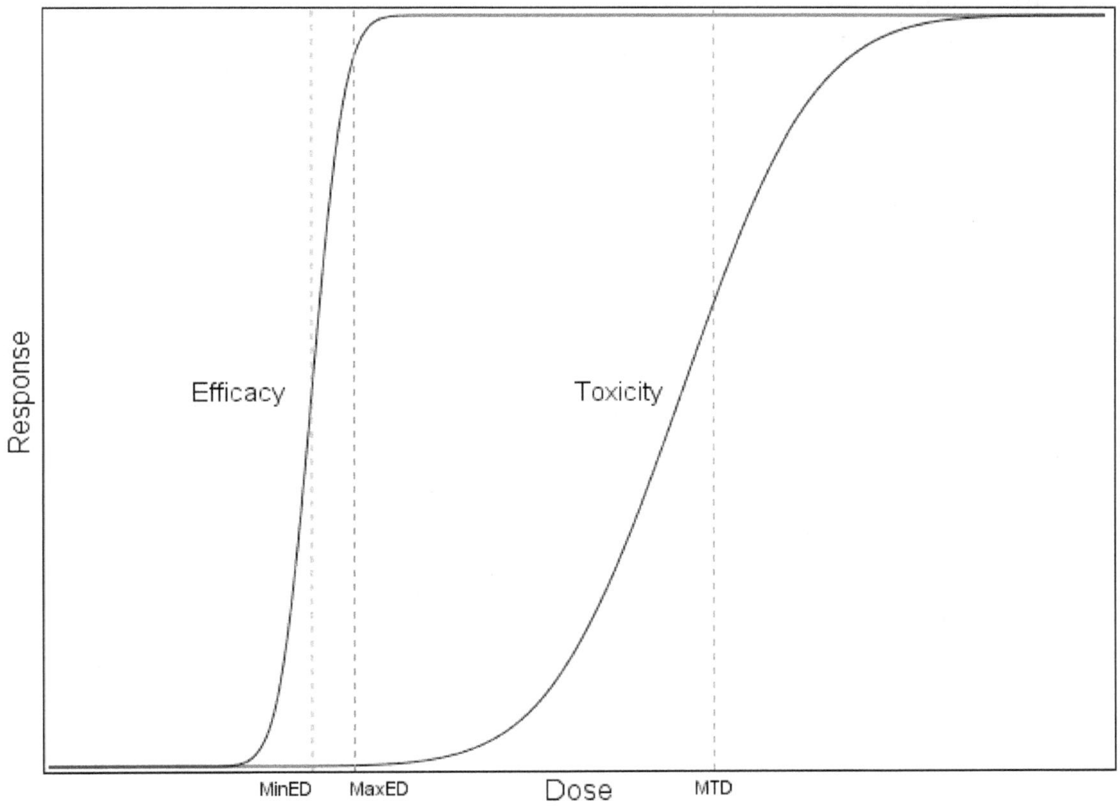

With certain products, the efficacy curve and the toxicity curve are widely separated. When this is the case, there is a wide range of doses for patients to take. In other cases, the two curves may be very close to each other and physicians have to dose patients very carefully so that while benefiting from the efficacy, patients do not have to be exposed to potential toxicity from the drug. This can be quantified by a so called therapeutic index (TI). The TI (also referred to as therapeutic window or safety window or sometimes as therapeutic ratio) is a comparison of the amount of a therapeutic agent that causes the therapeutic effect to the amount that causes toxicity [6]. Clearly, a drug with a wide therapeutic window (or a high TI) is preferred. If a drug has a narrow therapeutic window, then the drug will need to be developed even more carefully, and physicians will prescribe the drug with caution.

Oftentimes, products developed for life-threatening diseases (e.g., cancer) tend to have narrow therapeutic windows. On the other hand, drugs developed to treat chronic diseases (e.g., high blood pressure, depression, high cholesterol, or arthritis) are required to have wide therapeutic windows because these drugs are frequently used in older patients, or patients with other concurrent diseases, and sometimes used in children.

In clinical development, phase III trials are designed to confirm product efficacy. Results obtained from phase III studies provide evidence to help regulatory agencies make decisions on whether to approve a product, while the phase III program engaged significant resources. Therefore, it is critical that dose-ranging trials from phase II deliver the information to help with phase III design. In other words, if the appropriate dose or doses for product registration is not included in phase III trials, it is very likely that the product candidate will miss the opportunity of being approved for market authorization according to plan. Hence, information obtained from dose-ranging trials needs to provide sufficient support for dose selection in phase III study designs.

6.2.2 Finding the Minimum Effective Dose

ICH E4 defines the minimum effective dose (MinED) as the "smallest dose with a discernible useful effect" [4]. Finding the MinED is an important step in drug development. To illustrate, let's consider the following reported example. In a clinical development program for a test drug to treat osteoarthritis [7], the first dose-response study included a placebo, 80 mg, 120 mg, and 160 mg of the test drug. Results from this study indicate that all three doses are efficacious (the left panel of Figure 6.2 on page 167). These results also show that 80 mg may have already been at the high side of the dose-response curve. A second study was designed to explore the 40 mg dose, and results from this second study are given in the middle panel of Figure 6.2. With these findings, the project team started phase III studies using a dose of 120 mg to confirm the long-term efficacy of this drug.

An end-of-phase II meeting with the Food and Drug Administration (FDA) was held after the long-term phase III study started. The FDA commented that the minimum effective dose (MinED) was not found yet. The main issue here is that the efficacy response does not change as the dose level changes and all the three testing doses almost equally reach the full efficacy effect, so the dose-response relationship was not detected. Hence, the project team designed a third dose-response study to explore the lower dose range. Doses included in the third study are 2.5 mg, 10 mg, and 40 mg. As shown in the right panel of Figure 6.2 on page 167, the third study successfully established the dose-response relationship, i.e., the response increases as dose increases. Based on these results, it is clear that the phase III studies are designed with a dose being too high. The impact of this process can cause a major delay in the development program and considerable waste of resources.

Figure 6.2 *Dose-Response Results from the Three Studies of an Osteoarthritis Drug*

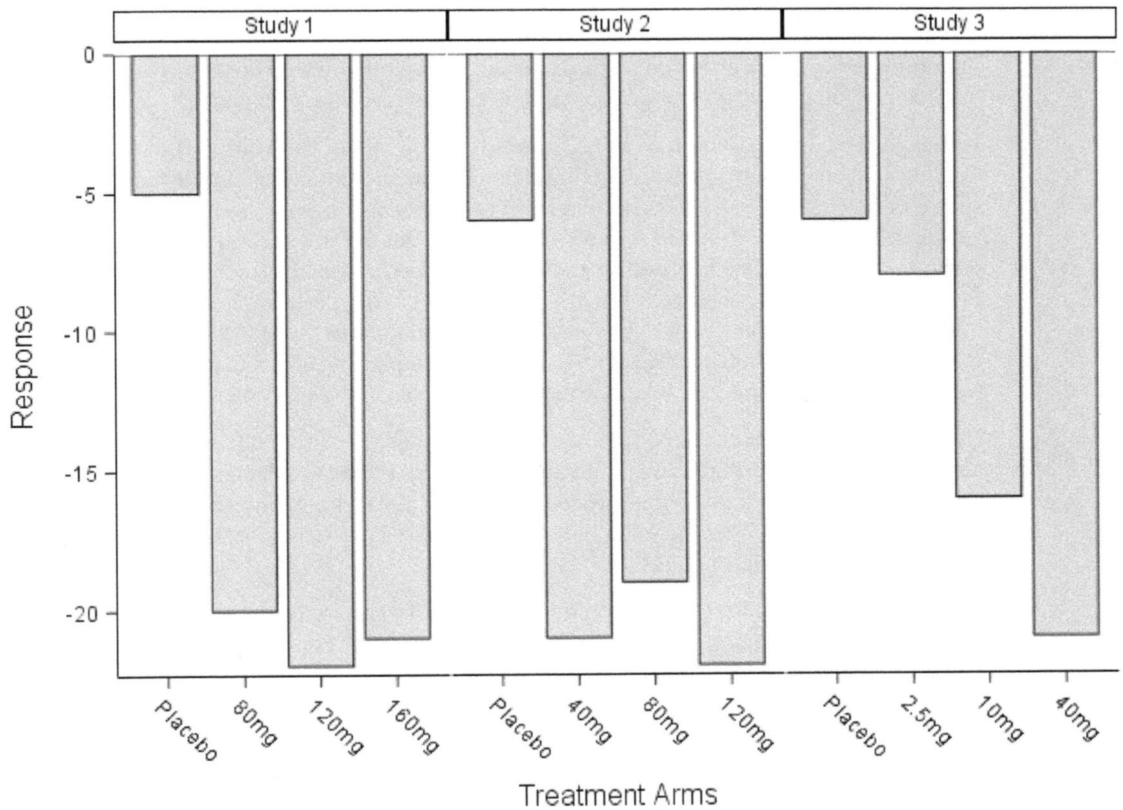

Therefore, the MinED is a very important concept in product development. Unfortunately, there is not a universally accepted definition of this term [8]. Finding MinED is critical because it is generally believed that toxicity increases as dose increases. Hence, a lower dose that is effective implies that it could be safer than higher doses.

Clinical results obtained from phase III studies are used to obtain an investigational product marketing authorization. Based on these data, if a dose is efficacious and safe, then that dose can be approved, and the product label specifies the dose or the range of doses that the product is approved for. However, after approval and broader use, if excessive adverse events are observed that impact the benefit-risk balance for patients, then a question as to whether the approved dose is low enough could be raised. At this time, it would be very challenging to ask what the MinED is for this product. Therefore, it is critical to find MinED in phase II, before it is too late.

Drug price in the US is not directly associated with dosage. However, in many other countries, the price of a medicinal product is linked to its dose. In other words, if the dose of the product is higher, then it is more expensive. Now suppose that a certain product is approved in such a country, and the price is set based on the lowest approved dose. If later it was detected that the MinED for the product is in fact, lower than the approved dose, then a dose reduction is needed at a post-market stage. Accordingly, the price of this product has to be lowered further. When this happens, there is a huge impact on the earnings of such a product. Therefore, from a marketing strategy point of view, it would be critical to identify the MinED before the product enters its phase III development.

Finding the MinED is a phase II practice. As discussed above, if the MinED was not identified at phase II, it would be very difficult and expensive to find the MinED at a later stage of product development. In fact, phase II could be the only opportunity to characterize the relationship between doses and product efficacy. Therefore, it is very important to pay more attention to phase II, and to carefully design dose-ranging clinical trials during this critical phase of clinical development for a new product.

Although there is a definition of MinED from ICH E4, in that the MinED is the "smallest dose with a discernible useful effect," the interpretation and implementation of such a definition varies a lot in practice [4]. The first question is the understanding of a "useful effect." It is difficult to achieve consensus about the smallest magnitude of an effect that is useful. One approach is to follow a well-established treatment effect such as lowering 5 mmHg of blood pressure in developing an antihypertensive drug. Another is to consider the concept of minimally clinically important difference (MCID). This is the magnitude of the treatment effect above and beyond a placebo effect that is large enough to be perceived by a subject. It is a commonly used concept in outcomes research.

However, the implementation of a discernible effect could be more difficult. Various authors recommend different ways of calling a dose as MinED based on the difference in treatment effect from a given dose as compared with a placebo. Some authors suggest the use of a dose-response model to help estimate MinED [9,10]. Others suggest the use of pairwise comparisons [11,12].

Even among those authors who recommend the use of pairwise comparisons to find MinED, there could be many differences in implementation. For example, some may argue that a multiple comparison adjustment could be necessary, and some may not. Whether adjustment for multiple comparisons is needed or not, the understanding of "a dose that delivers treatment effect which is different from placebo" could still vary a lot, depending on an individual's point of view. For example, let the useful effect defined above be denoted as δ, then for a given dose, a point estimate and a confidence interval can be constructed for δ. Suppose a positive value indicates a benefit effect, then the treatment response of the given dose of the test product subtracts the placebo response, which is expected to be positive. Hence, it is hoped that the point estimate of the treatment difference could be as much as δ. This leaves a wide range of interpretations – for MinED, should that dose be such that the point estimate is greater than δ? Should that dose be such that the lower confidence limit to be greater than 0? Should that dose be such that the upper confidence limit is greater than δ?

The implementation of this concept of the "smallest dose with a discernible useful effect" could be very difficult, depending on the various interpretations of this definition. However, in practice, one feasible way of finding the MinED in a dose-ranging clinical trial is to find a dose that is lower than MinED. Regardless of which practical definition the project team uses to identify the MinED, if there is a dose deemed to be not efficacious, and there is a higher dose that is efficacious, then it can be considered that the non-efficacious dose is below the MinED, and the efficacious dose is above the MinED. From a practical point of view, this information would usually be sufficient to help the team to design phase III clinical trials.

Of course in the selection of phase III doses, many other aspects will also have to be included in consideration; e.g., safety or toxicity findings, pharmacokinetic properties, formulations, etc. The information about MinED would be one of the most critical deliverables from phase II in supporting any phase III development plans.

6.2.3 Determining the Dose Range to Study

In non-adaptive design practice, usually the first dose ranging study covers a wide dose range, and then the next dose ranging study will be designed with a narrower dose range, filtering out the target doses to be assessed in phase III. Dose range in a clinical trial design is defined as the ratio of the highest dose divided by the lowest dose included in the design. For example, if the doses in trial A are a placebo, 20 mg, 40 mg, and 80 mg, then the dose range is 4 (= 80/20). If the doses in trial B are a placebo, 0.1 mg, 1 mg and 10 mg, then the dose range is 100 (= 10/0.1). Although the doses used in trial A are higher than doses used in trial B, in fact trial B has a much wider dose range – 25 times wider than trial A. It is critical to cover a wide dose range in the first dose ranging study. Inappropriate selection of dose range may result in a potential waste of study costs and resources and delay the time to market launch.

The key lesson learned from the above particular development program is that a very low dose was not explored in early phase II. In other words, if a dose at or below 10 mg was explored in the first study, a narrower dose range could have been established using the second study. Then the phase III studies could be designed with the appropriate dose range.

In general, the most difficult challenge in designing the first dose ranging trial in developing a new intervention is the selection of doses to be included. Generally, the study is designed with two very important assumptions:

1. The MTD was correctly estimated from earlier trials
2. Efficacy response is monotonic to ascending doses.

However, it is unclear what range of doses the efficacy activities would be in. At this stage, the best guidance available is the data obtained from pre-clinical experiments or from phase I using biomarkers. Even under the assumptions that the MTD was correctly estimated, and there is a monotonic efficacy dose-response relationship, there can still be many possible shapes of dose-response curves.

Figure 6.3 on page 170 presents an example of three dose-response curves. Dose-response curve 1 is based on the rabbit response models, curve 2 is based on mouse models, and curve 3 is from the dog models. The vertical dashed grey line (at the right side of Figure 6.3) represents the maximum tolerated dose (MTD). The primary challenge at this stage then becomes, what range of doses should be considered in the upcoming dose ranging clinical trial? From this perspective, the primary challenge in the dose ranging trial design is to consider which range of doses needs to be studied.

Figure 6.3 *Several Possible Dose-Response Curves*

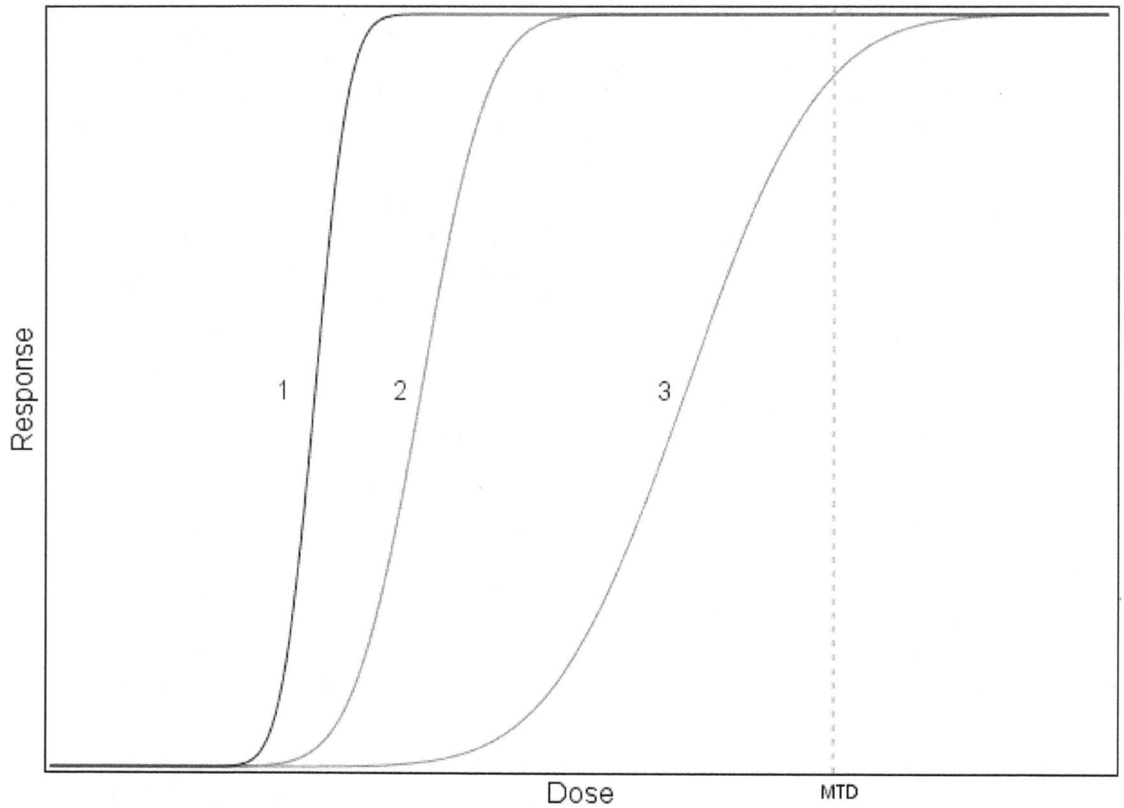

Given the discussion in the previous sections about MinED, it is critical to realize that in the first dose-ranging design, a wide dose range needs to be studied. The high dose is typically set at MTD or a dose below MTD to avoid any unacceptable toxicity. The real design challenge is to choose the lowest dose for this dose-ranging trial. If there is an interest in identifying a dose that is below MinED, then the difficult question would be "how low would be low enough?" Once the low dose is selected for the design, a dose range can be calculated as the ratio of the highest dose divided by the lowest dose.

6.2.4 Was the Concept Proven?

Sometimes it is desirable to combine the PoC and the dose-ranging studies into one single study with clearly defined objectives, hypotheses, and decision criteria. The advantage of such a design is to first make a "Go/No Go" decision based on PoC. If the decision is "Go", then the same study would sequentially provide dose-ranging information to identify the dose that could achieve the target treatment effect and help design the next study. When well designed and analyzed, the combined study saves development time by providing a range of efficacious doses going forward. The disadvantage is that more investment is at risk before the concept is proven.

Since a simple PoC is examined under a single hypothesis test, there is not much discussion about PoC study design with regard to statistical design principles. In contrast, there are a variety of design and analysis strategies for dose-ranging trials. There exist three major categories of dose ranging methods: multiple comparison procedures (MCP); modeling approaches; and MCP-Mod, which combines the first two [13,14].

The MCP method takes dose as a discrete factor and generally makes few assumptions about the underlying dose-response relationship. When there is no assumed ordering imposed on the testing of multiple doses, multiplicity adjustment is necessary to protect the family-wise-error rate (FWER). Popular procedures such as the Bonferroni, Dunnett, Holm and Hochberg require α splitting, which results in an increased sample size. The modeling approach treats dose as a continuous variable and assumes a functional relationship between the response and the dose. Sometimes the multiplicity issue is avoided as a result of the assumed functional relationship (e.g., non-decreasing dose-response relationship). The problem is that potential bias can be caused by model misspecification. A third approach, the MCP-Mod, addresses this issue by first selecting the dose-response model using MCP to protect the FWER; then the selected model is used to estimate the dose-response relationship. This approach is flexible in the sense of model selection; however, it pays the price of α split at the model selection step.

6.2.5 How to Space the Test Dosages

Hamlett et al. proposed to use a binary dose spacing (BDS) for dose allocation, since this method of dose allocation is based on dividing dose intervals into halves [15]. Over the years, BDS has been applied successfully in many dose ranging designs [12,16]. In order to determine the doses using the BDS approach, it is assumed that the MTD is T, thus the design space is $[0, T]$. Without loss of generality, T can be taken as 1. It is assumed that the dose-response relationship is monotonic. It is further assumed that the number of dose groups is known. Given this setting, doses are chosen from the interval [0,1]. Suppose we want a design with three treatment groups, including a placebo, a low dose and a high dose. The placebo dose is taken to be zero. The challenge then is to select a low dose and a high dose, keeping in mind that we may not want a high dose too close to 1 (the assumed MTD). An intuitive approach might be to split this interval into half, giving the two intervals $[0, 1/2]$ and $(1/2, 1]$ and select a dose in each of these intervals. A natural choice is to select the midpoint of each interval (split each interval in half), giving the test doses, $x_1 = 1/2^2 = 1/4$ and $x_2 = 3/2^2 = 3/4$. Note that if we choose doses in the upper end (greater than 1/2 and approaching 1) then these doses tend to be toxic and are generally not of primary interest in the dose-selection process. On the other hand, activities of the lower doses are very important information for drug development. Hence, the basic idea for BDS is to search for the lower end of the dose range.

In another case, suppose we want to consider a design with four treatment groups including a placebo, low, medium and high doses. In order to avoid selecting too high a dose, which can be toxic, we may want to keep $3/2^2$ as the high dose; that is, leave the interval $(1/2, 1]$ unchanged. Since we want to use of some low doses to help identify the MinED, we can divide the lower interval $[0, 1/2]$ in half, giving the new intervals $\left[0, 1/2^2\right]$ and $\left[1/2^2, 1/2\right]$. We select the midpoints of these two intervals and split the two intervals into halves – giving the three test doses $x_1 = 1/2^3$, $x_2 = 3/2^3$ and $x_3 = 3/2^2$. We continue in this fashion by splitting the lower interval into half and taking the midpoint of each interval, until all the doses are allocated. In general, let there be m test doses in addition to a placebo, then the test doses are given by $x_1 = 1/2^m$, $x_2 = 3/2^m$, $x_3 = 3/2^{m-1}$, $x_4 = 3/2^{m-2}$, … , $x_m = 3/2^2$.

Other ways of subdividing are also possible. Instead of splitting the initial interval into $[0, T/2]$ and $(T/2, T]$, we may use a $1/p$ cut – $[0, T/p]$ and $(T/p, T]$ – where $p \geq 2$ and then repeat the procedure described above. The BDS design is nonparametric because it does not depend on any underlying models other than the two assumptions: knowledge of MTD and a non-decreasing dose-response relationship. It provides a way to identify doses that are below the MTD and a means to potentially estimate the MinED.

In addition to BDS, other algorithms could be useful, e.g., log-dose spacing, the Fibonacci series, and the modified Fibonacci series approach can also be considered [17,18]. However, it is important to note that most of these methods propose dose spacing from lower doses to higher doses. In practice, dose spacing should be considered starting with the MTD, and move down to lower doses. Hence, when applying any of these algorithms, the dose allocation would be reversed (from high to low, instead of from low to high).

6.2.6 Number of Doses and Control Groups

As discussed in the previous sections, a wide dose range is critical in phase II dose ranging studies. Once the MTD is estimated from phase I and a wide dose range is considered, the natural questions to think about could be how many doses should be included in the study, whether a placebo control group is sufficient, or whether an active control group is also needed.

A single test dose plus a placebo arm design may be able to demonstrate the proof-of-concept, but cannot, by essence, characterize the dose-response relationship. Any attempt to interpolate a dose-response relationship between the placebo and the test dose would require very strong assumptions, which oftentimes are not realistic. Therefore, a dose-ranging study typically needs several test dose levels. One very commonly used design is a four-group study with a placebo, low dose, medium dose and high dose groups of the drug candidate under development. Some authors suggest that more doses could help; that is, in the first dose-ranging study, adding more doses to the study design [19]. However, the number of doses to be used might be limited by practical and logistical considerations (e.g., available formulations of test doses, dosing frequencies, convenience for outpatients to use on their own or blinding complexity, etc.). Given these many treatment groups already included in a study, it may not be practical to add very many test doses into the same study.

In an early phase II dose-ranging trial design, typically the total sample size is limited depending on budget, availability of patients, and difficulty in recruitment. Under this circumstance, more treatment groups in a design imply fewer patients per treatment group. A smaller sample size of each treatment group provides a less precise estimate of treatment effect. Hence, blindly adding dose groups to a study design does not necessarily make the design more likely to deliver more informative results. A well-thought-out design strategy is needed before the number of dose groups can be determined.

In our opinion, for the first dose-ranging study design, it is more important to cover a wide dose range, rather than simply adding more doses to a narrow range of doses. This is both practical, and scientifically sound. In practice, a trial with 4 to 5 test doses, plus a placebo control will deliver a good understanding of where the test medication is most active, if the dose range is wide enough, and if the dose spacing is reasonable. Some simulation studies suggest that among the number of treatment arms (4, 5, 6, or 7, placebo arm included), three test doses (the 4-arm design) could be insufficient in some cases because it significantly limits the space of potentially relevant models to fit to the data with clear potential impact on the ability to identify the optimal dose [16]. The performance increases when more than three doses are studied. On the other hand, six test doses (the 7-arm design) may not necessarily deliver better results than the four or five test doses (the 5-arm or 6-arm design) comparisons. When the total sample size is fixed, the 7-arm design offers a smaller sample size per group when an equal total sample size is used, and the precision would be sacrificed. It may also be a good idea to consider an unbalanced sample-size allocation, e.g., allocate more subjects to the extreme doses (i.e., higher dose(s) and a placebo arm).

Consequently, a dose ranging design including four to five test doses (in addition to a placebo) and covering a wide dose range provides a very useful and pragmatic basis in designing the dose ranging clinical trial [20].

6.2.7 Sample Size Considerations

6.2.7.1 Statistical Hypothesis for Determining PoC

Whenever sample size calculation is needed for a given study, the first point is to understand the hypothesis to be tested. In the process of designing a phase II dose ranging program, the initial statistical hypothesis is typically a proof of concept hypothesis. In the case when the study is designed with only two treatment groups – a placebo group is compared to the MTD of study product - the hypothesis can be expressed in a straight-forward fashion by comparing the response from the test treatment against the response from the placebo. If the comparison is based on means, then the hypothesis can be written as

$$H_0: \mu_T = \mu_P \text{ vs. } H_1: \mu_T > \mu_P$$

where μ_T is the test treatment group mean, and μ_P is the placebo treatment group mean. In other words, if the mean responses from the test treatment group are statistically significantly different from the mean responses from the placebo group, then the concept is considered proven.

However, in a dose-ranging trial design including more than two treatment groups, the PoC hypothesis is not necessarily straightforward. This is because it might not be the most efficient to just test the general hypothesis that at least one group is different than the others, but rather use a contrast as the primary objective. A typical dose-ranging design consists of the highest dose of the test product (could be the MTD) on the upper end, and it consists of the placebo representing the zero dose group. Ideally, such a design includes three or four different doses in between these two groups. Under this scenario, two possible contrast options could be considered in specifying the PoC hypothesis. One option is to use the contrast comparing two doses, keeping the hypothesis the same as that in the two-group setting – only test the highest dose (may be MTD) against a placebo, as expressed in the hypothesis above. Another option is to use a contrast that includes more than two treatment groups in order to perform the PoC hypothesis test. If the second option is selected, then there could be many varieties in writing such a contrast.

For example, in a four-group design with a placebo, low dose, medium dose and high dose, the PoC can only be based on the high dose versus a placebo (let μ_L be the mean response of low dose, μ_M be the mean response for the medium dose, and μ_H be the mean response of high dose):

$$H_0: \mu_H = \mu_P \text{ vs. } H_1: \mu_H > \mu_P.$$

Or, the contrast can be a trend test, which is based on all doses [12,16], assuming a monotonic dose-response relationship and equally spaced doses:

$$H_0: -3\mu_P - \mu_L + \mu_M + 3\mu_H = 0 \text{ vs. } H_1: -3\mu_P - \mu_L + \mu_M + 3\mu_H > 0.$$

Another possible PoC contrast may also include equal weight to each dose (i.e., testing the weighted sum of the three doses versus a placebo):

$$H_0: -3\mu_P + \mu_L + \mu_M + \mu_H = 0 \text{ vs. } H_1: -3\mu_P + \mu_L + \mu_M + \mu_H > 0.$$

Assuming only the high dose is effective (i.e., testing the highest dose versus the weighted sum of the other three groups):

$$H_0: -\mu_P - \mu_L - \mu_M + 3\mu_H = 0 \text{ vs. } H_1: -\mu_P - \mu_L - \mu_M + 3\mu_H > 0.$$

As can be found from the above examples, if a contrast (that includes more than two treatment groups) is used for the PoC hypothesis, then there could be many possible ways of writing such a contrast, but it is really important that the project team reflect on choosing the most meaningful one for the particular compound and therapeutic area.

In data analysis of dose-ranging studies, a modeling approach, or MCP-Mod method could also be used [13]. In these settings, there could be a parameter of interest – e.g., for a linear model, the parameter could be the slope, for an $E_{\max}$ model, the parameter could be $E_{\max}$. In these situations, sample sizes could be calculated using simulations, or using `proc power`. However, from a study design point of view, sample size may also be calculated using a PoC hypothesis. Again, this PoC can be based only on the highest dose against a placebo, or based on a contrast that includes more than just two treatment groups. Of course, if the interest is to write a contrast that reflects the underlying model, more variety of contrasts can be considered.

6.2.7.2 Selecting a Treatment Difference from a Placebo

The concept of identifying the MCID is necessary in designing dose-ranging clinical trials. Although, in practice, it is sometimes difficult to objectively establish a widely accepted MCID, it is critical to use a treatment difference (δ) as the target when calculating sample sizes for a clinical trial. In other words, without δ, sample size cannot be calculated. Hence, if there is a MCID for a given indication, it will be very helpful in clinical development of new products.

Typically in phase III clinical trials, the treatment differences used for trial design are mainly based on those observed from earlier studies from this product. But in early phase II, such a δ is not easily obtained. In general, there are three ways used in practice to obtain a δ for designing an early phase II clinical trial. One very popular way is to use data from other products. Especially when there are products already approved for general patient population use. In the US, after a product is approved, the Food and Drug Administration (FDA) publishes a summary basis for approval (SBA) for the product. In Europe, the European Medicinal Agency (EMA) publishes European Public Assessment Report (EPAR) to explain why a product is approved for public use. Typically, the treatment difference can be observed from either SBA or EPAR. In some situations, information on treatment difference of other products can be found from publications, product labels or a registries website, such as clinicaltrial.gov. Therefore, by using observed treatment differences from other products, a δ could be selected to help the design of this new study.

A second way of selecting a treatment difference is by evaluating earlier data observed from the products under development. Project team members use pre-clinical data, PK data, biomarkers, or other data obtained from this product and then propose a reasonable δ such that it is likely that the product candidate will be able to deliver. Usually, a δ obtained either from using other products (based on publications, labels, SBA or EPAR) or from the product itself, there could be long discussions among team members. The main reason is that in the early development phase, there is no direct efficacy data to support a clinical benefit of this candidate.

A third way to choose δ is to identify a value such that the sample size calculated using this δ is feasible. Typically, in the early phase of clinical development, the team does not have very strong confidence that the test product will be efficacious and safe. Hence, the investment, being a high risk, tends to be limited. The total number of patients to recruit would have to not exceed a certain number. On this basis, a δ can be inversely calculated using the number of patients and the pre-specified type I (α) and type II (β) errors. The mathematical formula used for sample size calculation indicates that the number of patients needed for the study is inversely related to the pre-specified δ. If the budget is limited, and hence the sample size is small, that implies a large δ will be necessary to have a reasonable likelihood to detect a treatment effect. The author understands that this may be happening in practice, but does not recommend this approach for informative decision making. When designing such early efficacy trial with a feasible sample size (which is not very large, indicating a greater δ is used or a higher α or a higher β in sample size calculation), the most important thing is to set-up Go/NoGo decision criteria prior to data access and data analysis, and understanding the risks that are associated to it (i.e., risk to stop a promising drug and risk to carry forward an ineffective drug).

6.2.7.3 Choice of Type I and Type II Errors

In clinical development of new products, it is well known that α is the probability of making a type I error; i.e., the probability of developing a placebo. β is the probability of making a type II error, or the probability of stopping development of a potentially good product. In most phase III development programs, Authorities generally expect the α to be set at a two-sided 0.05 (or one-sided at 0.025). In phase III, α can be thought of as a regulatory risk because it represents the risk of approving a product without sufficient efficacy for use in the targeted patient population, but could cause adverse events or other safety concerns. On the other hand, β can be thought of as the sponsor's risk because if a potentially good product was stopped for further development due to a wrong decision, then the sponsor's investment on this candidate would have been wasted. For this reason, regulatory agencies do not strictly require any particular β to be used in any phase of the clinical studies. Hence, the choice of β is usually left for the sponsor to determine. Usually in phase III, sponsors tend to choose a smaller β (or a higher power) for study designs so that a larger sample size will increase the likelihood of meeting the decision criteria with more accurate estimates (i.e., narrower confidence interval around the estimates).

However, the choice of α or β in phase II trial designs can be flexible. The two main reasons are: (i) decisions after a phase II clinical trial is primarily a sponsor decision rather than a regulatory decision and, hence, the sponsor gets to select the level of risks that they are willing to take; (ii) there is insufficient evidence at phase II for the sponsor to commit a huge amount of investment. Accordingly, the sponsor might accept higher risks (i.e., the α or β being larger) and contain the level of investment directly associated to the maximum sample size.

When designing a phase II study, if the δ has been determined, and the sample size is limited, then the only choice left with the project team would be whether to take a larger risk of making a type I error or a larger risk of making a type II error. This choice is critical because a discussion about probability of making a wrong decision should take place at the design stage, not after the study is unblinded and results are ready. From a frequentist point of view, the probability of observing a head or a tail of a coin toss can only be contemplated before the coin has landed. After the coin has landed, the observation is either a head, or a tail. There would be no probability associated with it. In clinical trials, the coin has landed when the blind is broken. At that time, clinical data are ready for statistical analysis, and statistics used to assess the Go/No Go criteria can be calculated (e.g., p-value, observed statistics, lower or upper limit of confidence interval). It is important to understand that such a Go/No Go statistic (e.g., p-value, confidence interval) is an observed statistic with the data in hand, and there is no uncertainty associated with it. The underlying truth – whether the test product is in fact efficacious or not – is still unknown. However, a Go or No Go decision will have to be made. What can be concluded at this stage is, using for instance the p-value, that if the observed p-value is small (less than α), and a Go decision is made, then the probability of making a type I error under such a decision is controlled at a level less than α. If an observed p-value is large (p greater than α) and a No Go decision is made, then the probability of making a type II error is smaller than β.

In phase III, the selection of β reflects the level of commitment of moving the candidate product forward (a smaller β implies a stronger commitment). It also represents the degree of investment that the sponsor is willing to spend. However, in phase II, the choice of β may need to be balanced with a choice of α. In most of situations, β is set at a higher level than α. For example, a typical α may be 0.05, while a β is set at 0.2 (indicating 80% power). This does not necessarily have to be the case in all phase II designs. In practice, phase II studies are designed with an α of 0.025, 0.05, 0.1, or sometimes a one-sided value of 0.15. A β value of greater than 0.2 is rare. But β values of 0.15, 0.1 or 0.05 are not uncommon. The project team must discuss and agree with the level of risk that the team is willing to take – either to give up a good product, or to develop a placebo. It is very important to note that these discussions should take place at the study design stage because after seeing the study results, the coin has landed, and it would be too late to discuss probabilities or risks.

6.2.7.4 Sample Size Calculation

Once the statistical hypothesis, the clinical difference, and the corresponding α and β have been determined, sample size for a given dose ranging trial can be calculated. Based on the above discussion, the sample size of a dose-ranging study can be calculated using the formula below [21]:

$$n = \left[\frac{\left(z_{1-\alpha} + z_{1-\beta}\right)\sigma}{\delta}\right]^2 \sum_{i=0}^{k} \frac{c_i^2}{f_i}$$

where

1. n is the total sample size of all treatment groups combined

2. $z_{1-\alpha}$ and $z_{1-\beta}$ are the critical values of the standard normal distribution corresponding to type I and type II error, respectively

3. δ is the weighted sum of the effect based on all doses

4. σ is the standard deviation

5. f_i is the fraction of number of patients in treatment group

6. c_i is the contrast coefficient that is associated with treatment group

7. k is the number of dose groups, plus placebo, where placebo is denoted as the 0 dose group.

In the calculation of sample sizes for a dose-ranging study, two popular types of patient allocation are possible – balanced allocation where each treatment group receives an equal number of patients, or imbalanced allocation where the highest dose and the placebo groups receive more patients, and other dose groups receive fewer patients per group. The sample size formula above works well with either type of patient allocation. Examples of these types of allocation can be found in [20]. The above formula applies to cases where the primary endpoint is a continuous variable. In fact, a sample size formula based on other types of response variables such as binary or time-to-event, can also be found in [21].

In order to demonstrate how an early phase II dose-ranging trial is designed, a real-world example is discussed in the next section. This example reflects three key features of the thinking process: (1) dose-range; (2) number of treatment groups; and (3) sample size. Note that in the real-world setting, other considerations are also important – selection of primary endpoints, choice of clinically meaningful differences (δ), determination of type I and type II error rates, as well as statistical hypothesis to be tested. However, all of these considerations are part of Step 3 – sample size calculation. Therefore, in dose-ranging study designs, once the dose-range and number of treatment groups are determined, the other design considerations are very similar to those for designing an ordinary clinical trial.

6.2.8 Example of the Design Stage

Rofecoxib® is a medication developed by Merck & Co. Inc. (Whitehouse Station, NJ, USA) for the treatment of rheumatoid arthritis (RA) and osteoarthritis (OA). In late 2004, Merck withdrew Rofecoxib® from the market because of concerns with excessive cardiovascular events. After this withdrawal, the drug development environment for any new anti-inflammatory agents became more and more challenging. For every new product developed to treat RA or OA, both drug safety and efficacy were followed very closely to ensure that the efficacy of this new product can be well established, while there is no signal of any safety concerns. Hence, in the clinical development plan, after the PoC and early dose-ranging studies to demonstrate drug efficacy, there will be large scale, long-term phase III studies to follow for efficacy, cardiovascular safety, and gastrointestinal (GI) safety.

A true case study of developing a drug to treat osteoarthritis (OA) is introduced here as an example [16]. This is a four-week study where OA patients first go through a screening visit. Then, after a wash-out of the current OA medication, patients are randomized between the treatment arms. Baseline measurements (demographic, medical history, background medications, efficacy, and other data) are collected prior to the first dose of the study drug. Thereafter, over the four-week treatment period, efficacy and safety measurements are continually collected at each visit. Note that at the early stage of clinical development, the maximum length of the study is constrained by the length of animal studies completed in the non-clinical experiments. In this case study, the animal toxicity studies are followed for up to 4 weeks, and hence, the current clinical study is designed with a four-week study period.

In order to offer the best opportunity for the new compound to show efficacy at the early phase II stage, the test dose to be used in the PoC should be as high as possible. In a typical clinical development program for drugs treating OA, both the efficacy dose response and the safety dose-response relationships are assumed to be monotonic. Hence, at the very high dose of this new product, if it does not demonstrate drug efficacy, the sponsor can stop developing this product, and then allocate investments and resources into developing other compounds that have greater potential to become successful.

Given the requirements of demonstrating long-term drug safety, it is critical for the new compound to offer doses low enough so that in the phase III studies where patients are exposed to long-term treatment, there is no safety concern, and patients can still experience the treatment benefit of efficacy. Hence, it is desirable that in the PoC study, some low doses of this new compound are explored to help detect a minimum effective dose (MinED). For these reasons, it is of interest to study a wide range of doses (so that the high dose that is close to MTD to help with PoC, and the low dose is low enough to help establish MinED).

In this example, the project team decides to study 5 parallel dose groups covering a wide dose range. In addition to these 5 dose groups, a placebo control and an active control are also used to help confirm the efficacy and explore drug safety. In some of the early phase II clinical studies, there is no active control group. Active controls are more likely to be used in phase III development. The reason to choose an active control in this case study is that, if the results fail to distinguish between a placebo and the tested doses, it will be unclear as to whether the test drug is truly ineffective, or there happens to be a very high placebo response (i.e. placebo effect). Under this situation, the comparison between an active control and the placebo helps the project team to differentiate the two conditions given above – if the active control is clearly superior to a placebo, then it can be concluded that the test drug is not efficacious. On the other hand, if the data cannot differentiate between the active control and the placebo, then this study is not informative because it is still unknown as to whether the test drug is beneficial or not. Hence, in this study, the active control is used for reference purposes only. When a treatment is already available on the market for the same indication and targeted population, it would be unethical to consider a placebo arm. In such circumstances, the choice of the low dose is important to demonstrate the dose response together with other pragmatic considerations to ensure patients' care.

For this test drug, the MTD was estimated from results observed in previous studies. Furthermore, the formulation group already prepared tablets with fixed drug strengths. Let the dose at MTD be 100% of the dose strength, and the formulated tablets be at the 2.5% and the 12.5% strengths of MTD. Given this, five doses are selected using the BDS approach (see section 6.2.5) by selecting the following doses: placebo, 2.5%, 5%, 12.5%, 25%, and 75% of MTD, plus an active control. Based on this design, the dose range is 30 (= 75%/2.5%). The active control group was selected to be a popular NSAID (non-steroidal anti-inflammatory drug).

Although osteoarthritis is considered an inflammatory disease, the symptom that brought an OA patient to the doctor is usually joint pain. Hence, in clinical studies of OA, the primary measure of efficacy focuses on pain, or symptoms related to pain. One of the widely accepted clinical measures for OA is the Western Ontario and McMaster University (WOMAC) Osteoarthritis index [22]. The WOMAC score includes 24 questions, 5 of these questions relate to the pain domain, 2 relate to the stiffness domain, and 17 relate to the function domain. In this true case study, the WOMAC pain domain is selected as the primary endpoint for efficacy analysis.

From the α-protection point of view, it is important that each study is designed with one primary efficacy endpoint, one primary comparison, one primary analysis set, and one primary time point. Under these pre-specified conditions, it is less likely that the probability of a type I error will be artificially inflated. In this case study, the primary endpoint is change in the pain domain of the WOMAC score from baseline to week 4 (the primary time point for analysis). The primary analysis set is the intent-to-treat set. Typically, this set is defined to include all patients who received at least one dose of the randomized study treatment.

At this point, one of the most important considerations in α control is the primary comparison. Given the design with five test doses plus placebo and an active control, the question is how to set the primary comparison so that the PoC decision can be made regarding this test drug.

In this case study, a trend contrast with discrete doses is proposed to serve as the primary comparison. In this contrast, the active control is not included in the comparison. As discussed earlier, the NSAID to be used in this study is only for validation purposes, in case the concept is not proven. Hence, the proposed trend contrast includes only the five dosing groups plus the placebo. Here only one contrast is used and, hence, there is no MCP adjustment. For a simple trend contrast with discrete doses, the treatment groups are simply ordered from low to high. The placebo response is assumed to be 0, the lowest dose (2.5% of MTD) is assumed to have 20% response, the next lowest dose (5% of MTD) is assumed to have 40% response, the medium dose (12.5% of MTD) is assumed to have 60% of response, the second highest dose (25% of MTD) is assumed to have 80% response, and the high dose (75% of MTD) is assumed to have 100% response. Then the coefficients -5, -3, -1, 1, 3, and 5 are assigned to these treatment groups [16]. Hence, the primary hypothesis to be tested is:

$$H_0: -5\mu_0 - 3\mu_1 - \mu_2 + \mu_3 + 3\mu_4 + 5\mu_5 \leq 0 \text{ vs.}$$

$$H_1: -5\mu_0 - 3\mu_1 - \mu_2 + \mu_3 + 3\mu_4 + 5\mu_5 > 0,$$

where μ_0 denotes the mean of placebo group, μ_1 denotes the mean of the 2.5% dose group, μ_2 denotes the mean of the 5% dose group, μ_3 denotes the mean of the 12.5% dose group, μ_4 denotes the mean of the 25% dose group, and μ_5 denotes the mean of the 75% dose group.

In the case of a dose-response study with k dose groups and a placebo, the sample size estimates based on a contrast can be derived as follows [21]. Let μ_i be the population mean for group i, $i = 0, \ldots, k$, where μ_0 is the mean from the placebo group, and let c_i be the corresponding coefficients in the contrast. The null hypothesis of no treatment effect (i.e., weight sum of treatment effect across all doses) can be written as:

$$H_0: L(\mu) = \sum_{i=0}^{k} c_i\mu_i \le 0 \text{ vs } H_1: L(\mu) = \sum_{i=0}^{k} c_i\mu_i = \delta > 0, \text{ with } \sum_{i=0}^{k} c_i = 0.$$

Under the alternative hypothesis and the condition of homogeneous variances, the sample size per group (i.e., equal sample size in each group) can be obtained as

$$n = \left[\frac{\left(z_{1-\alpha} + z_{1-\beta}\right)\sigma}{\delta}\right]^2 \sum_{i=0}^{k} c_i^2$$

where $z_{1-\alpha}$ and $z_{1-\beta}$ are the corresponding quantile points of a standard normal distribution.

The standard deviation used to generate these data is set as 4. From the observed placebo response, and the anticipated response from this test drug, possible targeted clinical differences (δ) can be considered, including 1.00, 1.25, or 1.50. From such a large standard deviation, and a relatively small delta (δ), the required sample size could be very large. For example, if a pairwise comparison is used, then under one-sided α of 0.05, with 90% power, and delta of 1.25, the sample size for each treatment group would be about 176 subjects. For a 7-arm study, this will take a total sample size of 1,232 subjects. To power the study using the trend contrast as specified above, the sample size would reduce to 126 per group (882 overall).

The study using the same assumptions is powered to detect a significant trend contrast test under a balanced design with equal number of subjects in each treatment group. In Table 6.1 on page 180, each of the scenarios is considered for different α and power. The standard deviation is assumed to be 4, and the 100% response is assumed to be 1, 1.25, or 1.5.

Because the test drug is at an early stage of clinical development, and the concept has not been proven, it is difficult to justify a huge budget of 882 subjects in an early phase II study. Upon review, the company decided that they were willing to take a higher risk on α, to reduce the sample size with a reasonable investment. The compromise was that the one-sided α can be increased to 0.1, and keep the power at 90%.

For this study, a treatment difference from a placebo of approximately 1.25 was selected. From Table 6.1 on page 180, a sample size of 97 per treatment group provides an estimated power of 90% for a one-sided α of 0.10 and, for this sample size, the power is over 80% for a one-sided α of 0.05.

A sample size of 100 subjects per treatment group is sufficient to detect differences larger than 1.25 in the mean change from baseline in the WOMAC OA Index Pain Subscale, using the aforementioned linear contrast. Since a single test for trend is employed, no adjustment for a multiple comparison is needed. If this test is significant at α of 0.1 (one-sided), the minimum effective dose (MinED) will be estimated.

Table 6.1 *Sample Sizes under Various α, Power, and δ*

One-sided α	Power	δ	*npergroup*	*ntotal*
0.10	0.9	1.00	151	1057
0.05	0.8	1.00	142	994
0.05	0.9	1.00	196	1372
0.10	0.9	1.25	97	679
0.05	0.8	1.25	91	637
0.05	0.9	1.25	126	882
0.10	0.9	1.50	67	469
0.05	0.8	1.50	63	441
0.05	0.9	1.50	87	609

npergroup is the number of subjects for each treatment group, *ntotal* is the total number of subjects that are needed for the study. The contrast that is used to perform this sample size estimation is $-5\mu_0 - 3\mu_1 - \mu_2 + \mu_3 + 3\mu_4 + 5\mu_5$. $\sigma = 4$.

It is worth noting that, in the above example, the chosen trend contrast coefficients are the ones assuming that the different doses are equally spaced which is actually not the case. Strictly speaking, in order to obtain the trend coefficients when the different doses are not equally spaced, using the **orpol** function in SAS/IML can be useful in calculating the orthogonal polynomial contrast coefficients and then integrating in a SAS macro (Example Code 6.1 on page 180). Figure 6.4 on page 181 shows an example for 6 doses.

Example Code 6.1 *SAS/IML Macro to Calculate Orthogonal Polynomial Contrast Coefficients*

```
%macro polyorth(fich_in=);
     data _null_;
          set &fich_in nobs=k ;
          call symput ("nlevel", put(k,8.0));
     run;
     data niv;
          length level $8. ;
          do i=1 to &nlevel. ;
             level="level " || trim(left(i));
             output niv;
          end;
     run;
     data deg;
          do i=1 to %eval(&nlevel.-1);
             degree="deg. " || trim(left(i));
             output deg;
          end;
     run;

     proc iml;
```

```
            start;
             use &fich_in. ;
             read all var{dose} into x;
             use niv ;
             read all var{level} into labco;
             use deg ;
             read all var{degree} into labro;
             degmax=nrow(x)-1;
             p=orpol(x,degmax);
             pp=p[,2:ncol(p)]`;
             create poly from pp [rowname=labro colname=labco];
             append from pp [rowname=labro];
             finish;
             run;
      quit;
      title1 "Orthogonal
      polynomial coefficient contrasts" ;
      title2 "------------------------------------------";
      title3 " ";
      proc print data=poly noobs label;
           label labro="Polynomial degree";
      run;
    %mend polyorth;

data pol ;
      input dose @@;
      cards;
      0 2.5 5 12.5 25 75
      ;
run;
%polyorth(fich_in=pol);
```

Figure 6.4 *Output for Example Code 6.1*

Polynomial degree	level_1	level_2	level_3	level_4	level_5	level_6
deg. 1	-0.31476	-0.27541	-0.23607	-0.11803	0.07869	0.86558
deg. 2	0.42306	0.25431	0.09689	-0.30741	-0.75471	0.28787
deg. 3	-0.49268	-0.01780	0.32207	0.64245	-0.48913	0.03509
deg. 4	0.49306	-0.34515	-0.56438	0.54868	-0.13485	0.00263
deg. 5	-0.26351	0.75721	-0.58819	0.10540	-0.01098	0.00006

Figure 6.4 on page 181 provides the contrast coefficients for the different degrees of a polynomial regression that would be adjusted between the doses and the response:

$$y = \alpha + \beta x + \gamma x^2 + \delta x^3 + \zeta x^4 + \eta x^5$$

The first row in the table of Figure 6.4 on page 181 provides the actual contrast coefficients for testing the linear trend ($H_0{:}\beta = 0, H_1{:}\beta \neq 0$) as opposed to the $(-5,\ -3,\ -1,\ 1,\ 3,\ 5)$ coefficients, which assumes that the different doses are equally spaced (which is not the case). The following rows provide coefficients for testing the subsequent polynomial degrees: quadratic (γ), cubic (δ), etc.

6.3 Considerations in the Design and Final Analysis Stages

Statistical thinking and considerations in the study-design stage (i.e., before data are available) could be different from those in the analysis stage (i.e., after the data are available). The main purpose of this chapter is to summarize our thinking on dose-response study design. Meanwhile, we think that it may be helpful to provide a few examples with relevant SAS code for readers to practice in the analysis stage after data are available. There are many analysis approaches in the analysis stage, this chapter is not intended to summarize all possible analysis approaches.

Therefore, "6.2 Statistical Design Considerations in a Classical Dose-Response Study" on page 164 demonstrates an example of thinking in the statistical design and clinical development stage, while the key focus in "6.4 Analysis Examples Using Simulated Data" on page 182 is the analysis stage, assuming that data are already collected and unblinded for the analysis. So the main purpose in the next section is to demonstrate two examples for analyzing unblinded data using SAS.

Please note that "6.2 Statistical Design Considerations in a Classical Dose-Response Study" on page 164 describes a factor type (ANOVA) model, which technically is a linear model. "6.4 Analysis Examples Using Simulated Data" on page 182 utilizes nonlinear regression models. Designing a study using nonlinear regression models is not the focus of this chapter, but it could be used and is often built on the asymptotic distributions. Complete coverage of this field has been presented in [23].

6.4 Analysis Examples Using Simulated Data

6.4.1 Brief Introduction to the Emax Model

This section describes two simulated practical examples for continuous and binary endpoints. The simulated data assume that there are 5 dose groups, 0mg (placebo), 2.5mg, 5mg, 10mg, and 20mg, in a phase II dose ranging trial. The sample size in each dose group is 60. The **nlmixed** procedure is used to fit 4-parameter E_{max} models to analyze the data. Note that **proc nlin** in SAS could be used to fit the 4-parameter model as well, which is dedicated to the nonlinear regression model. Both procedures produce very similar estimates and results. In addition, code for trend tests for PoC, using the contrast (generated with the **% polyorth** macro) accounting for equal or unequal dose spacing, are included for practical purpose for readers on both the continuous and binary endpoint cases.

The E_{max} model is one of the commonly used nonlinear models in dose response studies [24]. The model is shown below,

$$y_i = E_0 + E_{max} \times \frac{D_i^h}{ED_{50}^h + D_i^h} + \epsilon_i,$$

where

1. i is the subject ID

2. y_i is the observed continuous response variable for the ith patient

3. E_0 is the basal effect, i.e., the response when the dose is 0 mg

4. E_{max} is the maximum effect attributable to the drug

5. ED_{50} is the dose that produces half of E_{max}

6. h is the hill parameter, or slope, which measures the sensitivity of the response to the dose range of the drug, determining the steepness of the dose–response curve ($N > 0$)

7. D_i is the dose-level for the ith patient

8. ϵ_i is the random error for the ith patient. A standard assumption, adopted here, is that the ϵ_i terms are independent and identically distributed with a mean of 0 and a variance σ^2. An additional standard assumption is that the error terms are normally distributed.

Figure 6.5 on page 183, reproduced from [24], shows a typical dose-response curve, based on a monotonic increase assumption. Note that the E_{max} model dose-response curve can be either increasing or decreasing relative to an increase in dose. If the response is decreasing, the value of the E_{max} parameter will be negative.

Figure 6.5 *E_{max} Model Dose-Response Curve*

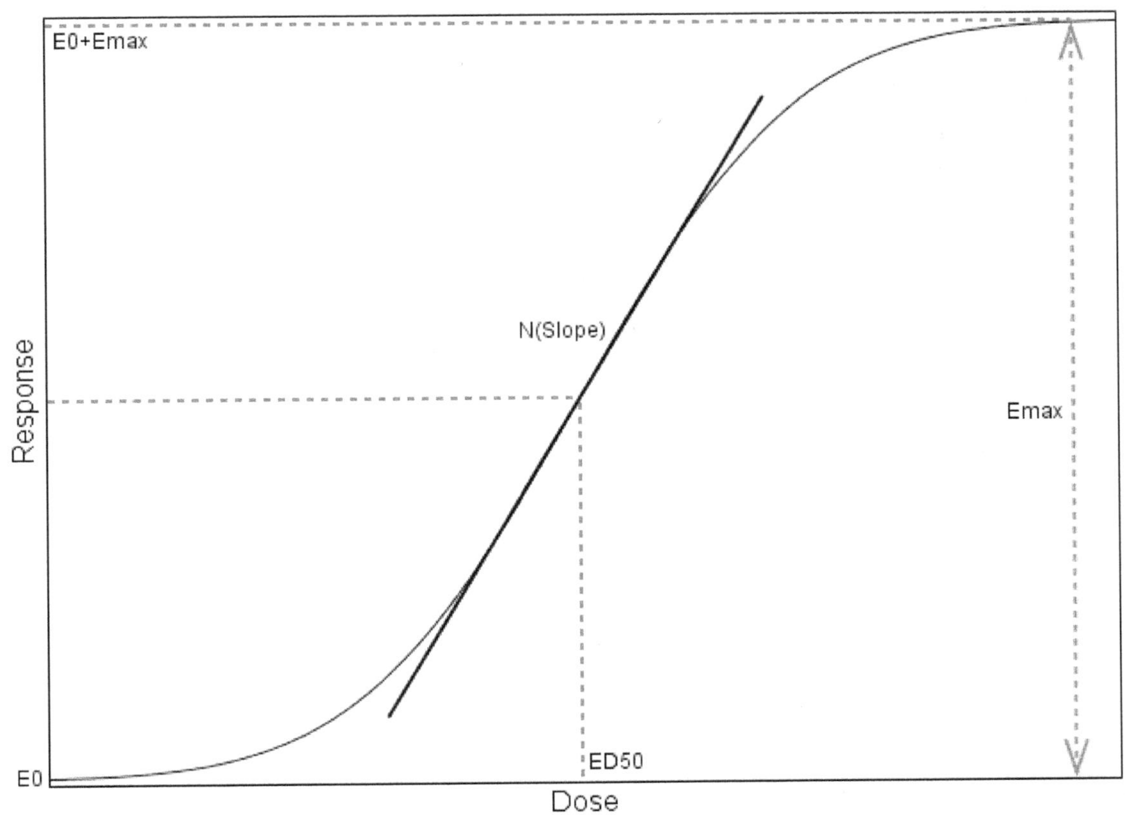

The above E_{max} model is a traditional 4-parameter E_{max} model (also called the sigmoidal E_{max} model) that is commonly used in dose-response study analysis. With 4 parameters (E_0, E_{max}, ED_{50} and h), the model provides great flexibility to fit various shapes of the dose-response relationship and makes it one of the popular dose-response models. However, there are some limitations in the applications of this model. First, because the model has 4 parameters, it requires at least 5 doses (could include a placebo as dose 0) and assumes a monotonic dose-response curve. Second, the 4-parameter E_{max} model sometimes does not converge. In the case that the 4-parameter E_{max} model does not converge or that a study is designed with only 4 dose levels, a common practice is to remove the hill parameter, e.g., set the slope parameter $h = 1$. The model then becomes a 3-parameter model (i.e., the so-called hyperbolic E_{max} model),

$$y_i = E_0 + E_{max} \times \frac{D_i}{ED_{50} + D_i} + \epsilon_i,$$

where the terms are defined as above for the sigmoidal E_{max} model.

The above model assumes that the response variable is continuous, but sometimes, the response variable could be binary, e.g., a response rate. In this case, the model can be readily revised to be a generalized E_{max} model using a logit link,

$$\log\left(\frac{\pi}{1-\pi}\right) = E_0 + E_{max} \times \frac{D_i^h}{ED_{50}^h + D_i^h},$$

where π is the observed response rate.

In the next two sections, we use the above described models to analyze the simulated data as a demonstration of applications. The data sets are simulated as **dstcon** (for a continuous endpoint) and **dstbin** (for a binary endpoint).

6.4.2 Continuous Endpoint

The sample SAS code for simulation and analysis are provided in Example Code 6.2, which simulates a data set that is based on the above E_{max} model.

Example Code 6.2 *Program to Simulate Continuous Data Using the E_{max} Model*

```
data dose;
    input dose@@;
    datalines;
0 2.5 5 10 20
;
run;

%macro simu(n=, sd=, e0=10, emax=80, ed50=5.5, h=1, outdst=dstcon);
    ** n is the sample size in each dose group;
    proc sql noprint;
       select count(dose)into:ngrp
       from dose;
    quit;
    %let ngrp= &ngrp.;

    data _null_;
        set dose;
        mean=&e0.+(&emax.*dose**&h.)/(dose**&h. + &ed50.**&h.);
        call symput(compress("mean"||put(_n_, 1.)), compress(mean));
        call symput(compress("dose"||put(_n_, 1.)), compress(dose));
    run;
```

```
    %do i=1 %to &ngrp.; %put **** Group &i. **** &&mean&i.; %end;

    data &outdst.;
      %do i=1 %to &ngrp.;
          group=&i.;
          mean=&&mean&i.;
          dose=&&dose&i.;
          do n=1 to &n.;
             resp=&&mean&i.+ &sd. *rannor(1500); **Seed number 1500 is used;
             output;
          end;
     %end;
    run;
%mend;

%simu(n=60, sd=10, e0=10, emax=80, ed50=5.5, h=1, outdst=dstcon);
```

The below **proc nlmixed** call in Example Code 6.3 on page 185 is used to fit a 4-parameter E_{max} model using the simulated data.

Example Code 6.3 *4-parameter E_{max} Model Fit Using proc nlmixed*

```
proc nlmixed data=dstcon alpha=0.05;
   ***set up initial values;
   parms  e0=10 emax=80 ed50=5.5 h=1 v=400;
   *****specify that ed50 must be positive;
   bounds ed50>0;
   ****define model;
   if dose=0 then eta = e0;
   else eta = e0 + ((emax*dose**h)/(ed50**h+dose**h));
   model resp ~ normal(eta, v);

   *****estimate the difference in means;
   estimate "Diff Means (dose 20mg -placebo)"
                        e0+((emax*20**h)/(ed50**h+20**h))-e0;
   estimate "Diff Means (dose 10mg -placebo)"
                        e0+((emax*10**h)/(ed50**h+10**h))-e0;
   estimate "Diff Means (dose 5 mg -placebo)"
                        e0+((emax*5**h)/(ed50**h+5**h))-e0;
   estimate "Diff Means (dose 2.5mg- placebo)"
                        e0+((emax*2.5**h)/(ed50**h+2.5**h))-e0;

   predict eta out=etahat;
   *****output estimations;
   *****dataset est has output for estimate of the mean differences;
   *****dataset parms has output for parameters: e0 emax ed50 h;
   ods output AdditionalEstimates=est
              ParameterEstimates=parms;
run;
```

The key results from Example Code 6.3 on page 185 are shown in Figure 6.6 on page 186 . The figure shows output for the model estimated mean difference of the test doses versus a placebo, as well as the 95% confidence intervals. The first row indicates that the mean difference between the dose level of 20mg versus the placebo is 60.8 with the 95% confidence interval (57.2, 64.4).

Figure 6.6 *Output for Example Code 6.3*

Additional Estimates								
Label	Estimate	Standard Error	DF	t Value	Pr > |t|	Alpha	Lower	Upper
Diff Means (dose 20mg -placebo)	60.8246	1.8422	300	33.02	<.0001	0.05	57.1993	64.4500
Diff Means (dose 10mg -placebo)	50.9201	1.6485	300	30.89	<.0001	0.05	47.6761	54.1642
Diff Means (dose 5 mg -placebo)	37.5029	1.6567	300	22.64	<.0001	0.05	34.2426	40.7632
Diff Means (dose 2.5mg- placebo)	23.7523	1.7872	300	13.29	<.0001	0.05	20.2353	27.2692

In case readers are interested in practicing the trend test using the contrast (generated with the SAS macro **%polyorth** in Example Code 6.1), sample code is provided below in Example Code 6.4 on page 186 using the simulated data set **dstcon**. The output for the polynomials is presented in Figure 6.7 on page 186. The trend test is performed in Example Code 6.5 on page 186, with the output presented in Figure 6.8 on page 187.

Example Code 6.4 *Program to Generate Orthogonal Polynomials for Trend Test*

```
data dose;
    input dose@@;
    datalines;
0 2.5 5 10 20
;
run;
%polyorth(fich_in=dose);
```

Figure 6.7 *Output for Example Code 6.4*

Polynomial degree	level_1	level_2	level_3	level_4	level_5
deg. 1	-0.47434	-0.31623	-0.15811	0.15811	0.79057
deg. 2	0.54596	0.03522	-0.33462	-0.65163	0.40507
deg. 3	-0.46999	0.42226	0.51435	-0.57050	0.10388
deg. 4	0.23672	-0.72143	0.63125	-0.15781	0.01127

Example Code 6.5 *PoC with Trend Contrast Accounting for Equal or Unequal Spacing*

```
title "General linear model for PoC hypothesis testing";
proc glm data=dstcon;
     class group;
     model resp = group ;
     contrast "Trend contrast" group
              -0.47434 -0.31623 -0.15811 0.15811 0.79057;
run;
```

Figure 6.8 *Output for Example Code 6.5*

Source	DF	Type I SS	Mean Square	F Value	Pr > F
group	4	136767.7035	34191.9259	328.46	<.0001

Source	DF	Type III SS	Mean Square	F Value	Pr > F
group	4	136767.7035	34191.9259	328.46	<.0001

Contrast	DF	Contrast SS	Mean Square	F Value	Pr > F
Trend contrast	1	109819.5017	109819.5017	1054.98	<.0001

Note that some procedures, like **proc genmod**, provide an option to evaluate the orthogonal polynomial contrasts. For example,

```
proc genmod data=dstcon;
     class dose / param=orthpoly;
     model resp = dose / scale=deviance;
run;
```

The use of the simple **%polyorth** macro helps in getting the actual coefficients, which can be used for sample size calculations.

6.4.3 Binary Endpoint

The sample SAS code for the simulation and analysis of a binary endpoint are provided here. The reader can use Example Code 6.6 on page 187 to simulate a data set based on the above E_{max} model.

Example Code 6.6 *Program to Simulate Binary Data Using the E_{max} Model*

```
data dose;
    input dose@@;
    datalines;
0 2.5 5 10 20
;
run;

%macro simu(n=, e0=-1.39, emax=3.54, ed50=5.5, h=1);

    proc sql noprint;
       select count(dose)into:ngrp
       from dose;
    quit;
    %let ngrp= &ngrp. ;

    data _null_;
         set dose;
         pai=exp(&e0.+((&emax.*dose**&h.)/(&ed50.**&h.+dose**&h.)))/
             (1+exp(&e0.+((&emax.*dose**&h.)/(&ed50.**&h.+dose**&h.))));
         call symput(compress( "pai" ||put(_n_, 1. )), compress(pai) ) ;
         call symput(compress( "dose" ||put(_n_, 1. )), compress(dose) ) ;
    run ;
    %do i=1 %to &ngrp.; %put *** Group &i. **** &&pai&i.; %end;

    proc iml ;
         prob= { %do i=1 %to &ngrp.; &&pai&i. %end; };
```

```
        p = repeat(prob,&n.);   /* repeat row n times: n/group */
        call streaminit( 321 ); /* call randseed(321) to set seed number; */
        x = rand( "Bernoulli" , p);
        create MyData from x;   /* create data set */
        append from x;          /* write data in vectors */
        close MyData;           /* close the data set */
    quit;

    data mydata;                /* add an observation number for transpose*/
         set mydata;
         id=_n_;
    run;

    proc transpose data=mydata out=mydatat ;
         var col1-col&ngrp. ;
         by id;
    run;

    data xdose;             /* add the different COLn to retreive the dose*/
         set dose;
         _name_= compress("COL" || put(_n_, 1. ));
    run;

    proc sql noprint;        /* retrieve the dose for the different groups*/
         create table dstbin as
          select a.id as obs, a.col1 as resp, b.dose
          from mydatat a left join xdose b
          on a._name_=b._name_
          order by b.dose, a.id;

         create table resp as
          select dose, sum(resp) as count, count(*) as n,
                 sum(resp)/count(*) as pai
          from dstbin
          group by dose ;
    quit;

    proc print data =resp;
    run ;
%mend;

%simu(n=60, e0=-1.39, emax=3.54, ed50=5.5, h=1);
```

There are two data sets created by the above simulation code, one is named **dstbin** which is based on the original scale, while the other is named **resp** which is based on the summarized scale (Figure 6.9 on page 189). Note that **proc nlmixed** uses the data set **resp** (and the procedure can also fit a model on individual-level data **dstbin** with **bernoulli** in the model statement). The below **proc nlmixed** call in Example Code 6.7 on page 189 is used to fit a 4-parameter E_{max} model using the simulated data in the previous program.

Figure 6.9 *Output for Example Code 6.6*

Obs	dose	count	n	pai
1	0.0	9	60	0.15000
2	2.5	22	60	0.36667
3	5.0	33	60	0.55000
4	10.0	42	60	0.70000
5	20.0	48	60	0.80000

Example Code 6.7 *4-parameter Binary E_{max} Model Fit Using proc nlmixed*

```
proc nlmixed data=resp alpha=0.05 ;
   *****specify that ed50 must be positive;
   bounds ed50>0;

   *****define models;
   if dose=0 then eta = e0;
   else eta = e0 + ((emax*dose**h)/(ed50**h+dose**h));
   expeta = exp(eta);
   p = expeta/(1+expeta);
   model count ~ binomial(n, p);

   *****estimate the difference in proportions (dose group-control group);
   estimate "Diff Props (20 mg - control group)"
            exp(e0+(emax*20**h/(ed50**h+20**h)))/(1+exp(e0+
            (emax*20**h /(ed50**h+20**h))))-exp(e0)/(1+exp(e0));

   estimate "Diff Props (10 mg - control group)"
            exp(e0+(emax*10**h/(ed50**h+10**h)))/(1+exp(e0+
            (emax*10**h /(ed50**h+10**h))))
            - exp(e0)/(1 + exp(e0));
   estimate "Diff Props (5 mg - control group)"
            exp(e0+(emax*5**h/(ed50**h+5**h)))/(1+exp(e0+
            (emax*5**h /(ed50**h+5**h))))- exp(e0)/(1 + exp(e0));
   estimate "Diff Props (2.5 mg - control group)"
            exp(e0+(emax*2.5**h /(ed50**h+2.5**h)))/(1+exp(e0+
            (emax*2.5**h /(ed50**h+2.5**h))))-exp(e0)/(1+exp(e0));

   predict p out=etahat;
   *****output estimations;
   *****data est will have output for estimate statement;
   *****data parms will have output for parameters;
   ods output AdditionalEstimates=est
              ParameterEstimates=parms;
run;
```

The key results from **PROC NLMIXED** are presented in Figure 6.10 on page 190 . The output shows the model estimated mean difference of the test doses versus the placebo with respect to the response rate, as well as the 95% confidence intervals. The first row indicates that the mean rate difference between the dose level of 20mg versus the placebo is 64.8% with the 95% confidence interval (47.2%, 82.5%).

Figure 6.10 *Output for Example Code 6.10*

Additional Estimates								
Label	Estimate	Standard Error	DF	t Value	Pr > |t|	Alpha	Lower	Upper
Diff Props (20 mg - control group)	0.6484	0.06850	5	9.47	0.0002	0.05	0.4723	0.8245
Diff Props (10 mg - control group)	0.5554	0.06310	5	8.80	0.0003	0.05	0.3932	0.7176
Diff Props (5 mg - control group)	0.3948	0.06914	5	5.71	0.0023	0.05	0.2171	0.5726
Diff Props (2.5 mg - control group)	0.2195	0.07436	5	2.95	0.0318	0.05	0.02834	0.4106

6.5 Summary

There are a lot of challenges in designing the first dose-ranging clinical trial. The two main problems are: (1) there is not much information about the efficacy of the candidate product available and; (2) too many answers are expected for this trial to deliver. Project team members tend to anticipate that such a study will establish the PoC, identify the MinED, characterize the dose-response relationship, and recommend doses for phase III designs. Fundamental statistical training points out that the best design is that one study answers only one question. Hence, the nature of a dose-ranging trial makes it a very difficult design in order to address so many scientific questions, and so little information to begin with.

In fact, there should be a logical sequence of thinking in addressing these questions. The first step is to consider how wide a dose range should be. This is also the most critical step. In order to approach this question, information about the drug candidate under development (pre-clinical and clinical phase I), other marketed drugs in a similar class, the indication that this study is designed for, and the target product profile, can all provide a better understanding of the potential dose range that needs to be explored. In practice, it is also important to have a good understanding of dosing frequency (from phase I results), formulation (from CMC), and other relevant issues.

Once the dose range is determined, the next step would be to consider the number of treatment groups – will there be a need of an active control? How many doses should be included in this design? What dose spacing should be considered? Basically speaking, a trial with 4 to 5 test doses, plus a placebo control will deliver a good understanding of where the test medication is most active, if the dose range is wide enough, and if the dose spacing is reasonable. But six or more test doses (in addition to a placebo) design may not necessarily deliver better results than the four or five test doses [20]. A study design with too many doses may introduce additional complexities from a practical and logistical point of view (e.g., formulation, blinding, or others).

Sample size calculation is needed for almost every clinical trial. Considerations in sample size calculations for a dose-ranging trial are very similar to those for other trials. However, because the nature of a dose-ranging trial is that it includes multiple treatment groups, this may cause some level of confusion – both to statisticians and non-statisticians. However, if the decision is to only use a single degree of freedom contrast test as the primary comparison, then the situation can be simplified a lot. In the case of one contrast, the two major challenges would be what assumptions of dose-response relationship that the team is willing to make, and sample size allocation – either a balanced approach or an imbalanced approach. After these decisions are made, the statistician would then follow up and calculate the sample size for the study.

Suppose a contrast with one degree of freedom is selected, and the sample size allocation is determined, the typical sample size considerations, such as choice of treatment difference, choice of alpha and beta can then be specified. With this information, sample size can be calculated using an existing formula. An example of a real study design in a test product developed for treatment of osteoarthritis is included in this manuscript to demonstrate how these methods can be applied in a real-world situation.

References

1. Ting N. (2006). Introduction and drug development process. In Ting N, ed. *Dose Finding in Drug Development*. New York: Springer.
2. Ting N. (2011). Phase 2 clinical development in treating chronic diseases. *Drug Information Journal* 45: 431–442.
3. International Conference of Harmonisation. (1997). E8: General Considerations for Clinical Trials. Available at: http://www.ich.org/fileadmin/Public_Web_Site/ICH_Products/Guidelines/Efficacy/E8/Step4/E8_Guideline.pdf (http://www.ich.org/fileadmin/Public_Web_Site/ICH_Products/Guidelines/Efficacy/E8/Step4/E8_Guideline.pdf).
4. International Conference of Harmonisation. (1994). E4: Dose–Response Information to Support Drug Registration. Available at: http://www.ich.org/fileadmin/Public_Web_Site/ICH_Products/Guidelines/Efficacy/E4/Step4/E4_Guideline.pdf (http://www.ich.org/fileadmin/Public_Web_Site/ICH_Products/Guidelines/Efficacy/E4/Step4/E4_Guideline.pdf).
5. Grieve AP. (2011). Adaptive trial designs: Looking for answers. *International Clinical Trials*, Issue 22, 16-20.
6. Trevor AJ, Katzung BG, Masters SB. (2010). *Katzung and Trevor's Pharmacology Examination & Board Review, Ninth Edition*. New York: McGraw Hill, 15.
7. Ting N. (2008). Confirm and explore, a stepwise approach to clinical trial designs. *Drug Information Journal* 42: 545-554.
8. Thomas N & Ting N. (2009). Minimum Effective Dose In D'Agostino RB, Sullivan L, Massaro J, eds. *Encyclopedia of Clinical Trials*. Hoboken, NJ: Wiley-Blackwell.
9. Fillon TG. (1995). Estimating the minimum therapeutically effective dose of a compound via regression modelling and percentile estimation. *Statistics in Medicine* 14: 925-932.
10. Pinheiro JC, Bornkamp B & Bretz F. (2006). Design and analysis of dose finding studies combining multiple comparisons and modeling procedures. *Journal of Biopharmaceutical Statistics* 16: 639–656.
11. Hochberg Y & Tamhane A. (1987). *Multiple Comparison Procedures*. New York: Wiley.
12. Wang X & Ting N. (2012). A proof-of-concept clinical trial design combined with dose-ranging exploration. *Pharmaceutical Statistics* 11: 403-409.
13. Pinheiro J, Bretz F & Branson. (2006). Analysis of dose-response studies-modeling approaches. In Ting N, ed. *Dose Finding in Drug Development*. New York: Springer.
14. Ting N, ed. (2006). *Dose Finding in Drug Development*. New York: Springer.
15. Hamlett A, Ting N, Hanumara C & Finman JS. (2002). Dose spacing in early dose response clinical trial designs. *Drug Information Journal* 36: 855-864.

16. Ting N. (2009). Practical and statistical considerations in designing an early phase II osteoarthritis clinical trial: A Case Study. *Communications in Statistics – Theory and Methods* 38: 3282-3296.

17. Penel N & Kramar A. (2012). What does a modified-Fibonacci dose-escalation actually correspond to? *BMC Medical Research Methodology* 12: 103.

18. Quinlan JA & Krams M. (2006). Implementing adaptive designs: logistical and operational considerations. *Drug Information Journal* 40: 437-444.

19. Krams M, Lees KR, Hacke W, Grieve AP, Orgogozo JM & Ford GA for the ASTIN Study Investigators. (2003). ASTIN: An adaptive dose-response study of UK-279,276 in acute ischemic stroke. *Stroke* 34: 2543-254.

20. Yuan G & Ting N. (2014). First dose ranging clinical trial design: More doses? Or a wider range? In Young WR & Chen DG, eds. *Clinical Trial Biostatistics and Biopharmaceutical Applications*. Boca Raton, FL: Chapman and Hall/CRC.

21. Chow SC, Shao J & Wang H. (2007). *Sample Size Calculations in Clinical Research, Second Edition*. Boca Raton, FL: Chapman & Hall/CRC.

22. Bellamy N, Campbell J, Stevens J, Pilcher L, Stewart C & Mahmood Z. (1997). Validation study of a computerized version of the Western Ontario and McMaster Universities VA3.0 Osteoarthritis Index. *Journal of Rheumatology* 24: 2413-2415.

23. Fedorov VV & Leonov SL. (2014). *Optimal Design for Nonlinear Response Models* Boca Raton, Florida: Chapman and Hall/CRC.

24. MacDougall J. (2006). Analysis of dose-response studies – Emax Model. In Ting N, ed. *Dose Finding in Drug Development*. New York: Springer.

Authors

Naitee Ting, Senior Principal Biostatistician, Boehringer-Ingelheim Pharmaceuticals Inc., Ridgefield, CT, USA.

Guojun Yuan, Director of Global Biostatistics, EMD Serono, Inc., a subsidiary of Merck KgaA, Billerica, MA, USA.

François Beckers, Head Global Biostatistics, Merck Serono, Inc., a subsidiary of Merck KgaA, Darmstadt, Germany.

Chapter 7

Implementing the MCP-Mod Procedure for Dose-Response Testing and Estimation

7.1 Introduction

A well-known problem of failed phase III programs is poor dose selection resulting from inappropriate knowledge of the dose-response relationship (efficacy and safety) at the end of the learning phase of drug development, i.e., phase II. Selection of a dose (or doses) to carry into confirmatory phase III trials is among the most difficult decisions in drug development. Although the exact numbers are unknown, it is believed that the high attrition rate plaguing the pharmaceutical industry in phase III studies are due, at least in part, to inadequate dose selection for confirming safety and efficacy in the intended patient population – doses that are too low to achieve adequate benefit, as well as doses that are too high and lead to dose-related safety events.

The basic difficulty in getting the right dose is the trade-off between wanted and unwanted effects. A prerequisite for informed decision making and dose selection at the end of phase II is, hence, a solid characterization of the dose-response relationships. Historically, dose finding studies were designed and analyzed based on multiple pairwise comparisons of the active doses against a placebo. Such traditional methods are mostly performed within the analysis-of-variance hypothesis testing paradigm and known to be inefficient in the sense that they fail to fully incorporate the available information across the doses [1]. Modeling approaches assume a functional relationship between response and dose, taken as a quantitative factor, according to a certain parametric model, such as the E_{max} model. The fitted model is then used to describe the dose-response relationship and estimate target doses of interest. Such an approach will often lead to more precise estimates of the dose-response relationship, due to the interpolation of information across doses. In addition, it also provides flexibility in investigating the effect of doses not used in the actual study. However, the validity of its conclusions will highly depend on an appropriate choice of the dose-response model, which in practice is often unknown.

The MCP-Mod approach considered in this chapter is an approach for dealing with this model uncertainty by combining principles of multiple comparisons with modeling techniques to overcome some of the shortcomings of applying either approach alone [2]. MCP-Mod has recently been qualified as an efficient statistical methodology for model-based design and analysis of phase II dose finding studies under model uncertainty [3]. The MCP-Mod approach impacts both the design and the analysis of dose-finding studies. At the trial design stage, a suitable set of candidate models is identified, which also impacts decisions on the number doses, required sample sizes, patient allocations, etc. At the trial analysis stage, dose-response is tested using suitable trend tests deduced from the set of candidate models. Once a dose-response signal is established, the best model out of the pre-specified candidate model set is then used for dose-response and target dose estimation. In the remainder of this chapter, we describe the core methodology of MCP-Mod in more detail, including an extension to general parametric models, illustrate its application with two examples, and provide the underlying SAS code.

7.2 Methodology

7.2.1 Original MCP-Mod Approach

In this section we first provide a short, technical description of the original MCP-Mod approach [2] for a single, normally distributed efficacy endpoint. Afterwards, we describe a recently developed variant of MCP-Mod that extends the core methodology to dose-finding studies for general parametric models (e.g. for binary, count, or time-to-event endpoints and including certain longitudinal modeling approaches), see [4].

The MCP-Mod procedure is implemented in five steps; see also Figure 7.1 on page 195 :

1. At the trial design stage, identify several candidate dose-response shapes, which are likely to represent the underlying true dose-response.
2. Derive optimum contrast coefficients, such that the marginal power to detect a specific dose-response shape that is associated with the respective candidate model is maximized.
3. At the analysis stage, evaluate the significance of the individual shapes in terms of a multiple contrast test based on the previously derived optimal contrast coefficients, to assess whether a dose-response signal can be established. This constitutes the MCP part of MCP-Mod.

4. Select a candidate model using a model selection criteria such as AIC or BIC or use model averaging.
5. Use the selected model(s) to produce inferences on adequate doses, employing a model-based approach. This constitutes the Mod part of MCP-Mod.

The results from this analysis may then form the quantitative basis for selecting the dose for the phase III program. In practice, selection of one or more doses to advance into phase III clinical trials is one of the most challenging decisions during drug development and will typically involve both qualitative and quantitative considerations. In the following sections we describe the individual steps of the MCP-Mod approach in more detail. We illustrate the original MCP-Mod approach with a numerical example and accompanying SAS code in the next section.

Figure 7.1 *High-Level Overview of the Original MCP-Mod Procedure*

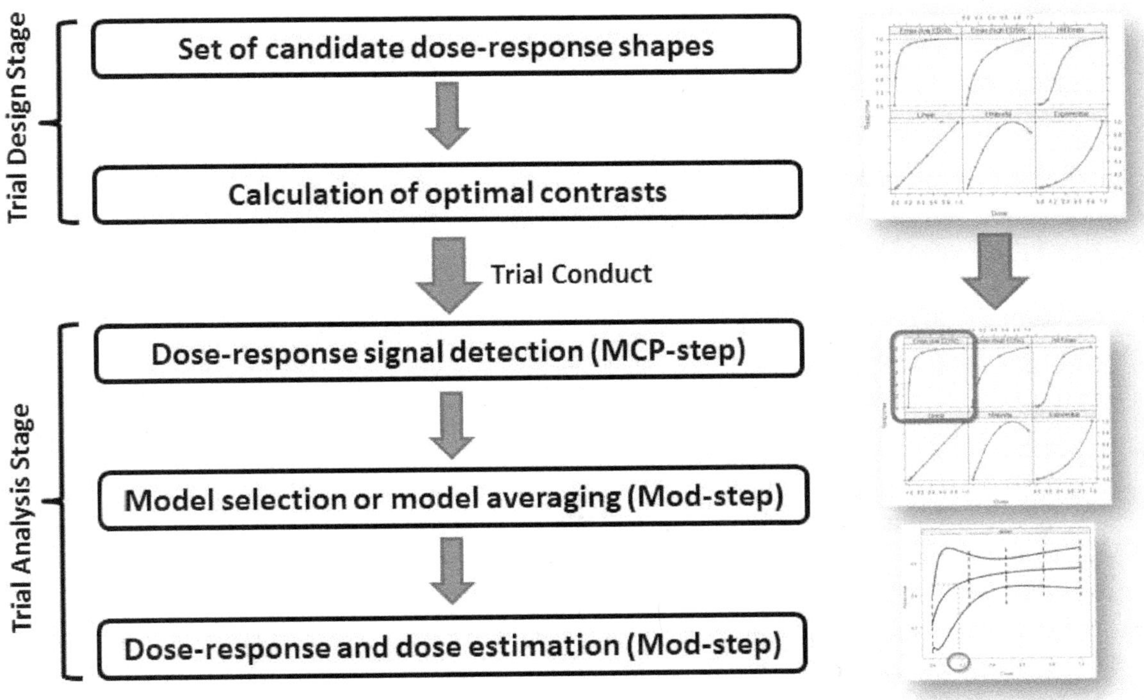

Assume a primary response variable y for a given set of parallel groups of patients corresponding to active doses $d_2, \ldots, d_k$ plus placebo d_1, for a total of k arms. For the purpose of dose-response signal testing and estimating target doses, we consider a one-way layout for the model specification $y_{ij} = \mu_i + \varepsilon_{ij}$, $\varepsilon_{ij} \sim N(0, \sigma^2)$ for $j = 1, \ldots, n_i$ and $i = 1, \ldots, k$, where the mean response at dose d_i can be represented as $\mu_i = \mu(d_i, \theta)$ for some dose-response model $\mu(.)$ parameterized by a vector of parameters θ, n_i denotes the number of patients allocated to dose d_i, and ε_{ij} is the error term for patient j within group i (assuming independent residuals). We note that most dose-response models used in practice can be written as $\mu(d, \theta) = \theta_0 + \theta_1 f^0(d, \theta_2)$ and $f^0(d, \theta_2)$ is typically a nonlinear transformation of the dose levels depending on θ_2. The parameters θ_0 and θ_1 determine location and scaling of the function f. An example for f^0 is $f^0(d, \theta_2) = d/(d + \theta_2)$, resulting in the (hyperbolic) $E_{\max}$ model where θ_2 denotes the

ED_{50} parameter. More dose-response models are given in Table 7.1 on page 196. Column θ_2 lists for each model the parameters that determine the shape of the model. For example, for the beta model $B(\delta_1, \delta_2) = (\delta_1 + \delta_2)^{\delta_1 + \delta_2} / \left(\delta_1^{\delta_1} \delta_2^{\delta_2}\right)$, where D is a constant larger than the highest dose in the study (e.g. 1.2 times the highest dose level), and for the quadratic model $\delta = \beta_2 / |\beta_1|$.

Table 7.1 *Example Dose-Response Models Often Used in Clinical Trials*

Model Name	$\mu(d, \theta)$	θ_2
linear	$E_0 + \delta d$	
linlog	$E_0 + \delta \log(d + c)$	
quadratic	$E_0 + \beta_1 d + \beta_2 d^2$	δ
E_{max}	$E_0 + E_{max} d / (d + ED_{50})$	ED_{50}
exponential	$E_0 + E_1(\exp(d/\delta) - 1)$	δ
sig E_{max}	$E_0 + E_{max} d^h / (d^h + ED_{50}^h)$	$(ED_{50}, h)'$
betaMod	$E_0 + E_{max} B(\delta_1, \delta_2)(d/D)^{\delta_1}(1 - d/D)^{\delta_2}$	$(\delta_1, \delta_2)'$

The first step of MCP-Mod is to identify a set of M parameterized candidate models together with prior parameter values for their standardized versions. When used with the doses planned for the trial, $d_1, \ldots, d_k$, these candidate models produce mean response vectors $\mu_m = (\mu_{m1}, \ldots, \mu_{mk})'$, where $\mu_{mi} = \mu_m(d_i, \theta_{2m})$ with a specified parameter θ_{2m} and μ_m is the mth dose-response function, $m = 1, \ldots, M$.

The second step is to test each of the dose-response shapes in the candidate set using a single contrast test, with coefficients chosen to maximize the power of the test when the true underlying mean response equals μ_m. This approach formulates the test for a dose-response trend in terms of a linear contrast $c'\mu$, where c is a contrast vector subject to $\sum_i c_i = 0$ and μ is the true mean at the dose levels. For a given vector μ, optimum contrast coefficients for model testing are proportional to $n_i(\mu_i - \mu^*)$, $i = 1, \ldots, k$, which after normalization lead to the unique solution (up to the sign) $c/||c||$, where $\mu^* = \mu' 1/k$. Each of M possible dose-response shapes is then represented by one contrast $c_m = (c_{m1}, \ldots, c_{mk})'$. The contrast coefficients for the mth shape are specified at the trial design stage, such that they maximize the power to detect the mth expected dose-response shape. For example, a linear contrast test for equally spaced doses and balanced patient allocation is defined such that the difference of any two adjacent contrast coefficients is a same constant. Assuming that the linear model has been included in the candidate model set, the linear contrast test is then a powerful test to detect the linear trend. Similarly, any dose-response relationship characterized through μ_m can be tested equally powerfully by selecting an appropriate contrast test, whose coefficients are defined in dependence of the assumed μ_m. Note that contrast tests are shift and scale invariant. The optimal contrast coefficient depend on the parameter(s) θ_2 in the f_0, but not on θ_0 and θ_1. The right column in Table 7.1 on page 196 displays the parameters, which need to be specified at the design stage for each model. Note that these prior guesses are only used for derivation of the contrasts. For example, for the $E_{\max}$ model, a prior guess is required for the ED_{50} parameter.

The third step is to test for an overall dose-response signal. The single contrast tests are defined as

$$T_m = \frac{\sum_{i=1}^{k} c_{mi}\bar{Y}_i}{S\sqrt{\sum_{i=1}^{k} c_{mi}^2/n_i}}, \qquad m = 1, \ldots, M,$$

where $S^2 = \sum_{i=1}^{k} \sum_{j=1}^{n_i} \left(Y_{ij} - \bar{Y}_i\right)^2 / \left(N - k\right)$ denotes the mean squared error and $N = \sum_i n_i$ the total sample size. Under the null hypothesis $H_0: c'\mu = 0$ of no dose-response effect, i.e., $\mu_1 = \ldots = \mu_k$, and under the distributional assumptions from above, $T_1, \ldots, T_M$ jointly follow a central multivariate t distribution with $N - k$ degrees of freedom, and the correlation matrix only depends on the sample sizes and the correlations between the different contrasts. Note, that for the data analysis step the critical value, contrast weights, etc. cannot be taken over from the design stage due to drop-outs, covariate effects, etc. In practice these computations have, therefore, to be re-done at this point.

The final test statistic $T_{\max}$ is based on the maximum contrast test, i.e., $T_{\max} = \max_m T_m$. A dose-response signal is verified if this maximum statistic $T_{\max}$, and thus at least one single contrast test, is statistically significant while controlling the familywise error rate (FWER) at pre-specified level α. Let $q_{1-\alpha}$ denote the multiplicity adjusted critical value. A dose-response signal is then established if $T_{\max} \geq q_{1-\alpha}$. In fact, any dose-response model with a test statistic larger than $q_{1-\alpha}$ can be declared statistically significant at level α. These models then form a reference set $\{M_1, \ldots, M_L\}$ of L significant models, provided $L \geq 1$. Every single contrast test thus translates into a decision procedure, whether a selected dose-response curve is significant given the observed data, while controlling the FWER at pre-specified level α. If no candidate model is statistically significant, the MCP-Mod procedure stops indicating that a dose-response signal cannot be established from the observed data. But such a result does not necessarily mean that the compound has no effect at all. In general we will assess that there was not enough evidence to get statistical significance. Possible reasons could include small sample sizes or high variance. In addition, the initial candidate set might have been poorly chosen, such that the candidate models do not fit the true curve (perhaps an umbrella-shaped curve) – although in such cases the compound has a pronounced effect and may be far from ineffective, as suggested by the insignificant p-value.

The fourth step is to select one or several weighted models out of the reference set of models. Information criteria like AIC or BIC can be used for this purpose.

The fifth and final step consists of fitting the selected model(s) to the data and estimating adequately the target dose(s) of interest using inverse nonlinear regression techniques. Note that in this step all parameters are estimated from the data for the different dose-response models (θ_0, θ_1 and θ_2).

7.2.2 MCP-Mod for General Parametric Models

In this section we describe an extension of the MCP-Mod procedure to acknowledge the fact that in practice the modeling situation and study design are more complex than described above for a normally distributed endpoint. For example, the response variable might be a count, binary, or time-to-event variable instead of being normally distributed. In addition, the final analysis usually has to be adjusted for relevant covariates (e.g. region, age, ...), patients' measurements are often recorded over time (necessitating the use of longitudinal models), and patients might receive more than one treatment (such as in cross-over or incomplete block designs). The core ideas of MCP-Mod remain applicable in these situations, as described here and laid out in [4] in more detail.

Let y denote the response vector of an experimental unit in the trial (e.g., a patient) which has been assigned a dose d (the formulation can easily be extended to the case of multiple doses). We assume that the residual distribution function is given by $y \sim F(z, \eta, \mu(d))$ where $\mu(d)$ denotes the dose-response parameter, η the nuisance parameters, and z possible covariates. The key features of MCP-Mod can then be formulated with respect to $\mu(d)$, including:

- accounting for uncertainty in the dose-response model via a set of candidate dose-response models
- testing for a dose-response signal via optimal contrasts based on plausible dose-response shapes
- model selection or model averaging to combine different models
- dose-response estimation and dose selection using nonlinear regression.

Because all dose-response information is assumed to be represented by $\mu(d)$, the interpretability of this parameter is critical for communicating with clinical teams, choosing candidate dose-response shapes, specifying clinically relevant effects, etc. As an example, consider the Weibull distribution: It is typically parameterized by a scale parameter λ and shape parameter α, neither of which is easily interpretable. For the purpose of interpretability, the model could be re-parameterized in terms of the median time to event $\mu = \log 2^{1/\alpha}/\lambda$ and α, and then use μ as an interpretable dose-response parameter.

Let $\widehat{\mu}$ denote the vector of estimated dose-response parameters under an analysis-of-variance (ANOVA) parameterization, obtained using the appropriate estimation method for the general parametric model above via maximum likelihood (ML), generalized estimating equations, partial likelihood, etc. The key assumption needed for this general version of MCP-Mod to work is that the response estimates $\widehat{\mu}$ at the doses are asymptotically multivariate normally-distributed with covariance matrix Σ. This approximation has been shown to hold for most parametric estimation problems, such as generalized linear models, parametric time-to-event models, mixed-effects models, etc. The MCP step consists of specifying a set of candidate models for the dose-response relationship $\mu(d)$. Similar to the original MCP-Mod approach, each of the candidate model shapes determines an optimal contrast for a trend test to evaluate the associated dose-response model signal. The optimal contrasts are applied to the previously described ANOVA-type estimates $\widehat{\mu}$, with the associated asymptotic distribution used for implementing the corresponding tests (i.e., critical values and p-values). It can be shown that the (optimal) contrast for testing the hypothesis that $c'\mu = 0$ with maximum power for a single given candidate model shape μ_m is proportional to $\Sigma^{-1}\left(\mu_m - \left(\mu_m'\Sigma^{-1}1\right)/\left(1'\Sigma^{-1}1\right)\right)$, which generalizes the formula given in "7.2.1 Original MCP-Mod Approach" on page 194 [4]. From the formula it can be seen that Σ does only have to be known up to proportionality. Once a dose-response signal has been established, one proceeds to the Mod step, fitting the dose-response profile and estimating target doses based on the models identified in the MCP step. There are many ways to fit the dose-response models to the observed data, including approaches based on maximizing the likelihood or the restricted likelihood. Pinheiro et al. suggested an alternative, two-stage approach to dose-response model fitting using generalized least squares to fit the dose-response models obtained from an ANCOVA model fit, which has some computational advantages [4]. Although this approach relies on asymptotic results, it has the appeal of being a general purpose application, because it depends only on $\widehat{\mu}$ and $\widehat{\Sigma}$. The generalized MCP-Mod approach can also be implemented in SAS, as shown later with an example.

7.3 Considerations for MCP-Mod at the Design Stage

One main consideration when implementing MCP-Mod is the choice of the candidate set of models. As a rule of thumb, often 3-7 dose-response shapes, corresponding to 2-4 dose-response models are appropriate. Note that multiple dose-response shapes might be used for each dose-response model because the shapes define the optimal contrasts to be used in the MCP step and the models are those to be fitted in the Mod step. While in general the candidate set should be broad, when there is large uncertainty, one should keep in mind that using a very broad and flexible candidate set does not come for free. Generally the sample size will increase with a broader candidate set of shapes (i.e., contrasts) as the critical value for the MCP step will increase. There is also a trade-off in terms of dose-response model fitting: A broader candidate set will decrease potential bias (in case of a misspecified model) but it will increase the variance of the estimates. To find a good trade-off the following considerations should be taken into account.

- General experience: Thomas et al. showed that in many situations an E_{max} or sigmoid E_{max} model can adequately describe the observed data [5].
- Drug-specific information: Dose-response curves of similar drugs, predictions from earlier phases of development (e.g. using a PK/PD model), or dose-response information of the same drug in a different indication can be used to suggest suitable dose-response shapes.
- Statistical considerations: If only a few active doses are available for use (say, three), it is difficult to fit more complex models (such as the sigmoid E_{max} or the beta model, which both have four parameters), which then would not be included in the candidate set. In these cases one would rather use dose-response models with fewer parameters to obtain an adequate breadth of potential dose-response shapes. Another consideration is to evaluate the consequences of omitting a dose-response shape from the set of candidate models in case it is the true one. This does not necessarily have severe consequences, as other model shapes may be able pick up the omitted model or shape. This can be evaluated for the MCP step (impact on power) using explicit calculations and for the Mod step (impact on precision for dose-response and dose estimation) using simulations [6].

Beyond identifying the candidate set of models, at least two other questions need to be addressed when designing a dose-finding study: (i) How many, and which doses to utilize and, (ii) how many subjects to allocate to the different doses.

Regarding (i) we suggest using 4-7 active dose levels as a rule of thumb and consider at least a tenfold dose range [7]. Equal spacing on the log-scale is commonly used for the dose strengths. More formally one can also consider optimal design theory to calculate doses and allocations to these doses. The essential idea is to use information on the anticipated dose-response curve and then to calculate doses and allocation to these doses so that the covariance matrix of the parameter estimates is minimized in a specified sense. When MCP-Mod is being utilized in a given study, a candidate set of dose-response models has then already been decided upon and this information can be used to calculate, for example, a model-averaged optimal design for calculation of the model parameters (D-optimal design) or estimation of a target dose (c-optimal design). Due to practical constraints in terms of production of the doses and logistics, it might not be possible to use the calculated optimal design directly. But one can also restrict the search for an adequate design to those that are feasible both in terms of logistics and production. Several authors discuss optimal design theory in the context of dose-finding studies [8,9]. Atkinson et al. provide a general background on optimal designs and discuss how to implement those in SAS [10].

Regarding question (ii) above, one can utilize two different approaches for calculating the total sample size, according to the two steps of MCP-Mod. One can consider the MCP step and calculate the sample size so that a specific power is achieved for the multiple contrast test; see [6] for a detailed description of this approach. Alternatively, one can calculate the sample size based on achieving a specified precision for the target dose or the dose-response curve estimate (e.g. by specifying a desired confidence interval width). This typically needs to be done using simulations because closed form expressions are not available. In general, however, one needs to keep in mind that the sample size for detecting a significant trend using the MCP step will often be much smaller than the one that is necessary to determine the dose-response curve and the target dose with sufficient precision (see also the conclusions of the PhRMA working group on adaptive dose-ranging studies in [1]).

Both the determination of dose, as well as sample size calculations, can be performed in SAS, but we do not provide example code for these calculations in this chapter. The related calculations can be performed using, for example, the **DoseFinding** R package, which contains extensive functionality for the design of dose-finding studies [11]. The commercial software package **ADDPLAN-DF** also contains extensive tools for designing dose finding studies using MCP-Mod [12].

7.4 Further Considerations on MCP-Mod

The original MCP-Mod procedure from Bretz et al. was motivated by the work of Tukey et al., who proposed to use several trend tests simultaneously based on different functional dose-response descriptions and subsequently to adjust the resulting p-values for multiplicity [2,13]. Since then, the methodology has been the subject of several investigations. Thomas and Wakana et al. investigated extensions to Bayesian methods for estimating or selecting the dose-response curve from a sparse dose design [14,15]. Klingenberg applied the MCP-Mod approach to proof-of-concept studies with binary responses [16]. Benda proposed a time-dependent dose finding approach with repeated binary data [17]. Akacha and Benda investigated the impact of dropouts on the analysis with recurrent event data [18]. Wouter extended the MCP-Mod approach to investigate longitudinal toxicological data [19]. Tao et al. incorporated both efficacy and safety endpoints through joint modeling [20]. Dette et al., Baayen et al., and Gutjahr and Bornkamp investigated the use of likelihood ratio tests instead of multiple contrast tests [21-23]. Miller, Tanaka, and Franchetti et al. extended the MCP-Mod approach to flexible, two-stage designs that include the possibility to perform adaptations (e.g. adding or dropping doses) under a strict FWER control [24-26]. Dragalin et al., Bornkamp et al., and Vandemeulebroecke et al. investigated the MCP-Mod procedure in response-adaptive designs, addressing two major challenges in dose-finding studies:

uncertainty about the dose-response models and large variability in parameter estimates [27-29].

7.5 Analysis Examples Using SAS

7.5.1 The optcont Macro

In this section we will illustrate the application of MCP-Mod with two examples and show how to implement it using SAS. The first example illustrates the original MCP-Mod procedure for normally distributed data, as described in "7.2.1 Original MCP-Mod Approach" on page 194, using a model selection approach. In this situation **proc glimmix** can be used for the MCP step, because it allows for the calculation of the required multiplicity adjusted p-values. **Proc nlmixed** can be used for fitting the associated nonlinear regression models and estimating target doses. The second example illustrates a more complex application of MCP-Mod in the context of a linear mixed-effect model. In this situation the generalized, two-step MCP-Mod methodology described in "7.2.2 MCP-Mod for General Parametric Models" on page 198 is used. In this example we also illustrate the application of a bootstrap model-averaging approach to perform inferences on the dose-response curve and target doses. **proc glimmix** is used for the MCP step and **proc iml** code is provided for the Mod step for the nonlinear model fit based on general nonlinear-optimization routines. Both examples rely on the calculation of optimal contrasts. For that purpose we first describe in detail a general SAS macro **% optcont** before discussing the specific examples.

The **% optcont** macro implements the optimal contrasts

$$c_{opt} \propto \Sigma^{-1}\left(\mu - \frac{\mu'\Sigma^{-1}1}{1'\Sigma^{-1}1}\right).$$

In order to calculate the optimal contrasts one needs the anticipated mean μ of the response at the individual doses [4]. Typically, the mean responses are determined using dose-response models with given "guesstimates" for the model parameters that determine the shape of the model (see the right column of Table 7.1 on page 196). Note that adding a constant to the mean vector μ or multiplying μ with a constant does not change the optimal contrast. That is, only the relative magnitude of the entries in μ are relevant for calculation of the optimal contrasts. Furthermore, the anticipated covariance matrix Σ needs to be specified as well. As seen from the formula above, the matrix Σ only needs to be known up to a multiplicative constant. To obtain a unique representation, the optimal contrast is standardized by its L_2 norm, i.e. $c_{opt}/\|c_{opt}\|$.

The input parameters of the **% optcont** macro are called **doses**, **models** (determining μ for the different models), **sigma** (determining the matrix sigma), **direction** (either equal to **incr** or **decr**, determining whether an increasing or decreasing value of the response is considered beneficial), and **dosevarname** (determining the name of the dose variable in the data set and the output). The input arguments **doses**, **models** and **sigma** need to be provided manually through a separate data set or extracted via **ODS** from a suitable SAS procedure. The **models** data set needs to be exactly in the format given in the example below, i.e., have columns **modnam**, **par1**, **par2** and **par3**, with missing values specified for the parameters when the models have less than three parameters. For the column names of the **sigma** data set no specific names need to be used. Given these input arguments, the macro generates a SAS data set called **optcontrasts** that contains the optimal contrasts for the different model shapes. In addition, it creates a global macro variable called **modcontr** that contains the string of the candidate models names and contrasts, which then can be used inside an **estimate** statement without re-typing them. The dose variable name that is used in the **modcontr** estimate statement is determined by the variable **dosevarname**. The code for the macro is provided in “Appendix A ” on page 213.

7.5.2 Example 1: biom Data with Normally Distributed Outcome and Model Selection

This example uses the **biom** data set from the **DoseFinding** R package [11]. The data set in Example Code 7.1 on page 202 has also been used in [2] to illustrate MCP-Mod. This was a randomized, double-blind parallel group trial with a total of 100 patients being allocated equally to either a placebo or one of four active doses coded as 0.05, 0.20, 0.60, and 1.

Example Code 7.1 *The biom Data*

```
data biom;
    input dose resp @@;
    datalines;
 0.05  1.3538
 0.05  0.1550
 0.05 -0.0708
 0.05  0.5837
 0.05  0.9626
 0.05  0.3814
 0.05 -0.0047
 0.05  0.5193
 0.05 -0.3633
 0.05  0.3389
 0.05  0.1456
 0.05  0.4428
 0.05 -0.0219
 0.05  0.3726
 0.05  1.5290
 0.05  0.1495
 0.05  0.3741
 0.05  1.0117
 0.05  0.2813
 0.05  0.9947
 0.20  1.1981
 0.20  1.5677
 0.20 -0.1556
 0.20  0.2066
 0.20  1.8535
 0.20  0.9957
 0.20  2.4522
 0.20 -0.5204
 0.20  0.0489
 0.20  0.6331
 0.20  0.5284
 0.20  0.4229
 0.20  1.2333
 0.20  1.8678
 0.20  1.0578
 0.20  0.3453
 0.20  0.4049
```

```
0.20  0.4842
0.20  0.5712
0.20  1.0107
0.60  1.1722
0.60  0.6676
0.60  1.7777
0.60  0.3097
0.60  0.0565
0.60  0.9001
0.60  0.7383
0.60  0.2279
0.60  1.3851
0.60  0.9124
0.60  0.2993
0.60  0.2789
0.60  0.2700
0.60  0.5696
0.60  1.6043
0.60  1.5769
0.60  2.9245
0.60  0.1715
0.60  2.1605
0.60  0.6856
1.00  2.2484
1.00  2.1737
1.00  1.2545
1.00  1.8646
1.00 -1.1131
1.00  1.1984
1.00  1.9749
1.00  0.6253
1.00  1.3303
1.00  0.1495
1.00  0.8871
1.00  0.5631
1.00  0.7309
1.00 -0.7715
1.00  0.4948
1.00  0.3031
1.00  0.4252
1.00  2.5578
1.00  1.1289
1.00  0.9483
0.00  0.3546
0.00  0.1365
0.00 -0.0172
0.00  0.3675
0.00  0.3951
0.00  0.3580
0.00  0.3129
0.00 -0.0449
0.00  0.6231
0.00  0.0395
0.00 -0.3084
0.00 -0.4530
0.00 -0.2017
```

```
    0.00  1.5609
    0.00  0.5613
    0.00  0.3362
    0.00 -0.1594
    0.00  0.9926
    0.00  0.8070
    0.00  1.2374;
run;
```

Compared to the original publication, for illustrative purposes we use a different set of candidate shapes here. Assume that it was decided to use the following shapes for the contrast test: Two E_{max} model shapes (one corresponding to $ED_{50} = 0.05$ and one corresponding to $ED_{50} = 0.2$), an exponential model shape with $\delta = 0.3$, a linear shape, a quadratic shape with $\delta = -0.8$ and a sigmoid E_{max} model shape with $ED_{50} = 0.2$ and Hill parameter, $h = 3$ (see Table 7.1 on page 196 for the general model definitions). Since we assume homogeneous variances across doses and the sample sizes are balanced, the covariance matrix Σ for contrast calculation is proportional to the identity matrix (Example Code 7.2 on page 204).

Example Code 7.2 *Contrasts for biom Data*

```
data doses;
   input dose @@;
   datalines;
      0 0.05 0.2 0.6 1
   ;
run;

/* equal sample size and variances: can use identity matrix
for calculation of optimal contrasts */
data scalemat;
   input c1-c5 @@;
   datalines;
      1 0 0 0 0
      0 1 0 0 0
      0 0 1 0 0
      0 0 0 1 0
      0 0 0 0 1
   ;
run;

data models;
    length modnam $25;
    input modnam par1-par3;
    datalines;
        emax 0.05 . .
        emax 0.2  . .
        exponential 0.3 . .
        linear  . . .
        quadratic -0.8 . .
        sigEmax 0.2 3 .
        ;
run;

/*Write optimal contrasts in data set optcontrasts and in global
macro variable modcontr */
```

```
%optcont(models=models, doses=doses, sigma=scalemat, direction=incr,
dosevarname=dose);

proc print data=optcontrasts label noobs;
   title "Optimal contrasts for defined models";
run;

data _null_;
   call execute ("
      proc glimmix data=biom;
         class dose;
         model resp = dose  /NOINT solution COVB ;
         estimate &modcontr.
         / adjust=simulate(nsamp=1000000 seed=1) uppertailed;
      run;
   ");
run;
```

Running this **% optcont** macro once generates the optimal contrasts given in Table 7.2 on page 205, rounded to 2 digits. One can directly use those contrasts to calculate the test statistics and multiplicity adjusted p-values using the **proc glimmix** call at the bottom of Example Code 7.2 on page 204.

Table 7.2 *Optimal Contrasts for the Candidate Shapes for the biom Data*

Dose	E_{max} $(ED_{50} = 0.05)$	E_{max} $(ED_{50} = 0.2)$	**Exponential** $(\delta = 0.3)$	**Linear**	**Quadratic** $(\delta = -0.8)$	**Sigmoid** E_{max} $(ED_{50} = 0.2, h = 3)$
0	-0.80	-0.64	-0.30	-0.44	-0.59	-0.51
0.05	-0.17	-0.36	-0.29	-0.38	-0.39	-0.49
0.2	0.21	0.06	-0.26	-0.20	0.09	0.01
0.6	0.36	0.41	-0.02	0.27	0.67	0.48
1	0.40	0.53	0.87	0.74	0.22	0.51

The **call execute** function is necessary, because the contrasts are stored in the **modcontr** macro variable and need to be resolved before **proc glimmix** gets executed. This call produces the test statistics and adjusted p-values in Table 7.3 on page 205. In this case, all models produce relatively small p-values, indicating a strong evidence for existence of a dose-response effect.

Table 7.3 *Results of the Contrast Test for the biom Data*

Model Shape	**Test Statistic**	**Adjusted p-value**
$E_{max}(ED_{50} = 0.05)$	3.34	0.0018
$E_{max}(ED_{50} = 0.2)$	3.46	0.0012
Exponential $(\delta = 0.3)$	2.26	0.0323

Model Shape	Test Statistic	Adjusted p-value
Linear	2.97	0.0053
Quadratic ($\delta = -0.8$)	3.29	0.0021
Sigmoid E_{max} $(ED_{50} = 0.2, h = 3)$	3.41	0.0014

Fitting the individual models can be done with `proc nlmixed`. In “Appendix B” on page 216 we provide SAS code to fit all nonlinear regression models that are used in the `biom` data example and compare them using the AIC criterion. The AIC values for the different models are given in Table 7.4 on page 206. It can be seen that the E_{max} model provides the lowest AIC and is therefore selected.

Table 7.4 AIC Values for Fitted Models for the biom Data

Model	AIC
E_{max}	219.1
Exponential	223.1
Linear	220.5
Quadratic	219.7
Sigmoid E_{max}	220.8

The final step consists of fitting the E_{max} model and estimating the target dose of interest. In our example, the dose achieving a target effect of 0.4 over the placebo is given by 0.16. A plot of the fitted model shown as a difference to the placebo with confidence intervals, and the estimated target dose achieving an effect of 0.4 are given in Figure 7.2 on page 207. The code for this figure is presented in “Appendix C” on page 218.

Figure 7.2 *Estimated Dose-Response Curve for the biom Data*

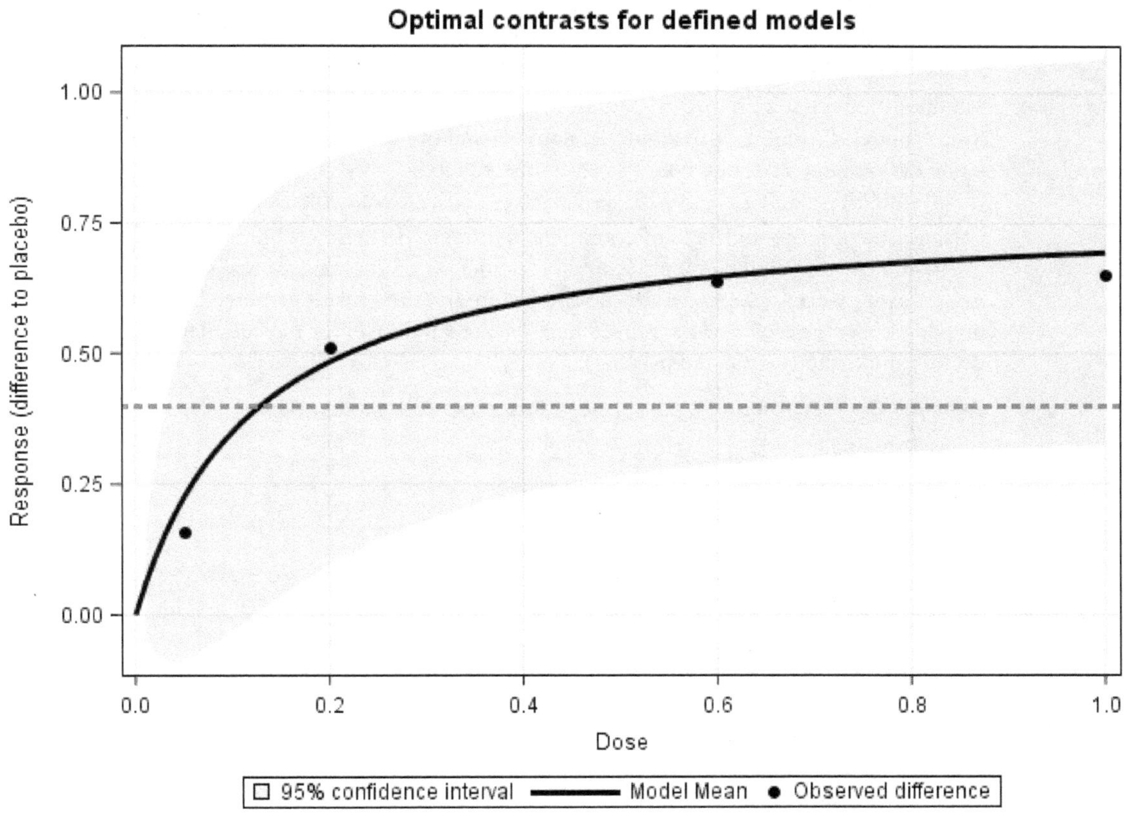

7.5.3 Example 2: neurodeg Data for Generalized MCP-Mod Approach with Model Averaging

The second example concerns simulated data from [4] to illustrate the use of the generalized MCP-Mod approach. The data set is available under the name **`neurodeg`** from the **`DoseFinding`** R package. The SAS code used for the computations and summarization of all results can be found in "Appendix D" on page 219.

This example refers to a phase II clinical study for a neurodegenerative disease. The disease status is measured through a functional scale, with smaller values corresponding to more severe neurodegeneration. The goal of the drug is to reduce the rate of disease progression, which is measured by the linear slope of the functional scale over time.

The trial design includes a placebo and four doses: 1, 3, 10, and 30 mg, with balanced allocation of 50 patients per arm. Patients are followed up for one year, with measurements of the functional scale being taken at baseline and every three months thereafter. The study goals are to (i) test for a dose-response signal, (ii) estimate the dose-response, and (iii) select a dose to be brought into the confirmatory stage of the development program.

The functional scale response is assumed to be normally distributed and, based on historical data, it is believed that the longitudinal progression of the functional scale over the one year of follow up can be modeled by a simple linear trend. A mixed model is assumed for the functional scale for the measurement y_{ij} of patient i at time j,

$y_{ij} = (\beta_0 + b_{0i}) + (\mu(x) + b_{1i})t_{ij} + \epsilon_{ij}$, $[b_{0i}, b_{1i}] \sim N(0, \Omega)$ and $\epsilon_{ij} \sim N(0, \sigma^2)$.

Consequently, the dose-response parameter of interest in this situation is $\mu(d)$, the slope of disease progression associated with the dose d. Assume that the candidate models for $\mu(x)$ in this example include an $E_{\max}$ model with $ED_{50} = 1.11$, a quadratic model with maximum effect at 23 mg ($\delta = -0.022$), an exponential model with $\delta = 8.867$ and a linear model. Fitting the mixed model above using the **proc glimmix** call in Example Code 7.3 on page 208, one obtains the estimated slopes $\widehat{\mu} = (-5.099, \ -4.581, \ -3.220, \ -2.879, \ -3.520)'$ with corresponding estimated variance-covariance matrix $\widehat{\Sigma}$ of compound symmetry structure with diagonal elements 0.149 and off-diagonal elements 0.0094. Calculation of the contrast test statistics and p-values using **proc glimmix** for the MCP step gives the result displayed in Table 7.5 on page 208. **proc glimmix** is used here because it allows for the calculation of the desired multiplicity-adjusted p-values.

Example Code 7.3 *Mixed-Model of Dose Response for neurodeg Data*

```
proc glimmix data=neurodeg;
   class dose id;
   model resp= dose*time/solution COVB ;
   random intercept time / type=UN subject=id;
   estimate &modcontr. / adjust=simulate(nsamp=1000000 seed=1) uppertailed;
run;
```

Table 7.5 *Contrast Test Statistics for the neurodeg Data*

Model	Test Statistic	Adjusted p-value
$E_{\max}(ED_{50} = 1.11)$	4.56	<.0001
Quadratic $\delta = -0.022$	3.68	0.0003
Exponential ($\delta = 8.867$)	1.28	0.1826
Linear	2.27	0.0252

It can be seen that all models, apart from the exponential one, achieve a small p-value. Thus, there is evidence for the existence of a dose-response effect, with the $E_{\max}$ and the quadratic shape obtaining the highest test statistics.

The Mod step in this example implements a bootstrap model averaging approach. The idea is to simulate a large number B of values $\boldsymbol{\mu}^{(b)}$ from the 5-dimensional normal distribution with mean $\widehat{\boldsymbol{\mu}}$ and covariance matrix $\widehat{\boldsymbol{\Sigma}}$. For each of the generated bootstrap data sets, each of the four dose-response models are fitted to the simulated summaries per group using the generalized least squares estimation approach discussed in [4]. That is the function $\Psi_{\mathrm{m}}(\boldsymbol{\theta_m}) = \left(f_m(d, \boldsymbol{\theta_m}) - \boldsymbol{\mu}^{(b)}\right)'\widehat{\boldsymbol{\Sigma}}^{-1}\left(f_m(d, \boldsymbol{\theta_m}) - \boldsymbol{\mu}^{(b)}\right)$ is minimized with respect to $\boldsymbol{\theta}$ for all candidate models. An AIC-type value to compare the model adequacy can be calculated by using $\Psi_{\mathrm{m}}(\widehat{\boldsymbol{\theta}}_{\boldsymbol{m}}) + 2\dim(\widehat{\boldsymbol{\theta}}_{\boldsymbol{m}})$. At the end one can select for each simulated replication b the dose-response model that provides the best fit and use this to predict the quantity of interest (for example a target dose or the dose-response estimate at specific doses). The bootstrapping approach is implemented in **proc iml**, and details can be found in "Appendix D" on page 219. In some of the bootstrap resamples for some models the optimization fails with a warning message. We suspect this happens for models that cannot be fit or are inadequate for the current bootstrap resample. In this case these error messages had no impact on the overall results.

In Figure 7.3 on page 209 one can observe the bootstrapped dose-response curve based on 5,000 boostrap samples. One can see that the estimated curve shows a slight unimodality, which is introduced because the point estimate for the slope at dose 30mg is slightly smaller than for 10mg and 3mg. Looking at how often each model was selected in the bootstrap resamples, one obtains 54% of for the E_{max} model and 46% for the quadratic model. For the **neurodeg** data set the linear and exponential model can clearly be ruled out, but both the E_{max} as well as the quadratic model seem to describe the data adequately. Selecting one model over another model in such a situation is potentially problematic, because it does not represent the underlying uncertainty adequately. Using a model-averaging approach seems more realistic in this example.

Figure 7.3 *Estimated Dose-Response Curve for Slopes of Disease Progression for neurodeg Data*

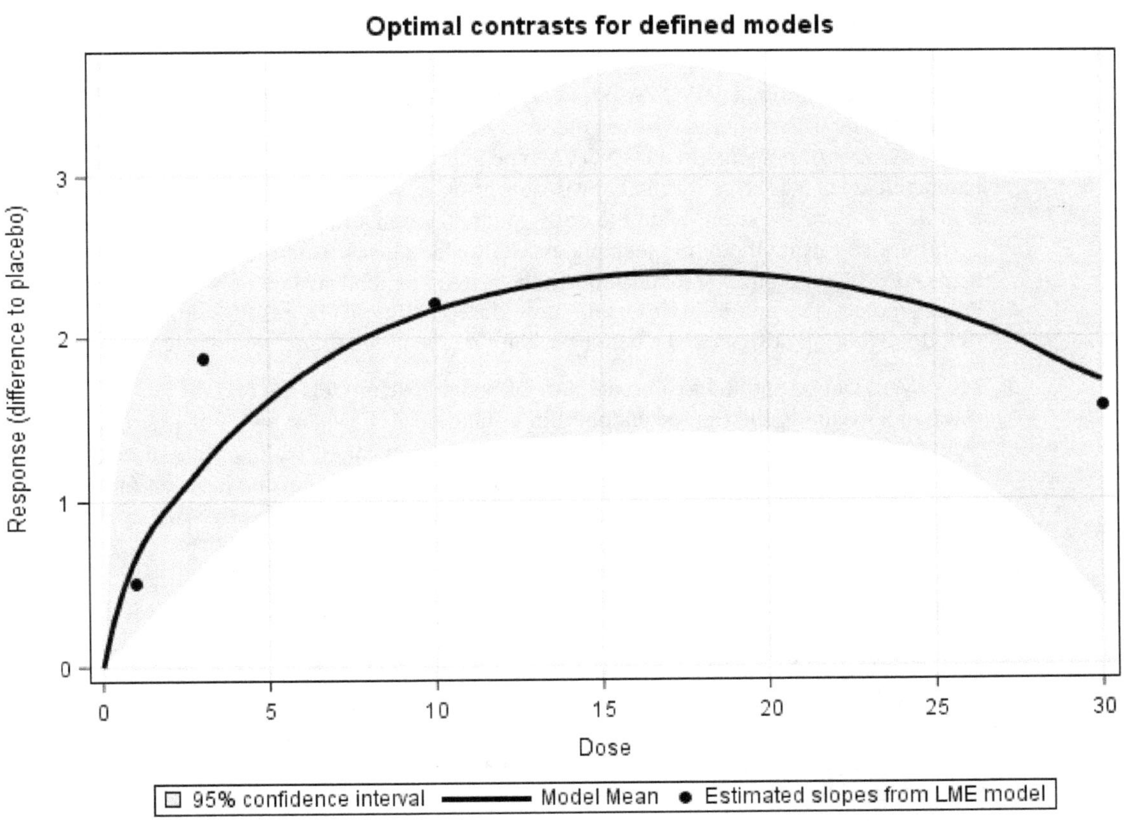

7.6 Conclusions

Current dose-finding practices often are not satisfactory: Many dose-finding studies are not properly designed (too few doses, dose-ranges too narrow, sample sizes not large enough, etc.) and the inferences drawn from them are not adequately accurate, thus leading to major consequences in drug development that are undesirable (e.g., high failure rate in phase III, need for label changes after approval, etc.).

Here, we have described a unified strategy for analyzing dose-finding studies, including the testing for a dose-response signal and the selection of one or more doses to take into further development. The proposed methodology combines the advantages of the multiple comparison and modeling approaches, consisting of a multistage procedure. Dose-response is tested in the first stage, using multiple comparison methods to identify statistically significant contrasts corresponding to a set of candidate models. If a dose-response signal is established in the first stage, the best model is then used for dose-response and target-dose estimation. Different model-based dose selection methods, incorporating both statistical significance and clinical relevance, were presented and evaluated via the analysis of real and simulated data.

The MCP part of the proposed method is seen to maintain the FWER at its nominal level, has power comparable to the standard trend tests under monotone dose-response settings, and is better under non-monotone scenarios, provided the set of candidate models is broad enough. The clear advantage of this new approach, in comparison to more traditional multiple comparison dose-finding methods, is its added flexibility in searching for and identifying an adequate dose for future drug development through the use of modeling techniques. Several variants of the proposed methods are possible and have been investigated in the literature.

Compared to traditional ANOVA-based pairwise multiple comparisons, MCP-Mod has the advantage of enabling the use of more doses in the design, without requiring a much larger number of patients. In an ANOVA-type approach, only the information from the respective dose is used to estimate the dose-response, which means that the required sample size depends strongly on the doses studied, when a fixed precision is required at each dose. By using modeling techniques MCP-Mod allows us to interpolate information across dose-levels, and the total sample size will not depend strongly on the number of doses studied. The possibility of using more doses will typically result in information-rich dose-finding designs and a better basis for decision making at end of phase II.

MCP-Mod can be applied to a broad class of parametric models beyond the standard setup of a normally distributed endpoint in a standard ANOVA model. For example, the response variable might be a count, binary, or time-to-event variable instead of being normally distributed. For the generalized MCP-Mod all that is needed is an estimate of the response at the doses, as well as the associated covariance matrix. In SAS, different methods can be used to produce these estimates. `proc glimmix` is probably the most general procedure and might thus be recommended for most situations. Another advantage is that it produces the adequate multiplicity adjusted p-values. The Mod step of the procedure can then be performed using the `proc iml` code provided, which is quite flexible, and does not depend on the underlying distribution of the endpoint. Of course, other procedures, such as `proc nlin` or `proc nlmixed` could also be used for the Mod step. In addition, the final analysis has usually to be adjusted for relevant covariates (e.g. region, age, etc.), patients' measurements are often recorded over time (necessitating the use of longitudinal models), and patients might receive more than one treatment (such as in cross-over or incomplete block designs). In this chapter we have illustrated with two real data sets, how to use the MCP-Mod approach in practice. Furthermore, we have provided relevant SAS code that should enable the interested reader to implement and perform the MCP-Mod approach in many situations of practical relevance. An alternative possibility to implement MCP-Mod is via the **`DoseFinding`** R package [11], which contains extensive functionality both for the design and the analysis of dose-finding studies. The commercial software package **`ADDPLAN-DF`** contains extensive tools for designing dose-finding studies using MCP-Mod [12]. In addition, Cytel has developed **`PROC MCPMOD`** as an add-on to SAS that focuses on the analysis of dose-finding studies using MCP-Mod.

References

1. Bornkamp B, Bretz F, Dmitrienko A, Enas G, Gaydos B, Hsu CH, Koenig F, Krams M, Liu Q, Neuenschwander B, Parke T, Pinheiro J, Roy A, Sax R, & Shen F. (2007). Innovative approaches for designing and analyzing adaptive dose-ranging trials (with discussion). *Journal of Biopharmaceutical Statistics* 17: 965-995.

2. Bretz F, Pinheiro J & Branson M. (2005). Combining multiple comparisons and modeling techniques in dose-response studies. *Biometrics* 61: 738-748.

3. European Medicines Agency. (2014). Qualification opinion of MCP-Mod as an efficient statistical methodology for model-based design and analysis of Phase II dose-finding studies under model uncertainty. Available at: http://www.ema.europa.eu/docs/en_GB/document_library/Regulatory_and_procedural_guideline/2014/02/WC500161027.pdf (http://www.ema.europa.eu/docs/en_GB/document_library/Regulatory_and_procedural_guideline/2014/02/WC500161027.pdf).

4. Pinheiro J, Bornkamp B, Glimm E & Bretz F. (2014). Multiple comparisons and modeling for dose finding using general parametric models. *Statistics in Medicine* 33: 1646-1661.

5. Thomas N, Sweeney K & Somayaji V. (2014). Meta-analysis of clinical dose response in a large drug development portfolio. *Statistics in Biopharmaceutical Research* 6: 302-317.

6. Pinheiro J, Bornkamp B & Bretz F. (2006). Design and analysis of dose finding studies combining multiple comparisons and modeling procedures. *Journal of Biopharmaceutical Statistics* 16: 639-656.

7. European Medicines Agency. (2015). Report from Dose Finding Workshop. Available at: http://www.ema.europa.eu/docs/en_GB/document_library/Report/2015/04/WC500185864.pdf (http://www.ema.europa.eu/docs/en_GB/document_library/Report/2015/04/WC500185864.pdf).

8. Dette H, Bretz F, Pepelyshev A & Pinheiro JC. (2008). Optimal designs for dose finding studies. *Journal of the American Statistical Association* 103: 1225-1237.

9. Bretz F, Dette H, & Pinheiro J. (2010). Practical considerations for optimal designs in clinical dose finding studies. *Statistics in Medicine* 29: 731-742.

10. Atkinson A, Donev A & Tobias R. (2007). *Optimum Experimental Design with SAS.* Oxford, UK: Oxford University Press.

11. Bornkamp B, Pinheiro J & Bretz F. (2014). DoseFinding: Planning and analyzing dose finding experiments, R package, version 0.9-12, Available at: http://CRAN.R-project.org/package=DoseFinding (http://cran.r-project.org/package=DoseFinding).

12. ADDPLAN DF. (2013). Adaptive Designs – Plans and Analysis. DF Version 3.1. (Software Documentation.) Cologne: ADDPLAN GmbH. http://www.addplan.com (http://www.addplan.com/).

13. Tukey JW, Ciminera JL & Heyse JF. (1985). Testing the statistical certainty of a response to increasing doses of a drug. *Biometrics* 41: 295-301.

14. Thomas N. (2006). Hypothesis testing and Bayesian estimation using a sigmoid Emax model applied to sparse dose response designs. *Journal of Biopharmaceutical Statistics* 16: 657-677.

15. Wakana A, Yoshimura I & Hamada C. (2007). A method for therapeutic dose selection in a phase II clinical trial using contrast statistics. *Statistics in Medicine* 26: 498-511.

16. Klingenberg B. (2009). Proof of concept and dose estimation with binary responses under model uncertainty. *Statistics in Medicine* 28: 274-292.

17. Benda N. (2010). Model-based approaches for time-dependent dose finding with repeated binary data. *Statistics in Medicine* 29: 1096-1106.

18. Akacha M & Benda N. (2010). The impact of dropouts on the analysis of dose-finding studies with recurrent event data. *Statistics in Medicine* 29: 1635-1646.

19. Wouter W. (2012). The power and type I error of statistical analysis approaches for longitudinal toxicological data. M.Sc. thesis, University of Gent.

20. Tao A, Lin Y, Pinheiro J & Shih WS. (2015). Dose finding method in joint modeling of efficacy and safety endpoints in phase II studies. *International Journal of Statistics and Probability* 4: 33-45.

21. Dette H, Titoff S, Volgushev S & Bretz F. (2015). Model identification for dose response signal detection. *Biometrics*. DOI: 10.1111/biom.12357.

22. Baayen C, Hougaard P & Pipper B. (2015). Testing effect of a drug using multiple nested models for the dose-response. *Biometrics* 71: 417-427.

23. Gutjahr G & Bornkamp B. (2015). Likelihood ratio tests for a dose-response effect using multiple nonlinear regression models. *Technical Report, Cornell University Library.* Available at: http://arxiv.org/abs/1510.06253 (http://arxiv.org/abs/1510.06253).

24. Miller F. (2010). Adaptive dose-finding: Proof of concept with type I error control. *Biometrical Journal* 52: 577-589.

25. Tanaka Y. (2011). An adaptive two-stage dose-response design method for establishing proof of concept in drug development. PhD thesis, University of Pittsburgh.

26. Franchetti Y, Anderson S & Sampson A. (2013). An adaptive two-stage dose-response design method for establishing proof-of-concept. *Journal of Biopharmaceutical Statistics* 23: 1124-1154.

27. Dragalin V, Bornkamp B, Bretz F, Miller F, Padmanabhan SK, Patel N, Perevozskaya I, Pinheiro J & Smith JR. (2010). A simulation study to compare new adaptive dose-ranging designs. *Statistics in Biopharmaceutical Research* 2: 487-512.

28. Bornkamp B, Bretz F, Dette H & Pinheiro J. (2011). Response-adaptive dose-finding under model uncertainty. *Annals of Applied Statistics* 5(2B): 1611-1631.

29. Vandemeulebroecke M, Bretz F, Pinheiro J & Bornkamp B. (2011). Adaptive dose-ranging studies. In: Pong A & Chow SC, eds. *Handbook of Adaptive Designs in Pharmaceutical and Clinical Development.* Boca Raton, Florida: CRC Press.

Authors

Björn Bornkamp, Senior Expert Statistical Methodologist, Novartis, Basel, Switzerland.

Vladimir Bezlyak, Senior Principal Biostatistician, Novartis, Basel, Switzerland.

Frank Bretz, Global Head of the Statistical Methodology and Consulting Group, Novartis, Basel, Switzerland.

Appendix

Appendix A

Example Code 7.4 *Code for %optcont Macro*

```
%macro optcont(doses=,
   models=,
   sigma=,
   direction=,
   dosevarname=);
   /***********************************************************************
   Reading in models
   ***********************************************************************/
   data &models;
      set &models;
      length modspec $ 50;

      if compress(modnam)="emax" then
         do modelnum=1;
            modspec="emax "!!compress("(ed50="!!par1!!")");
         end;
      if compress(modnam)="exponential" then
         do modelnum=2;
            modspec="exponential "!!compress("(delta="!!par1!!")");
         end;
      if compress(modnam)="linear" then
         do modelnum=3;
            modspec=modnam;
         end;
      if compress(modnam)="linlog" then
         do modelnum=4;
            modspec="linlog "!!compress("(off="!!par1!!")");
         end;
      if compress(modnam)="quadratic" then
         do modelnum=5;
            modspec="quadratic "!!compress("(delta="!!par1!!")");
         end;
      if compress(modnam)="sigEmax" then
         do modelnum=6;
            modspec="sigemax "!!compress("(ed50="!!par1!!", h="!!par2!!")");
         end;
      if compress(modnam)="betaMod" then
         do modelnum=7;
            modspec="betamod "!!compress("(del1="!!par1!!", del2="!!par2!!",
               scal="!!par3!!")");
         end;
   run;

   proc sql noprint;
```

```
   select count(distinct(dose))format=1.0 into :n_dose_ from &doses;
quit;

proc sql noprint;
   select count(modelnum) into :n_mod_ from &models;
quit;

proc sql noprint;
   select modnam into :mod1 - :mod%left(&n_mod_) from &models;
quit;

proc sql noprint;
   select modspec into :modspec1 - :modspec%left(&n_mod_) from &models;
quit;

%if &direction=incr %then %do; %let dir=1; %end;
%if &direction=decr %then %do; %let dir=-1; %end;

/**********************************************************************
Calculation of contrasts
 **********************************************************************/
proc iml ;
   /* read in doses, covariance mat, models/guesstimates and model names*/
   use &doses var {dose };
   read all into dose;
   use &sigma;
   read all into sigma;
   use &models;
   read all var{modelnum par1 par2 par3} into par;
   use &models;
   read all var{modnam} into modlist;

   /* Unity matrix */
   unity=j(&n_dose_, 1, 1);

   /* Empty matrix for calculated mean vectors and contrasts */
   meanmat=j(&n_dose_, &n_mod_+1, -88);
   meanmat[, 1]=dose;

   /* row labels */
   contmat=j(&n_dose_, &n_mod_, -88);

   /* calculation of stand. mean-vector for each model*/
   do j=2 to &n_mod_+1;
      modnum=par[j-1, 1];
      do i=1 to &n_dose_;   /* for each dose*/
         if modnum=1 then
            meanmat[i, j]=dose[i]/(par[j-1, 2] + dose[i]);
         if modnum=2 then
            meanmat[i, j]=exp(dose[i]/par[j-1, 2]) - 1;
         if modnum=3 then
            meanmat[i, j]=dose[i];
         if modnum=4 then
            meanmat[i, j]=log(dose[i] + par[j-1, 2]);
         if modnum=5 then
            meanmat[i, j]=dose[i] + par[j-1, 2]*dose[i]**2;
```

```
         if modnum=6 then
            meanmat[i, j]=dose[i]**par[j-1, 3]/(par[j-1, 2]**par[j-1,
               3] + dose[i]**par[j-1, 3]);
         if modnum=7 then
            do;
               maxDens=(par[j-1, 2]**par[j-1, 2]) * (par[j-1,
                  3]**par[j-1, 3])/((par[j-1, 2] + par[j-1,
                  3])**(par[j-1, 2] + par[j-1, 3]));
               standdose=dose[i]/par[j-1, 4];
               meanmat[i, j]=1/maxDens * (standdose**par[j-1, 2]) *
                  (1 - standdose)**par[j-1, 3];
            end;
      end;
   end;
   invsigma=inv(sigma);

   do j=2 to &n_mod_+1;      /* calculation of contrasts*/
      mean_t=t(meanmat[, j]);
      _1=mean_t*invsigma*unity;
      _2=t(unity)*invsigma*unity;
      _3=_1/_2;
      _4=_3*unity;
      _5=meanmat[, j]-_4;
      contrast=invsigma*_5;
      c_norm=sqrt(ssq(contrast));
      contmat[, j-1]=&dir*contrast/c_norm;
   end;
   create optcontrasts from contmat;

   /* Export the final contrasts to dataset*/
   append from contmat;
   quit;

data &models;
   set &models;
   i=_n_;
run;

data _null_;
   set &models;
   do j=1 to &n_mod_;
      if j=i then
         do;
            call execute ("
data optcontrasts; set optcontrasts;
attrib col"!!compress(j)!!" label='"!!compress(modnam)!!"';
  run;");
         end;
   end;

data optcontrasts;
   merge &doses(keep=dose) optcontrasts;
run;

/************************************************************************
Add labels to contrast matrix and
```

```
    create string of the contrasts to be used in estimate statement
    *********************************************************************/
    %global modcontr;
    %let modcontr=;

    %do i=1 %to &n_mod_;
       %let k=%eval(&i);

       data optcontrasts;
          set optcontrasts;
          attrib col&i label="&&modspec&k.";

       proc sql noprint;
          select col&i.
        into :cont_&i. separated by '   ' from optcontrasts;
       quit;

       %let type = &&modspec&k;

       %if %eval(&i < &n_mod_) %then
          %do;
             %let modcontr = &modcontr. %str(%'&&modspec&i.%') &dosevarname
             &&cont_&i.%str(,);
          %end;
       %else %if %eval(&i=&n_mod_) %then
          %do;
             %let modcontr = &modcontr. %str(%'&&modspec&i.%') &dosevarname
             &&cont_&i. ;
          %end;
    %end;
%mend;
```

Appendix B

Example Code 7.5 *Code to Fit Dose-Response Models in Example 1*

```
/***********************************************************************
Fit all models & compare AIC values
 ***********************************************************************/

/* emax model */
proc nlmixed data=biom;
   ods output FitStatistics=fitem;
   parms e0=0.3 emax=1 ed50=1 sigma=1;
   bounds 0.001 < ed50 < 1.5;   /* bound for ed50: [0.001,1.5]*maxDose */
   mn=e0 + emax*dose/(dose + ed50);
   model resp ~ normal(mn, sigma**2);
run;

data fitem;
   set fitem(where=(descr='AIC (smaller is better)'));
   model="emax";
   drop descr;
run;

/* exponential model */
```

```
proc nlmixed data=biom;
   ods output FitStatistics=fitexpo;
   parms e0=0.3 e1=1 delta=1 sigma=1;
   bounds 0.1 < delta < 2;   /* bound for delta: [0.1,2]*maxDose */
   mn=e0 + e1*(exp(dose/delta)-1);
   model resp ~ normal(mn, sigma**2);
run;

data fitexpo;
   set fitexpo(where=(descr='AIC (smaller is better)'));
   model="expo";
   drop descr;
run;

/* linear model (could also be fit with other procedures!) */
proc nlmixed data=biom;
   ods output FitStatistics=fitlin;
   parms e0=0.3 delta=1;
   mn=e0 + delta*dose;
   model resp ~ normal(mn, sigma**2);
run;

data fitlin;
   set fitlin(where=(descr='AIC (smaller is better)'));
   model="lin";
   drop descr;
run;

/* quadratic model (could also be fit with other procedures!) */
proc nlmixed data=biom;
   ods output FitStatistics=fitquad;
   parms e0=0.3 b1=1 b2=1 sigma=1;
   mn=e0 + b1*dose + b2*dose**2;
   model resp ~ normal(mn, sigma**2);
run;

data fitquad;
   set fitquad(where=(descr='AIC (smaller is better)'));
   model="quad";
   drop descr;
run;

/* sigmoid Emax model */
proc nlmixed data=biom;
   ods output FitStatistics=fitsig;
   parms e0=0.3 emax=1 ed50=1 h=1 sigma=1;
   bounds 0.001 < ed50 < 1.5, 0.5 < h < 10;   /* bound for h: [0.5,10] */
   if dose=0 then
      mn=e0;
   if dose > 0 then
      mn=e0 + emax*dose**h/(dose**h + ed50**h);
   model resp ~ normal(mn, sigma**2);
run;

data fitsig;
   set fitsig(where=(descr='AIC (smaller is better)'));
```

```
   model="sigemax";
   drop descr;
run;

data aics;
   set fitem fitexpo fitlin fitquad fitsig;
run;
/* compare AICs of different fitted models */
proc print data=aics;
run;

/* emax model has best AIC value */
```

Appendix C

Example Code 7.6 *Code to Produce Plot for Example 1*

```
/**********************************************************************
Create a plot showing the results
 **********************************************************************/
/* data set containing where to predict dose-response curves */
data biompredict;
   do i=1 to 100;
      dosepred=(i-1)/99;
      output;
   end;
   drop i;
run;

data biompredict;
   merge biom biompredict;
run;

/* model fit */
%let deltadiff=0.4;

/* fit emax model and predict at specified grid of dose values */
proc nlmixed data=biompredict;
   ods output FitStatistics=fitem;
   parms e0=0.3 emax=1 ed50=1 sigma=1;
   bounds 0.001 < ed50 < 1.5;
   mn=e0 + emax*dose/(dose + ed50);
   model resp ~ normal(mn, sigma**2);
   predict emax*dosepred/(dosepred + ed50) out=predout;
   estimate 'TD' &deltadiff * ed50/(emax - &deltadiff);
run;

/* create adjusted raw means for plot */
proc sql;
  create table adj_means as
  select distinct(dose), mean(resp) as mean_resp
  from biom
  group by dose;
run;

data adj_means;
```

```
   set adj_means;
   if dose=0 then mean0=mean_resp;
   retain mean0;
   if dose ne 0 then diff=mean_resp-mean0;
run;

data predout;
   set predout adj_means;
   refline=0.4;
run;

/* plot dose-response curve confidence intervals and adjusted raw means */
proc sgplot data=predout;
   xaxis grid label="Dose";
   yaxis grid label="Response (difference to placebo)";
   band x=dosepred lower=lower upper=upper /transparency=0.5
      legendlabel="95% confidence interval";
   series x=dosepred y=pred /legendlabel="Model Mean" lineattrs=(thickness=3);
   scatter x=dose y=diff / markerattrs=(symbol=circlefilled)
      legendlabel="Observed difference";
   refline refline / lineattrs=(thickness=2 color=red pattern=shortdash)
      legendlabel="Target Difference";
run;
```

Appendix D

Complete data are available in the supplemental materials.

Example Code 7.7 *Code to Produce Results for Example 2*

```
data neurodeg;
   input resp id dose time @@;
   datalines;
191.70155   1    0    0 178.39954   1    0    3 167.33850   1    0
6 149.50935   1    0    9 131.45853   1    0   12

…

205.09590 250   30    0 175.24421 250   30    3 152.41340 250   30
6 113.48094 250   30    9  84.95754 250   30   12
;

   /* # of doses */
proc sql noprint;
   select count(distinct(dose))format=1.0 into :n_dose from neurodeg;
quit;

/* initial model to obtain the matrix for calculation of the contrasts */
ods output CovB=Omega (keep=effect col2-col6)
   ParameterEstimates=beta (where=(Effect ne "Intercept"));

proc glimmix data=neurodeg;
   class dose id;
   model resp=dose*time/solution COVB;
   random intercept time / type=UN subject=id;
run;
```

```
data omega;
   set omega;
   where effect ne "Intercept";
   drop effect;
run;

data models;
   length modnam $25;
   input modnam par1-par3;
   datalines;
emax 1.11 . .
quadratic -0.022  . .
exponential 8.867 . .
linear  . . .
;
run;

data doses;
   input dose @@;
   datalines;
      0 1 3 10 30
      ;
run;

/* calculate optimal contrast based on candidate models and
covariance matrix */
%optcont(models=models, doses=doses, sigma=omega, direction=incr,
dosevarname=dose*time);
%put &modcontr;

data _null_;
   call execute ("
proc glimmix data=neurodeg;
   class dose id;
   model resp= dose*time/solution COVB ;
   random intercept time / type=UN subject=id;
   estimate &modcontr.
      / adjust=simulate(nsamp=1000000 seed=1) uppertailed;
run;");
run;

/* Run bootstrap simulations to get estimates and CI for dose-response
estimates*/
proc iml ;
   /*initiation step*/
   call randseed(1);
   nsim=10000;

   /* read-in data */
   use omega;
   read all var {col2 col3 col4 col5 col6} into cv;
   use beta;
   read all var {Estimate} into mn;
   read all var {dose} into dose;
```

```
/* model fitting */
/* additional variables needed later on */
invs=inv(cv);
nd=nrow(dose);
predmn=mn;
resp=mn;

/* define functions to optimize for different models */
start fnglsemax(par) global(dose, resp, invs, predmn, nd);

do i=1 to nd;
   predmn[i]=par[1]+par[2]*dose[i]/(dose[i] + par[3]);
end;
dif=(predmn-resp);
return(dif`*invs*dif);
finish fnglsemax;
start fnglsexpo(par) global(dose, resp, invs, predmn, nd);

do i=1 to nd;
   predmn[i]=par[1]+par[2]*(exp(dose[i]/par[3])-1);
end;
dif=(predmn-resp);
return(dif`*invs*dif);
finish fnglsexpo;
start fnglslin(par) global(dose, resp, invs, predmn, nd);

do i=1 to nd;
   predmn[i]=par[1]+par[2]*dose[i];
end;
dif=(predmn-resp);
return(dif`*invs*dif);
finish fnglslin;
start fnglsquad(par) global(dose, resp, invs, predmn, nd);

do i=1 to nd;
   predmn[i]=par[1]+par[2]*dose[i]+par[3]*dose[i]**2;
end;
dif=(predmn-resp);
return(dif`*invs*dif);
finish fnglsquad;

/* macro to fit models */
%macro gfitmod(savestart=);
   optn={. . . . . . . . . . . .};

   /* emax */
   con={. . 0.03, . . 45};      /* bounds: [0.01,1.5]*maxDose for ED50 */
   call nlpqn(rc, xr, "fnglsemax", stemax, optn, con);
   dim=ncol(xr);
   gaicemax=2*fnglsemax(xr)+2*dim;
   paremax=xr;

   if &savestart=1 then
      stemax=xr;

   /* exponential */
```

```
    con={. . 3, . . 60};       /* bounds: [0.1,2]*maxDose for delta */
    call nlpqn(rc, xr, "fnglsexpo", stexpo, optn, con);
    dim=ncol(xr);
    gaicexpo=2*fnglsexpo(xr)+2*dim;
    parexpo=xr;

    if &savestart=1 then
       stexpo=xr;

    /* linear */
    start={0 0};
    con={. . , . .};
    call nlpqn(rc, xr, "fnglslin", start, optn, con);
    dim=ncol(xr);
    gaiclin=2*fnglslin(xr)+2*dim;
    parlin=xr;

    /* quadratic */
    start={0 0 0};
    con={. . . , . . . };
    call nlpqn(rc, xr, "fnglsquad", start, optn, con);
    dim=ncol(xr);
    gaicquad=2*fnglsquad(xr)+2*dim;
    parquad=xr;
%mend;

/* fit to original data to get good starting values*/
stemax={-5 2 10};
stexpo={-5 1.5 40};
%gfitmod(savestart=1);

/* sample from multivariate normal distribution and fit models */
emaxdat=j(nsim, 4, 0);
expodat=j(nsim, 4, 0);
quaddat=j(nsim, 4, 0);
lindat=j(nsim, 3, 0);

do i=1 to nsim;
   resp=t(randnormal(1, mn, cv));
   %gfitmod(savestart=0);
   emaxdat[i, ]=gaicemax||paremax;
   expodat[i, ]=gaicexpo||parexpo;
   quaddat[i, ]=gaicquad||parquad;
   lindat[i, ]=gaiclin||parlin;
end;
create emaxdat from emaxdat[colname={'emax_gaic' 'emax_e0' 'emax_emax'
   'emax_ed50'}];
append from emaxdat;
close emaxdat;
create expodat from expodat[colname={'expo_gaic' 'expo_e0' 'expo_e1'
   'expo_delta'}];
append from expodat;
close expodat;
create quaddat from quaddat[colname={'quad_gaic' 'quad_e0' 'quad_b1'
   'quad_b2'}];
append from quaddat;
```

```
   close quaddat;
   create lindat from lindat[colname={'lin_gaic' 'lin_e0' 'lin_delta'}];
   append from lindat;
   close lindat;
   quit;

   /* postprocessing in data step */
data simresults;
   merge emaxdat expodat quaddat lindat;
   min_gaic=min(emax_gaic, expo_gaic, quad_gaic, lin_gaic);
   array doseresp(101);

   if(emax_gaic=min_gaic) then
      do;
         do i=1 to 101;
            dose=(i-1)/100*30;
            doseresp(i)=emax_emax*dose/(emax_ed50+dose);
         end;
      bestmod='emax';
      end;

   if(expo_gaic=min_gaic) then
      do;
         do i=1 to 101;
            dose=(i-1)/100*30;
            doseresp(i)=expo_e1*(exp(dose/expo_delta)-1);
         end;
      bestmod='exponential';
      end;

   if(lin_gaic=min_gaic) then
      do;
         do i=1 to 101;
            dose=(i-1)/100*30;
            doseresp(i)=lin_delta*dose;
         end;
      bestmod='linear';
      end;

   if(quad_gaic=min_gaic) then
      do;
         do i=1 to 101;
            dose=(i-1)/100*30;
            doseresp(i)=quad_b1*dose+quad_b2*dose**2;
         end;
      bestmod='quadratic';
      end;
   drop i dose;
run;

/* which model is selected how often?  */
proc freq data=simresults;
   tables bestmod;
run;

/* create plot of boostrap quantiles */
```

```
proc univariate data=simresults noprint;
   var doseresp1-doseresp101;
   output out=quant25 pctlpts=2.5 pctlpre=dose1-dose101 pctlname=P5;
   output out=quant50 pctlpts=50 pctlpre=dose1-dose101 pctlname=P5;
   output out=quant975 pctlpts=97.5 pctlpre=dose1-dose101 pctlname=P5;
run;

data quant;
   set quant25 quant50 quant975;
run;

proc transpose data=quant out=tquant;
run;

data dosevar;
   do i=1 to 101;
      dose=(i-1)/100*30;
      output;
   end;
   drop i;
run;

data tquant;
   set tquant;
   set dosevar;
run;

data rawest;
   input doseobs diff;
   datalines;
1 0.518
3 1.879
10 2.220
30 1.579
;
run;

data tquant;
   set tquant rawest;
run;

proc sgplot data=tquant;
   xaxis grid label="Dose";
   yaxis grid label="Response (difference to placebo)";
   band x=dose lower=col1 upper=col3 /transparency=0.5
      legendlabel="95% confidence interval";
   series x=dose y=col2 /legendlabel="Model Mean" lineattrs=(thickness=3);
   scatter x=doseobs y=diff / markerattrs=(symbol=circlefilled)
      legendlabel="Estimated slopes from LME model";
run;
```

Chapter 8
Bayesian Dose Response

8.1 Introduction and Background

Phase II is an exciting and challenging phase where efficacy is initially tested for a new drug. This may include efficacy assessments for a single dose or multiple doses, possibly in separate studies (traditional phase IIa and IIb studies) or in a single study, such as a seamless phase IIa or IIb study.

When testing multiple doses, one of the key strategic decisions is how wide of a dosing range will be tested and what doses should be tested across that interval. Though many dose-ranging studies are powered for pairwise comparisons, the strength of dose-response modeling is in the ability to better understand the drug effect across the dosing interval. A wide dose range or higher dosing ratio helps adequately characterize the dose-response curve and enable better evaluation of doses not tested in a phase II study.

For example, assume that the first study is designed with 3 doses and a placebo where the doses are selected in the following manner: two near the maximal dose effect (E_{max}) and one around the dose that produces 50% of the effect (ED_{50}); however, it does not incorporate any doses near the minimally effective dose. The second study designed includes a placebo and two doses with one near the minimally effective dose and one close to the ED_{50}. These two studies may be combined in the Bayesian framework to adequately characterize the full dose response. The first study data could be incorporated as an informative prior when analyzing the second study. This will help to characterize the dose response of the compound adequately through borrowing information. This requires the assumption of exchangeability for this analysis, i.e. the data from the first and the second trial are exchangeable. While dose ranging studies are not often designed with multiple doses near a minimally or maximally effective dose, the results of phase II studies may appear to indicate that more than one dose achieved a minimal or maximum effect. The Bayesian dose-response design enables the seamless combination of study results.

Consider a second example that uses the information on the dose response of the compound in a pre-clinical study using a biomarker or a pre-clinical assay for determining efficacy of the compound. The next clinical study is designed to estimate the same dose-response curve. If there is confidence on the translatability of the pre-clinical assay, a weakly informative prior based on the pre-clinical data can be utilized to calculate the posterior distribution of the dose response of the compound.

Another example where Bayesian dose-response analysis can be helpful is when testing compounds with the same endpoints in the same indication. If another internal compound has been tested for a particular indication, information from this compound could be utilized to construct an informative prior distribution for the next dose-response study in the same indication and endpoint. If there is reluctance to use the other compound's dose response, prior results could be used as informative priors for modeling the placebo response. These examples are a few of the ways Bayesian techniques allow the use of prior information so the dose-response curve is characterized with either fewer patients or is estimated with greater precision.

The ICH E4 Dose response information to support drug registration guidelines state that "knowledge of the relationship among dose, drug concentration in blood, and response (effectiveness and undesirable effects) is important for the safe and effective use of drugs in individual patients" [1]. The guidelines further state that "agencies should also be open to the use of various statistical and pharmacometric techniques such as Bayesian and population methods, modeling, and pharmacokinetic-pharmacodynamic approaches." This further emphasizes the importance and value of Bayesian dose-response analysis.

In the case of dose-response studies with limited doses and small sample size designs, the asymptotic-based maximum likelihood estimators (MLE) may not estimate the parameters of the $E_{\max}$ model adequately, whereas the Bayesian $E_{\max}$ model does not have such a drawback. There are some examples of sparsely designed dose response clinical studies where the ED_{50} parameter estimates using the asymptotic-based maximum likelihood were negative [2]. However, a Bayesian sigmoid model utilizing adequate prior information was able to obtain reasonable estimates for the ED_{50} and $E_{\max}$ parameters.

During the learning phase of the clinical trial, i.e. phase II, implementation of a Bayesian dose-response analyses allows for appropriate decisions by utilizing external belief and/or data and provides precise estimates for the dose response relation even with smaller sample sizes.

Typically, responses for clinical trials in the inflammation and immunology area are binary in nature, i.e. a success or failure of the outcome. Although there are continuous scales that are available in these disease areas, the clinicians prefer to define success on the basis of whether a subject has responded or remitted. Apart from a model for continuous endpoint we also provide an example for a Bayesian $E_{\max}$ model for binary data.

8.2 Statistical Model for Bayesian Dose-Response

In this chapter we will only provide examples of a Bayesian hyperbolic $E_{\max}$ model (Chapter 6). The sigmoid model or other non-linear models are out of scope [3,4]. It may be noted though that the sigmoid model can easily be implemented by adding a hill parameter to the hyperbolic model. From Section 6.4.1, the Bayesian hyperbolic E_{max} model is written as

$$y_i = E_0 + E_{max} \times \frac{D_i}{ED_{50} + D_i} + \epsilon_i,$$

where

1. i is the subject ID
2. y_i is the observed continuous response variable for the ith patient
3. E_0 is the basal effect, the response when the dose is 0mg
4. E_{max} is the maximum effect attributable to the drug
5. ED_{50} is the dose that produces half the effect of E_{max}
6. D_i is the dose level for the ith patient
7. ϵ_i is the random error for the ith patient. A standard assumption, adopted here, is that the ϵ_i terms are independent and identically distributed with a mean of 0 and variance σ^2. An additional standard assumption is that the error terms are normally distributed.

Further, assume that $y_i \sim N(\mu_i, \tau)$, where $\tau = 1/\sigma^2$ is the precision. For the Bayesian analysis, prior assumptions are made around the distribution of the parameters of the hyperbolic E_{max} model, i.e., by assuming some distributions around the parameters of the model (E_0, ED_{50}, E_{max} and the precision parameter τ).

For a binary outcome, the model can be readily revised to be a generalized hyperbolic E_{max} model using a logit link,

$$\log \frac{\pi}{1-\pi} = E_0 + E_{max} \times \frac{D_i}{ED_{50} + D_i},$$

where π is the observed response rate.

8.3 Analysis Examples for a Continuous Endpoint

8.3.1 Asthma Trial with 75 Patients Per Group

Consider a phase IIb study in asthma assessing the response of a new entity in a clinical trial. The typical phase II endpoint of interest is FEV_1 (forced expiratory volume in 1 second) which is a common spirometry test that is used in asthma studies. An advantage of the FEV_1 endpoint is that the length of follow-up required to observe changes is much shorter than the typical phase III endpoint of exacerbations. The FEV_1 endpoint is continuous and can be assumed to be normally distributed. The sponsor ran a couple of phase IIa studies for this experimental drug; the first study tested the effect of the maximum tolerated dose (MTD), the second study tested another dose closer to the MTD and a low dose. Based on these two previous clinical studies we do have some understanding of the E_{max}. The pre-clinical studies on this compound and the two phase II studies provide some understanding of the ED_{50}.

```
prior e0: ~normal(mean=0, precision=10);
prior emax: ~normal(mean=0.20, precision=10);
prior tau: ~gamma(shape=0.001, scale=0.001);
prior lned50: ~normal(mean=0.69, precision=0.4);
```

Due to knowledge around the maximum effect and the ED_{50} we assume an informative prior around the E_{max} and a vaguely informative prior around ED_{50}. For a Bayesian analysis, the precision $\tau = 1/\sigma^2$ is modeled instead of the variance. For all the parameters in the above code we notify the precision around the parameter rather than the variance. The prior distribution for E_{max} is assumed to be normal with a mean of 0.2 (closer to the maximum effect) and precision equal to 10. Instead of the ED_{50} we model the exponential logarithm of ED_{50} in order to restrict the parameter space for ED_{50} to be positive. The prior distribution for the exponential logarithm of ED_{50} also follows a normal distribution with mean equal to 0.69. This would correspond to an ED_{50} of 2. Assuming that a gamma distribution for τ is a standard distribution to model the precision parameter. It is a conjugate prior on the precision.

The current study with the experimental drug explores a wide dosing range with a dosing ratio of 81. Let us assume that the trial data are available from this study and we will analyze the data in light of the knowledge that we gained in the previous trials; i.e. utilizing some prior data. For purposes of this example, code for simulating sample data is provided in Example Code 8.1 on page 228.

Example Code 8.1 *Simulated Data for Asthma Trial with 75 Patients Per Group*

```
%macro conemaxsim(ntrt=,r0=,r1=,r2=,r3=,r4=,r5=,r6=,r7=,r8=,
npergrp=,pdrop=,seed=);
  data sims (keep = subject treatment dose response);
    format treatment $8.;
      subject = 0;
      %do trt = 0 %to &ntrt;
      do i = 1 to &npergrp;
          subject = subject + 1;
        if &trt = 0 then do;
          treatment = "Placebo";
              dose = 0;
            end;
          else do;
          treatment = "Active";
              dose = 3**(&trt -1);
            end;
         response = 0.35*rannor(floor(&seed)) + &&r&trt;
            dropout = ranbin(floor(&seed), 1, &pdrop);
            if dropout = 0 then output;
        end;
     %end;
  run;

  proc sort data = sims;
    by dose;
  run;

  proc means data = sims;
```

```
    var response;
    output out=sumstat mean=mean sum = sum n=n std=sd;
    by dose;
  run;

  data sumstat(keep = mean dose n sd);
    set sumstat;
  run;
%mend;

%conemaxsim(ntrt=5, r0=0.02, r1=0.075, r2=.10, r3=.16, r4=.20, r5=.25,
npergrp=75, pdrop=.10, seed=35123);
```

The summary data for the doses as a result of this simulation are provided below in Table 8.1 on page 229. Once the trial data has been generated, the **proc mcmc** statement is used to proceed with the Bayesian analysis in Example Code 8.2 on page 229.

Table 8.1 *Dose Summary of Asthma Trial with 75 Patients Per Group*

Dose	N	Mean	Standard Deviation
0	62	0.011	0.38
1	74	0.091	0.36
3	69	0.093	0.35
9	70	0.122	0.34
27	67	0.215	0.35
81	67	0.246	0.39

Example Code 8.2 *Analysis of Asthma Trial with 75 Patients Per Group*

```
/** Proc MCMC syntax sets the data set to output posterior summaries, sets
number of monte carlo iterations along with the seed, parameters to monitor,
plots to monitor autocorrelation and thining ***/

proc mcmc data = sims outpost = emax_out nmc = 50000 nbi = 1000 seed = 3746
   monitor = (_parms_ var_subj std_subj ed50 lned50)
   nthin = 3 stats(percent=2.5 5 10 15 50 75 95 97.5) dic;
   ods output PostSummaries=summaries PostIntervals=intervals;
   parm e0 emax tau lned50; /** sets parameters **/
   /** Setting prior for each parameter ***/
   prior e0~normal(mean=0, precision=10);
   prior emax~normal(mean=0.20, precision=10);
   prior tau ~gamma(shape=0.001, scale=0.001);
   prior lned50 ~normal(mean=0.69, precision=0.4);
   beginnodata;
      /** Setting residual variance ***/
      var_subj = 1/tau;
      std_subj = sqrt(var_subj);
      /** Ed50 ***/
```

```
        ed50 = exp(lned50);
        /** Calculating the posterior predictive distribution ***/
        Preddist outpred=predout nsim=5000 covariates=Sumstat;
    endnodata;
    mu = e0 + (emax*dose)/(ed50 + dose);
    model response ~ normal(mean=mu, precision=tau );
    title;
run;
```

The **proc mcmc** statement uses the input data set **sims** (**data =**) that we have generated using the macro **conemaxsim** in Example Code 8.1 on page 228. The posterior samples will be saved in the **emax_out** data set using the **outpost** option. In this example, 50,000 markov chain simulations (**nmc**) are planned with 1,000 burn-in samples (**nbi**) and a thinning rate of 3 (**thin**), implying that every 3rd simulation sample is kept with the remaining samples discarded. The model parameters and the initial values are specified in the **parms** statement (unspecified initial values are determined from the prior specified in the **prior** statement), the priors are specified in the **prior** statement, and the distribution of the response variable conditioned on the parameters is specified in the **model** statement. For ED_{50}, the natural logarithm transformation has been applied and a normal prior is specified for the transformed variable. Even though a normal prior distribution is specified, the transformation ensures that the ED_{50} estimates are positive.

Once the posterior distributions are computed, **proc mcmc** computes the point estimates of the parameters, along with the standard deviation and percentiles. By default, only the quantiles are provided but one can specify percentiles using the **stats(percent =)** option in the **proc mcmc** step. **proc mcmc** also generates deviance information criterion (**dic**), which could be used as a model diagnostic tool when multiple chains are used (not shown), and highest posterior density (HPD) intervals (not shown). The **mcmc** procedure also generates graphs of the posterior samples such as trace plots, auto-correlation plots, and kernel density plots. These are generated by default with **ods graphics on**, as shown in Figure 8.1 on page 231, Figure 8.2 on page 232, Figure 8.3 on page 233, Figure 8.4 on page 234, and Figure 8.5 on page 235. The trace and auto-correlation plots provide a good visualization of the convergence. The trace plots for the parameters **e0**, **emax** and **ed50** indicate that the Markov chain has stabilized and that the chain has good mixing properties. The auto-correlation plot shows a low degree of auto-correlation among posterior samples for the three parameters (potentially due to the thinning of the posterior samples).

Figure 8.1 *Diagnostic Plots for e0*

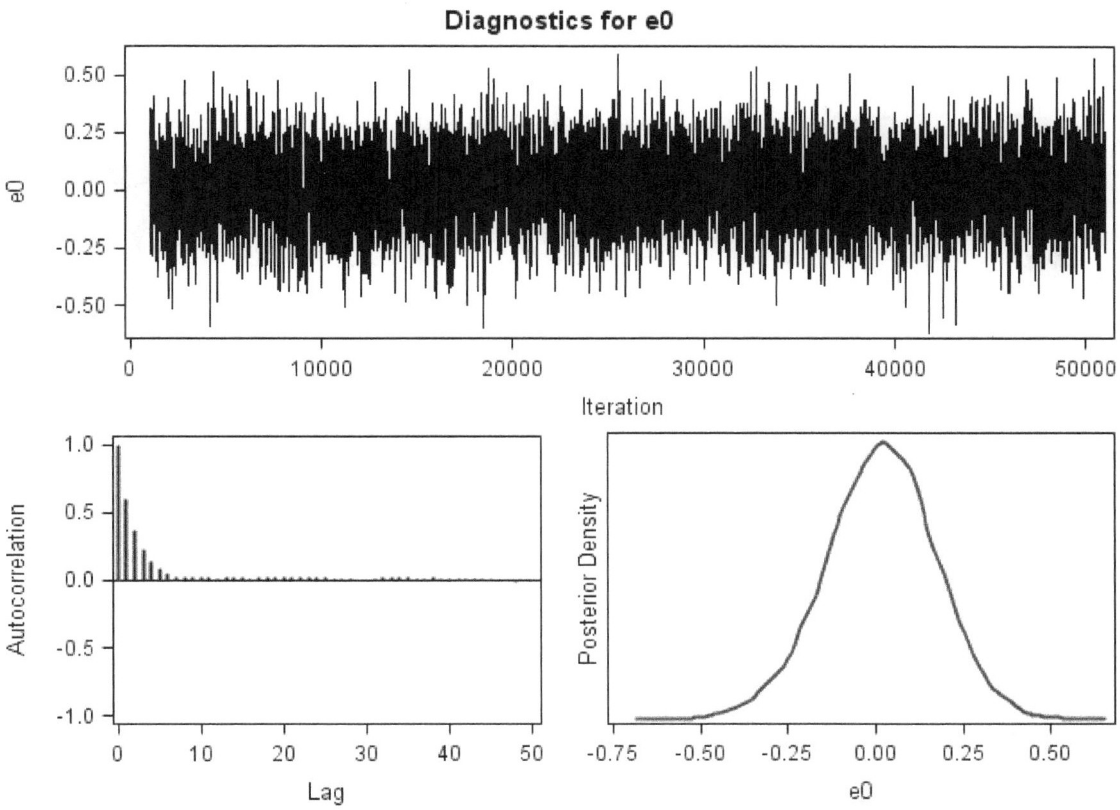

Figure 8.2 *Diagnostic Plots for E_{max}*

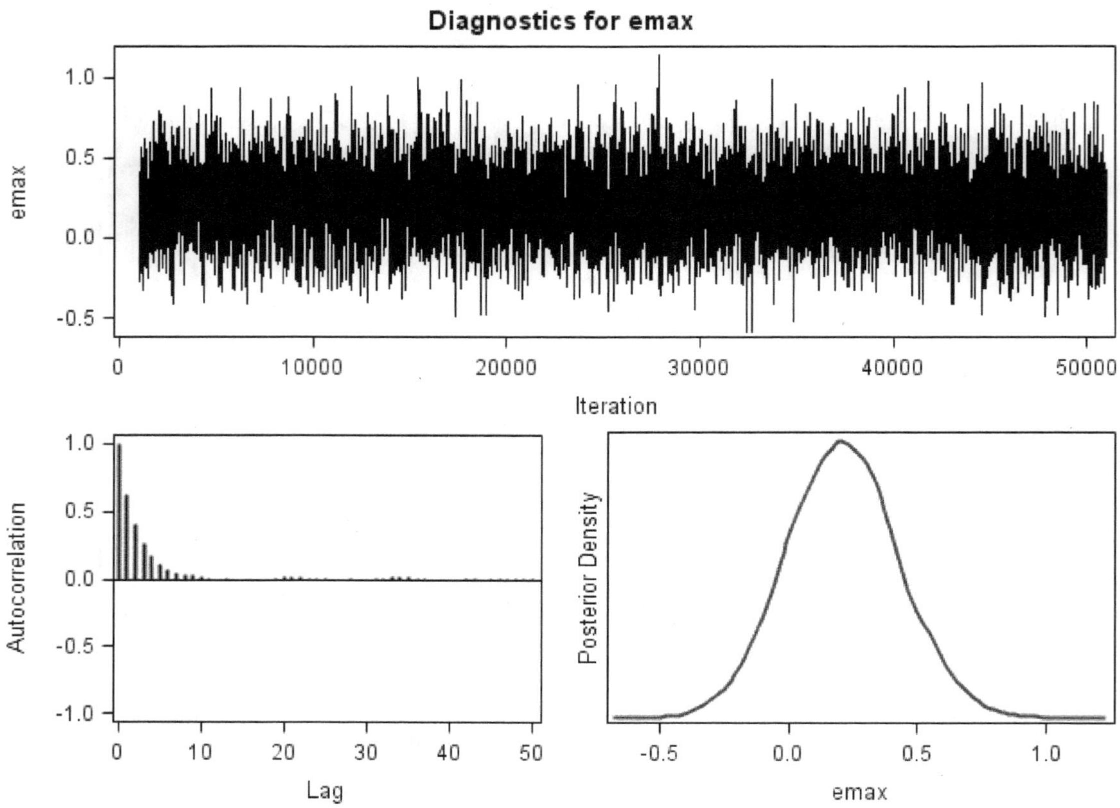

Figure 8.3 *Diagnostic Plots for tau*

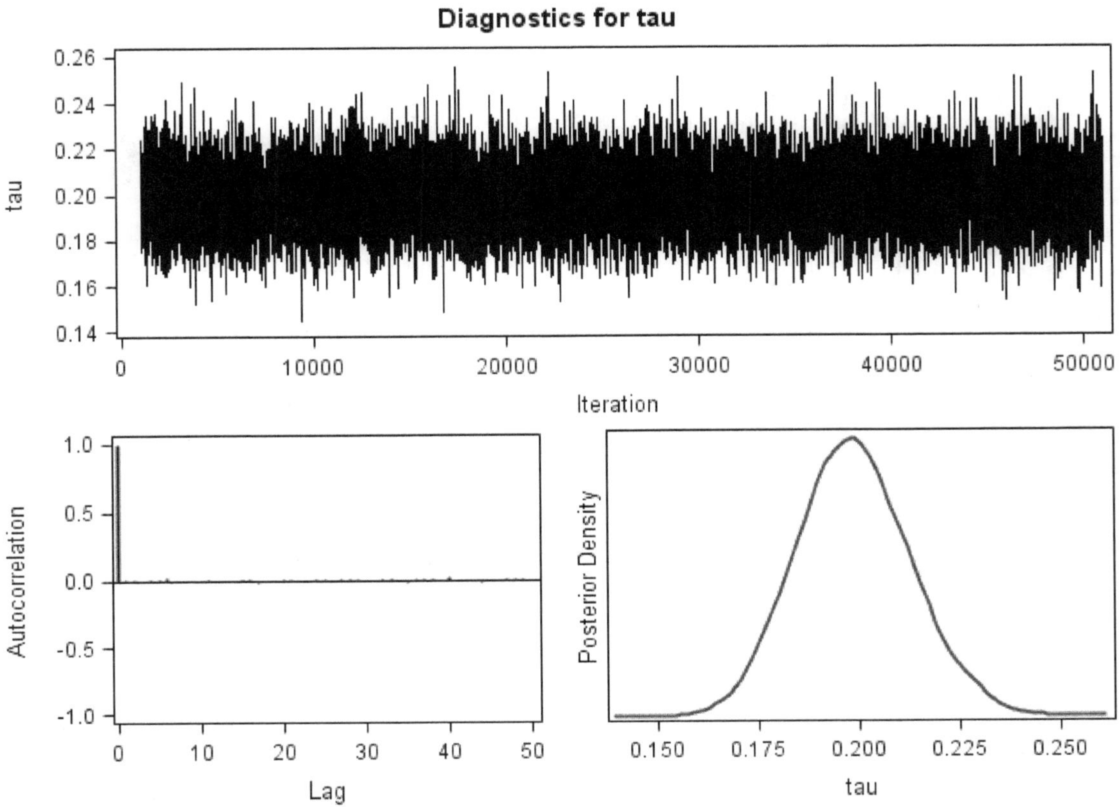

Figure 8.4 *Diagnostic Plots for lned50*

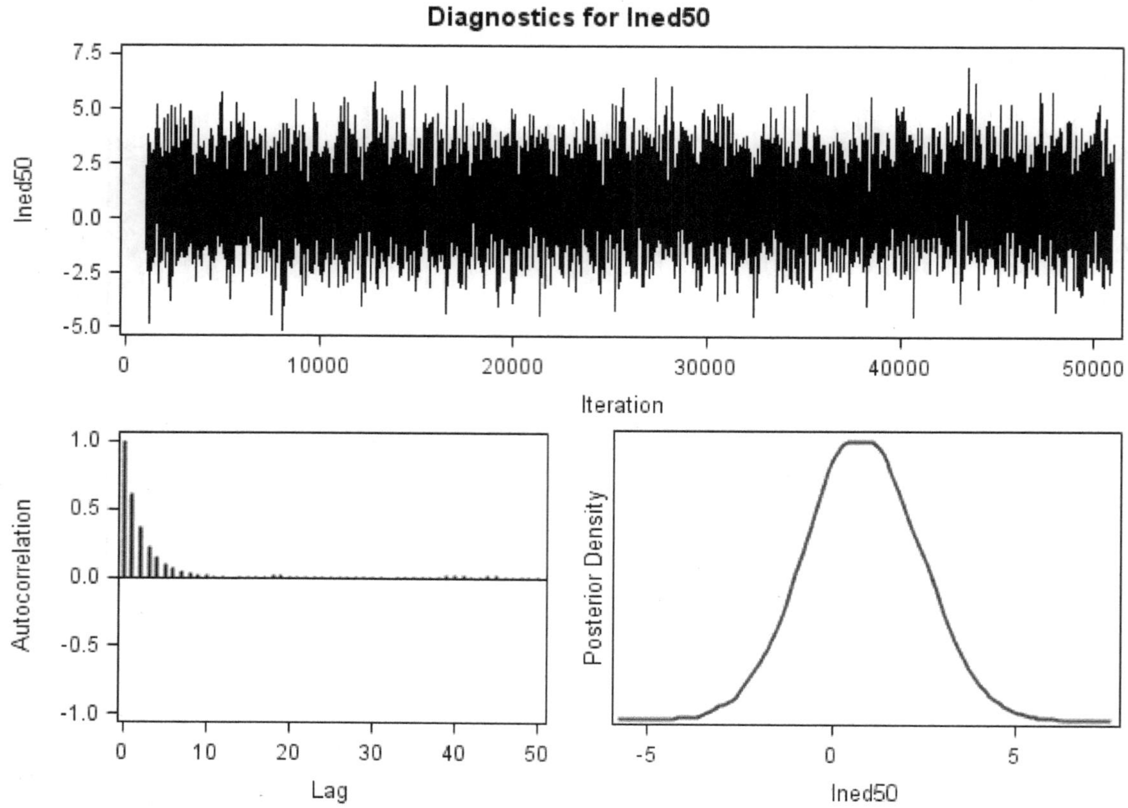

Figure 8.5 Diagnostic Plots for var_subjid

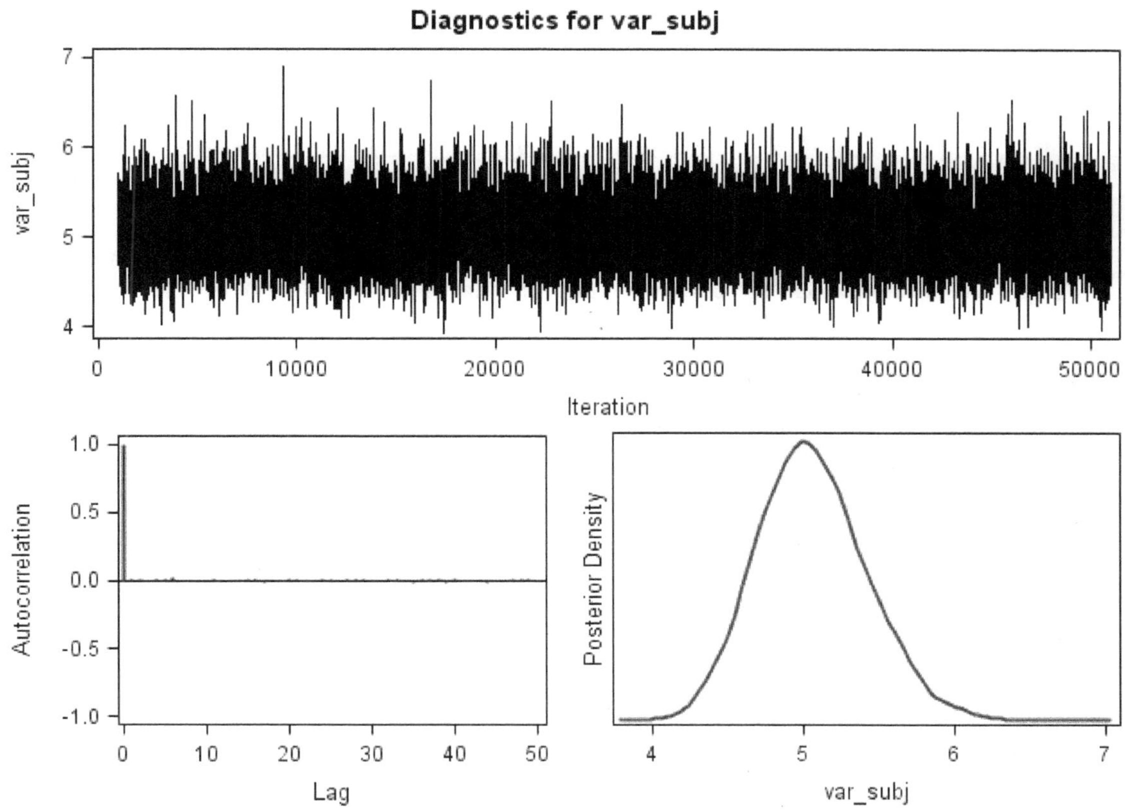

Figure 8.6 Posterior Summaries for Example Code 8.2

Posterior Summaries											
				Percentiles							
Parameter	N	Mean	Standard Deviation	2.5	5	10	15	50	75	95	97.5
e0	16667	0.0147	0.1559	-0.3080	-0.2472	-0.1867	-0.1437	0.0177	0.1181	0.2656	0.3118
emax	16667	0.2086	0.2169	-0.2097	-0.1412	-0.0650	-0.0163	0.2067	0.3510	0.5699	0.6442
tau	16667	0.1986	0.0140	0.1723	0.1760	0.1807	0.1840	0.1984	0.2080	0.2224	0.2272
lned50	16667	0.8417	1.5442	-2.1455	-1.6612	-1.1240	-0.7450	0.8279	1.8811	3.4085	3.8775
var_subj	16667	5.0597	0.3595	4.4012	4.4965	4.6102	4.6905	5.0407	5.2887	5.6808	5.8028
std_subj	16667	2.2480	0.0797	2.0979	2.1205	2.1471	2.1658	2.2452	2.2997	2.3834	2.4089
ed50	16667	7.7147	22.0391	0.1170	0.1899	0.3250	0.4747	2.2884	6.5609	30.2185	48.3035

The **emax** posterior mean (standard deviation) estimate equals 0.21 (0.22) and indicates that the maximum effect of the drug is at 0.21 (Figure 8.6 on page 235). Although in this study the estimates of the two higher doses are greater, the combined information from the previous studies combined with this study indicates that the maximum effect for the experimental drug will be around 0.21. The prior information on the maximum effect has more influence on the posterior estimate. The posterior mean (standard deviation) of **ed50** is estimated to be around 22.04 (0.12). However, there appears to be a higher variability around the **ED50** estimate. The prior information on **ed50** was not strong, hence the likelihood of this study drives the estimate of the posterior density. Note that the median is 2.29 (since **ed50** is a skewed distribution). Due to the skewed nature of the **ed50** distribution, 2.29 appears to be a more realistic estimate of the **ed50**.

8.3.2 Asthma Trial with 100 Patients Per Group

For the previous example consider the situation that the sponsor did not conduct phase IIa studies for the experimental drug. The pre-clinical data for the experimental drug will shed light on the potential ED_{50} and the maximum effect of the drug. Due to the lack of clinical data, the pre-clinical data (after applying some uncertainty around them) is posed as diffused priors for the analysis.

The code for the simulated data remains the same as above in the previous example, except that the planned sample size per group is 100 instead of 75, and the seed changes. The **conemaxsim** macro was rerun after updating **npergrp = 100** and **seed = 9865** (Example Code 8.3 on page 236).

The summary data for the doses as a result of this simulation are provided in Table 8.2 on page 236. The **proc mcmc** call with new priors is provided in Example Code 8.3 on page 236. The prior for E_0 remains unchanged. The E_{max} is a diffused prior assumed to be normally distributed with mean 0.15 and a low precision of 1 (as opposed to a precision of 10 for the previous example). The ED_{50} is also diffused assuming a flat uniform prior between 0 and 20. In this example there is no prior clinical information on the drug, hence we assume a flat uniform prior from 0 to 20. If we had more information on the drug (similar to the previous example), we could have assumed a bounded beta distribution - for example, bounded at 20 and tweaking the parameters of the beta distribution to make it informative. In general, to choose the priors judiciously the priors should be adequately discussed with clinical and/or pre-clinical colleagues.

Table 8.2 *Dose Summary of Asthma Trial with 100 Patients Per Group*

Dose	N	Mean	Standard Deviation
0	87	0.008	0.29
1	93	0.080	0.34
3	89	0.064	0.33
9	96	0.138	0.38
27	95	0.234	0.35
81	90	0.236	0.37

Example Code 8.3 *Analysis of Asthma Trial with 100 Patients Per Group*

```
%conemaxsim(ntrt=5, r0=0.02, r1=0.075, r2=.10, r3=.16, r4=.20, r5=.25,
npergrp=100,pdrop=.10,seed=9865);

proc mcmc data = sims outpost = emax_out nmc = 80000 nbi = 1000 seed = 3746
monitor = (_parms_ var_subj std_subj ed50) nthin =3
stats(percent=2.5 5 10 15 50 95 97.5) dic;
ods output PostSummaries=summaries PostIntervals=intervals;
   parm e0 emax tau  ed50; /** sets parameters **/
   /** Setting prior for each parameter ***/
   prior e0 ~normal(mean=0, precision=.01);
```

```
        prior emax ~normal(mean=0.15, precision=1);
        prior tau ~ gamma(shape=0.001, scale=0.001);
        prior ed50 ~ uniform(0, 20);
        beginnodata;
           /** Setting residual variance ***/
           var_subj = 1/tau;
           std_subj = sqrt(var_subj);
           /** Calculating mean for each dose ***/
           Preddist outpred=predout nsim=5000 covariates=Sumstat;
        Endnodata;
        mu = e0 + (emax*dose)/(ed50 + dose);
        model response ~ normal(mean=mu, precision=tau);
        title;
    run;
```

Figure 8.7 *Posterior Summaries for Example Code 8.3*

Posterior Summaries										
				Percentiles						
Parameter	N	Mean	Standard Deviation	2.5	5	10	15	50	95	97.5
e0	26667	0.0225	0.1428	-0.2694	-0.2177	-0.1591	-0.1209	0.0258	0.2537	0.2958
emax	26667	0.2433	0.2544	-0.2646	-0.1777	-0.0786	-0.0166	0.2442	0.6581	0.7372
tau	26667	0.2653	0.0160	0.2348	0.2396	0.2450	0.2487	0.2650	0.2924	0.2976
ed50	26667	10.3736	5.7192	0.6038	1.1897	2.3341	3.3789	10.5813	19.0393	19.5264
var_subj	26667	3.7829	0.2295	3.3604	3.4203	3.4969	3.5471	3.7735	4.1730	4.2583
std_subj	26667	1.9441	0.0589	1.8331	1.8494	1.8700	1.8834	1.9426	2.0428	2.0636

This trial had larger sample sizes per group; however, the assumed prior was weaker than the previous example. The trace and auto-correlation plots provide a good visualization of the convergence of the parameters (not shown). If we compare the mean estimate of the **e0**, **emax** and **ed50** parameters with the posterior distribution they are quite comparable for both examples, except for **ed50** (Figure 8.7 with Figure 8.6). The **e0** mean estimate is 0.01 (75 patients per group) compared to 0.02 (100 patients per group), and the **emax** mean estimate is 0.24 (75 patients per group) compared to 0.24 (100 patients per group), but the **ed50** mean estimate is 22.04 (75 patients per group) compared to 10.37 (100 patients per group). Further, the posterior distributions for **ed50** differ substantially: for 75 patients per group the 95% credible interval equals (0.12, 48.30) as compared to the **ed50** for 100 patients per group, which is (0.60, 19.53). The **ed50** prior for 100 patients per group is flat between 0 and 20; this upper bound is reflected in the posterior distribution of **ed50**. As a sensitivity analysis, the same priors were run on the same simulated data but only changing the **ed50** prior. The **ed50** prior was set to uniform (0, 81) indicating the complete dosing range instead of the uniform (0, 20), all other priors remaining the same. With the new prior, the mean (standard deviation) of the posterior distribution for **ed50** was 53.24 (8.81) with a 95% credible interval (37.96, 68.82). This further elucidates the fact that priors may have influence on the results and careful discussion, as well as understanding that the clinical endpoint or the biological justification around the prior is critical.

8.4 Analysis Example for a Binary Endpoint

Planning for a phase IIb study in the indication of systemic lupus erythematosus (SLE) has begun. This study will use the systemic lupus erythematosus responder index (SRI) as the primary endpoint. The SRI is a composite binary endpoint. In order to be considered a responder, a subject must show a 4-point reduction on the primary symptom score (SLEDAI-2K), have no worsening symptoms based on a physician's assessment, and no new organ domain scores in the two highest categories of a secondary symptom score (BILAG). All three criteria must be met in order to be considered a responder. It has been decided that three active dose groups and one placebo group will be included in this study, with 60 subjects in each dosing group. Initial sample size estimates assumed a placebo response of 0.4, a treatment response of 0.65 at $\alpha = 0.05$ and 80% power using a two-sample test of proportions. The dose response of the new compound will be evaluated after 24 weeks of dosing to estimate the optimal dose to carry into phase III testing, assuming the study is successful. A Bayesian E_{max} model has been proposed for this analysis.

The last drug approved in SLE was belimumab, which used the binary endpoint of SRI for registration. Across two phase III studies, 218 placebo subjects were SRI responders out of 562 subjects tested or a response rate of 0.388. Assuming that placebo subjects in the new trial will respond at the same rate as seen in these phase III trials, this estimate of 0.388 can be used for the prior distribution of E_0. Thus, logit(0.388) will be used as the estimate of central tendency for an informative normal prior on the E_0 parameter. The proposed study for a new compound is smaller than these studies and assumed to be more variable. Also, only two studies are being used to inform the expected placebo response, so a weak informative prior will be used. In order to make the prior distribution fairly diffuse, a variance of 4 is employed. In **proc mcmc**, this could be parameterized as **sd = 2**, **var = 4** or **precision = 0.25** for the normal distribution.

The prior belief in the drug is that a change of 25% in SRI responders can be shown for subjects taking this drug. It would be possible to construct an informative prior on the E_{max} using this information, though this is not illustrated in the example code below. A non-informative prior (i.e., with mean 0) has been implemented using the same assumed standard deviation that was used for the E_0 parameter.

The information on the ED_{50} parameter only comes from non-clinical studies. A uniform (0, 12) scaled to just a little more than the dose range will be used for as a non-informative prior distribution.

Example Code 8.4 on page 238 is used to simulate the data for this study, including assuming a 15% dropout rate.

Example Code 8.4 *Simulated Data for Binary Endpoint*

```
%macro binemaxsim(ntrt=,p0=,p1=,p2=,p3=,p4=,p5=,p6=,p7=,p8=,npergrp=,pdrop=,seed=);
  data sims (keep = subject treatment dose response);
    format treatment $8.;
   subject = 0;
   %do trt = 0 %to &ntrt;
      do i = 1 to &npergrp;
       subject = subject + 1;
        if &trt = 0 then do;
          treatment = "Placebo";
```

```
          dose = 0;
        end;
         else do;
            treatment = "Active";
          dose = 3**(&trt -1);
        end;
          response = ranbin(floor(&seed), 1, &&p&trt);
        dropout = ranbin(floor(&seed), 1, &pdrop);
        if dropout = 0 then output;
      end;
    %end;
   run;

   proc freq data = sims noprint;
     table response * dose / norow nopercent out=sum_dt outpct;
   run;

   data sum_dt (keep = response dose count total pct_col);
     set sum_dt;
     total = round((count / pct_col)*100,1);
     if response = 1;
   run;
 %mend;

 %binemaxsim(ntrt=3,p0=.35,p1=.4,p2=.5,p3=.55,npergrp=60,pdrop=.15, seed=1234);
```

The summary data for the doses as a result of this simulation are provided below in Table 8.3 on page 239 , and an analysis is performed in Example Code 8.5 on page 239.

Table 8.3 *Dose Summary of SLE Trial*

Dose	Response Rate	Percent
0	10/46	21.7
1	21/52	40.4
3	25/51	49.0
9	24/49	49.0

Example Code 8.5 *Analysis of SLE Trial*

```
proc mcmc data = sum_dt outpost = emax_out nmc = 150000 nbi = 10000 seed = 123456
  monitor = (_parms_ ed50 preddose1 preddose3 preddose9 pipred0 pipred1 pipred3 pipred9)
  stats(percent = 2.5 5 10 50 90 95 97.5)=(interval summary);
  ods output PostIntervals = intervals;
  ods output PostSummaries = summaries;
  parm e0 emax ed50;
  prior e0 ~normal(mean=-0.45,var=4);
  prior emax ~normal(mean=0,var=4);
  prior ed50 ~uniform(0,15);

  beginnodata;
     preddose1 = exp(e0+(emax*1)/(ed50+1))/(1+exp(e0+(emax*1)/(ed50+1)))
```

```
                    - exp(e0+(emax*0)/(ed50+0))/(1+exp(e0+(emax*0)/(ed50+0)));
        preddose3 = exp(e0+(emax*3)/(ed50+3))/(1+exp(e0+(emax*3)/(ed50+3)))
                    - exp(e0+(emax*0)/(ed50+0))/(1+exp(e0+(emax*0)/(ed50+0)));
        preddose9 = exp(e0+(emax*9)/(ed50+9))/(1+exp(e0+(emax*9)/(ed50+9)))
                    - exp(e0+(emax*0)/(ed50+0))/(1+exp(e0+(emax*0)/(ed50+0)));

        pipred0 = exp(e0+(emax*0)/(ed50+0))/(1+exp(e0+(emax*0)/(ed50+0)));
        pipred1 = exp(e0+(emax*1)/(ed50+1))/(1+exp(e0+(emax*1)/(ed50+1)));
        pipred3 = exp(e0+(emax*3)/(ed50+3))/(1+exp(e0+(emax*3)/(ed50+3)));
        pipred9 = exp(e0+(emax*9)/(ed50+9))/(1+exp(e0+(emax*9)/(ed50+9)));
    endnodata;

    eta = e0 + ((emax*dose)/ (ed50+dose));
    expeta = exp(eta);
    p = expeta/(1+expeta);
    model count ~ binomial(total, p);
  run;
```

Figure 8.8 *Diagnostic Plots for e0*

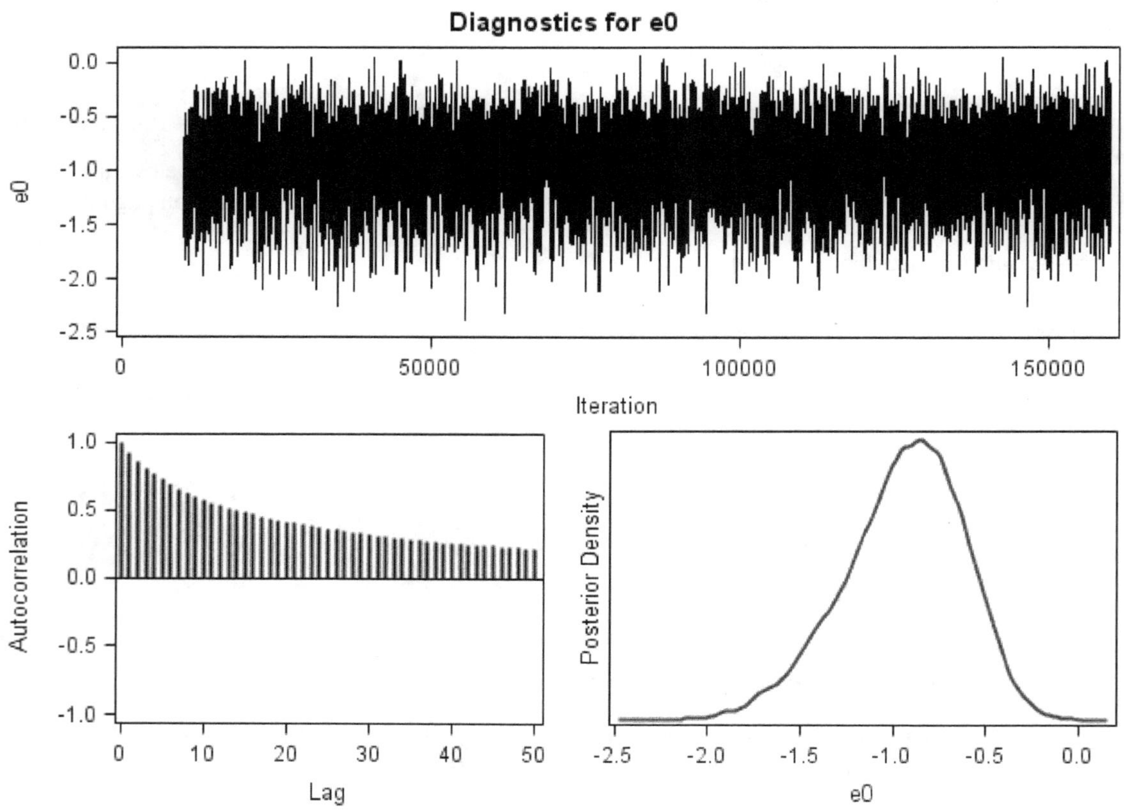

Figure 8.9 *Diagnostic Plots for* E_{max}

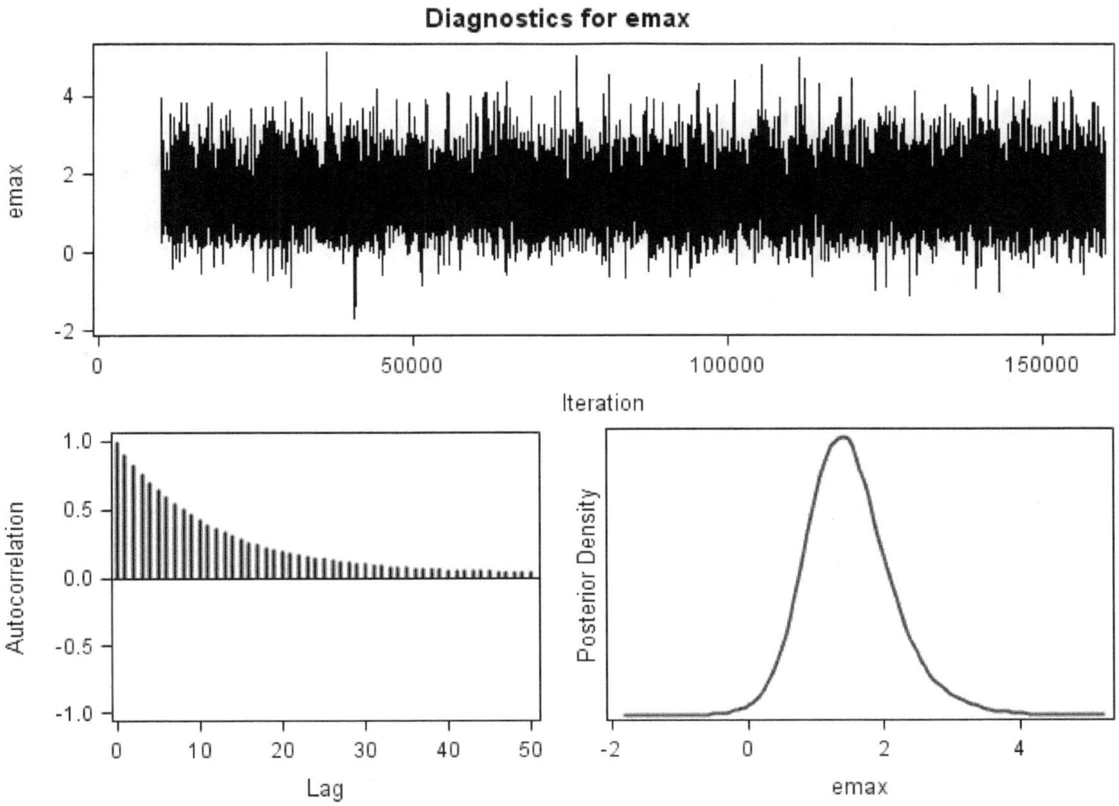

Figure 8.10 *Diagnostic Plots for ed50*

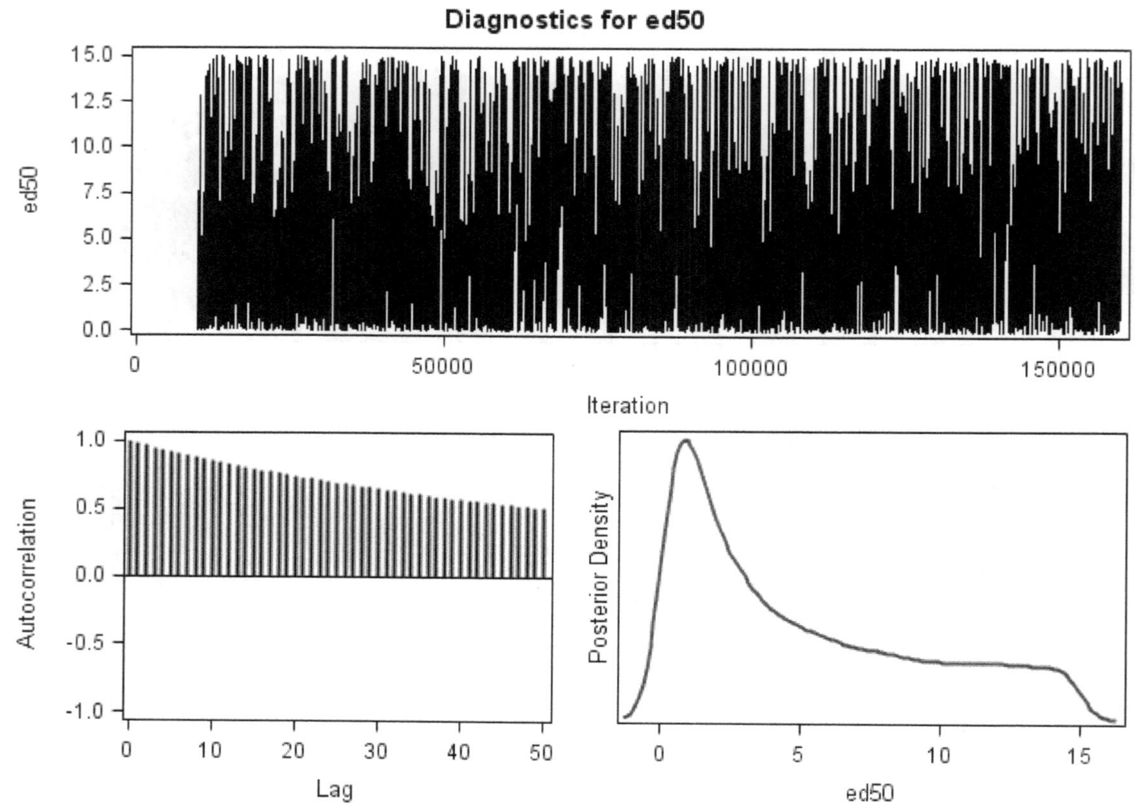

Figure 8.11 *Output for Example Code 8.5*

Posterior Summaries										
				Percentiles						
Parameter	N	Mean	Standard Deviation	2.5	5	10	50	90	95	97.5
e0	150000	-0.9451	0.3239	-1.6574	-1.5247	-1.3857	-0.9176	-0.5524	-0.4641	-0.3934
emax	150000	1.4995	0.6418	0.3591	0.5399	0.7410	1.4572	2.3141	2.6254	2.9269
ed50	150000	4.9940	4.3295	0.1646	0.2836	0.5123	3.5133	12.1170	13.5584	14.2935
preddose1	150000	0.0865	0.0637	0.0106	0.0166	0.0241	0.0664	0.1823	0.2169	0.2438
preddose3	150000	0.1549	0.0790	0.0265	0.0419	0.0605	0.1448	0.2665	0.2969	0.3217
preddose9	150000	0.2330	0.0910	0.0506	0.0801	0.1151	0.2347	0.3479	0.3795	0.4046
pipred0	150000	0.2845	0.0630	0.1601	0.1788	0.2001	0.2854	0.3653	0.3860	0.4029
pipred1	150000	0.3709	0.0444	0.2880	0.3007	0.3150	0.3689	0.4286	0.4479	0.4625
pipred3	150000	0.4393	0.0436	0.3578	0.3701	0.3840	0.4382	0.4960	0.5132	0.5277
pipred9	150000	0.5174	0.0585	0.4046	0.4229	0.4436	0.5161	0.5934	0.6154	0.6341

The **pipred0** to **pipred9** statements could also be programmed using the **preddist** statement in **proc mcmc**. Because the **pipred** variables are included in the **monitor** statement, posterior summaries and intervals are calculated for them. Diagnostic plots for selected parameters are included in Figure 8.8 on page 240, Figure 8.9 on page 241, and "Figure 8.10 on page 242." The posterior estimates of **e0** and **emax** are stable as indicated by the trace plot and show little autocorrelation. The estimates of **ed50** may not be as stable, as shown in the diagnostic plots. The trace plot does not look like a fuzzy caterpillar and may indicate that the chains are not mixing fully. Additionally, the posterior density is somewhat irregularly shaped, and high autocorrelation persists beyond the first few lags. Also note that the posterior distribution tails off abruptly around 15. This is the effect of choosing a prior distribution in the range of 0 to 15. If the prior was less informative, the credible interval for the `ed50` would likely be larger. The only caution is that the `ed50` is a function of the independent variable (dose in this case). The evaluation of diagnostics plots corresponding to the independent variable needs to be more nuanced than the evaluation of diagnostic plots for the dependent variable. Potential ways to understand and evaluate the stability of the `ed50` estimates include:

1. Rerunning `proc mcmc` using the log of `ed50`. (See "8.3 Analysis Examples for a Continuous Endpoint" on page 227 where `lned50` is modeled using an appropriately transformed and scaled prior distribution and `ed50 = exp( lned50)`).

2. Utilize a different prior (a scaled beta distribution or a less informative prior) for the `ed50` , which may help stabilize the estimation.

The posterior mean (standard deviation) estimate of the `ed50` is 4.99 mg (4.33), with a 95% credible interval of (0.16, 14.29) (Figure 8.11 on page 242). This implies that the study may not have covered the dose range of interest. If the actual `ed50` is above 9 mg, then no doses will have been tested at or above `ed50` and the model may not be representative of the true dose-response relationship above these values. The placebo-corrected effect of the first dose is an approximate 8.7% increase in the SRI for the 1 mg dose (95% credible interval of 1.1-24.4), a 15.5% increase in SRI response for the 3 mg dose (95% credible interval of 2.7-32.2), and 23.3% for the 9 mg dose (95% credible interval of 5.1-40.5). The dose-response model indicates a less than 25% increase in the SRI response, though a separation from the observed placebo response based on the credible intervals is present.

The placebo response was not highly influenced by the prior information since the observed data and the prior data show some concordance. The modeled response at 1 mg was highly influenced by the structure of the E_{max} model since the 3 and 9 mg doses exhibited a strong response on the SRI. Sensitivity analyses should be performed to better understand their effect on PROC MCMC estimation. These analyses may include varying the prior distributions or running multiple chains to test for convergence, which leads to better understanding of the robustness of the model conclusions.

A plot of the observed proportions, posterior estimates, and 95% HPD intervals, which are the narrowest intervals including 95% of the posterior samples, is shown in Figure 8.12 on page 244. This shows graphically that the whole dose range may not have been properly explored given the fact that no doses appear to have approached the estimated maximum response from the model.

Figure 8.12 *Observed and E_{max} Posterior Estimates for SRI Response*

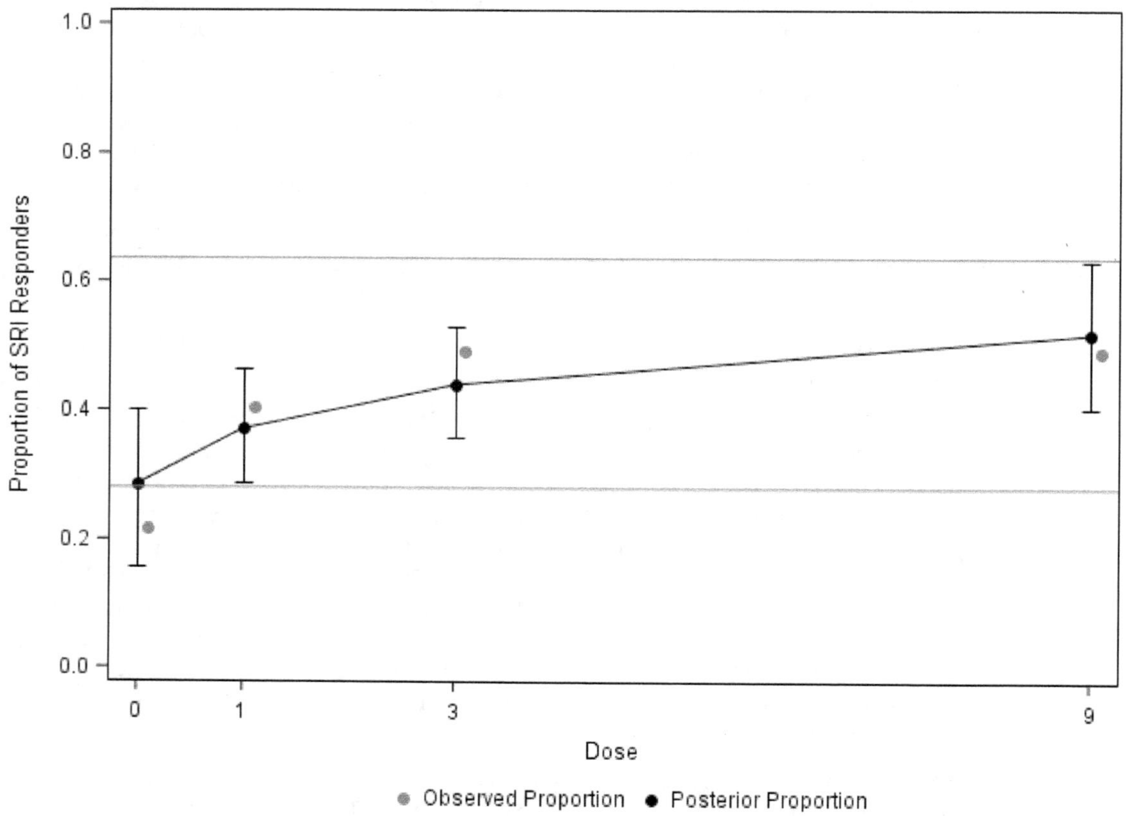

The code to produce Figure 8.12 is presented in Example Code 8.6 on page 244.

Example Code 8.6 *Code to Produce Figure of Observed and Posterior Estimates for SRI Response*

```
proc sort data = summaries;
  by parameter;
run;

proc sort data = intervals;
  by parameter;
run;

data combined (drop=alpha);
  merge summaries intervals;
    by parameter;
run;

data _plot;
  retain logite0 .;
  set combined;
  if parameter = 'e0' then do;
    logite0 = mean;
    e0 = exp(mean)/(exp(mean)+1);
    call symput("e_0", put(e0, best8.));
  end;
  else if parameter = 'ed50' then call symput("ed_50", put(mean, best8.));
```

```
  else if parameter = 'emax' then do;
    temp = (exp(mean+logite0)/(exp(mean+logite0)+1));
    call symput("maxeffect", put(temp, best8.));
  end;
  else if parameter = 'pipred0' then dose = 0;
  else if parameter = 'pipred1' then dose = 1;
  else if parameter = 'pipred3' then dose = 3;
  else if parameter = 'pipred9' then dose = 9;
  if parameter in ('pipred0', 'pipred1', 'pipred3', 'pipred9');
run;

data plot_dt;
  label pct_col = "Observed Proportion";
  label mean    = "Posterior Proportion";
  merge _plot sum_dt;
    by dose;
  dose_jit = dose + 0.1;
  pct_col = pct_col / 100;
run;

proc sgplot data = plot_dt;
  *title1 "Observed and Emax Posterior Estimates for SRI Response";
  *title2 "with 95% Highest Posterior Density Intervals";
  scatter x = dose_jit y = pct_col /
     markerattrs=(symbol=circlefilled color=red) name="scat1";
  scatter x = dose y = mean / yerrorlower = hpdlower yerrorupper = hpdupper
   markerattrs=(symbol=circlefilled color=black)
   errorbarattrs=(color=black) name = "scat2";
  series  x = dose y = mean / lineattrs=(pattern=solid color = black);
  xaxis values = (0 1 3 9 ) label = "Dose" offsetmin=0.03 offsetmax=0.03;
  yaxis values = (0 to 1 by 0.2) label = "Proportion of SRI Responders";
  refline &e_0 &maxeffect / axis = y;
  keylegend "scat1" "scat2" / title = " " noborder;
run;
```

8.5 Summary

The Bayesian E_{max} model is a flexible tool that can be used to better understand the dose response. In some cases, it may converge where a traditional maximum likelihood model may not converge [2]. Moreover, there may be examples where the maximum likelihood E_{max} model converges but estimates for the parameters such as ED_{50} may be nonsensical. In such situations, a Bayesian E_{max} analysis may yield robust estimates of the E_{max} model parameters. Like all Bayesian analyses, the results are dependent on the assumed priors, so careful consideration should be given to the center and spread of the prior distribution. For clinical trials, this means that the prior range should make biological and/or clinical sense. In small studies or studies with few doses, frequentist estimation utilizing an E_{max} model may not yield robust estimates [2]. A Bayesian model could be explored in these cases to see if the convergence properties may be improved. As stated in the ICH E4, dose-response information to support drug registration, the agency is open to Bayesian techniques of analysis and it reiterates the importance of Bayesian dose-response analysis [1]. Bayesian inference is particularly well suited to clinical trial development because prior clinical and pre-clinical studies may be included in the estimation of the effect of the most recent trial, though reconciliation may be required if there are variable effects from trial to trial. Being able to change the prior information also provides an opportunity to assess the robustness of the conclusions that may be drawn for the current study.

References

1. International Conference of Harmonisation. (1994). E4: Dose–Response Information to Support Drug Registration. Available at: http://www.ich.org/fileadmin/Public_Web_Site/ICH_Products/Guidelines/Efficacy/E4/Step4/E4_Guideline.pdf (http://www.ich.org/fileadmin/Public_Web_Site/ICH_Products/Guidelines/Efficacy/E4/Step4/E4_Guideline.pdf).
2. Thomas N. (2006). Hypothesis testing and Bayesian estimation using a sigmoid Emax model applied to sparse dose-response designs. *Journal of Biopharmaceutical Statistics* 16: 657-677.
3. Bretz F, Pinheiro JC & Branson M. (2005). Combining multiple comparisons and modeling techniques in dose-response studies. *Biometrics* 61: 738-748.
4. MacDougall J. (2006). Analysis of dose-response studies-Emax model. In Ting N, ed. *Dose Finding in Drug Development*. New York: Springer.

Authors

Anindita Banerjee, Director, PharmaTherapeutics Clinical Research, Pfizer Inc., Cambridge, MA, USA.

Jared Christensen, Senior Director, PharmaTherapeutics Clinical Research, Pfizer Inc., Cambridge, MA, USA.

Chapter 9
Overview of Adaptive Randomization

9.1 Introduction

Randomized clinical trials are the gold standard to differentiate effects of different treatments. To ensure an objective comparison of different treatments, patients' allocation should be random or unpredictable so that both known and unknown prognostic factors and potential confounders can be balanced out. In practice, selection bias should be prevented as much as possible by using randomization and blinding, including single- or double-blind schemes. A single-blind study only blocks the identity of the treatments to patients, while a double-blind study blocks both patients and clinicians. Most clinical trials attempt to balance the treatment assignment by restricting the allocation probability equally across arms, but it may not be effective and ethical. Adaptive randomization schemes, which modify the probability of treatment assignment according to the accumulated information in the trial, have become increasingly common nowadays. Several factors affect the design of a randomized clinical trial. On one hand, the effects of different treatments should be differentiated quickly, so that more patients outside of the trial would benefit from the more efficacious treatment sooner. For this purpose, patients' allocation should be (nearly) balanced across the comparative arms. On the other hand, each trial participant should be treated the most effectively for his/her own best health, and patients themselves also hope that they would be assigned to the arm that is more beneficial. This often leads to the allocation probabilities being skewed toward favoring the potentially better treatment. Therefore, randomized clinical trials need to strike a balance between individual and collective ethics.

Randomization can effectively reduce bias and confounding effects. Clinical trials with well-balanced prognostic variables can provide a more efficient and cleaner comparison. In general, randomization can be classified into five major types depending on the study objectives, as summarized below in Table 9.1 on page 248 [1].

Table 9.1 *Different Types of Randomization Schemes*

Type of Randomization	Description	Example
Simple randomization	Fixes randomization probabilities but may lead to an imbalance among treatment arms.	Equal randomization
Restricted randomization	Aims to balance the numbers of subjects among treatment arms.	Permuted block design, Biased coin design
Covariate-adaptive randomization (CAR)	Desires to balance the treatment assignments across selected covariates.	Stratified scheme, CAR by minimization, Model-based optimal CAR
Response-adaptive randomization (RAR)	Allows the allocation probability to change as the trial proceeds, so that the chance for a patient to be assigned to a better arm increases.	Play-the-winner rule, Optimal RAR, Bayesian RAR
Covariate-adjusted response-adaptive randomization	Combines CAR and RAR, which skews the randomization probability to the potentially better treatment, as well as controlling patient heterogeneity.	Bayesian CARA

9.2 Simple Randomization

As the simplest way of randomization, simple randomization fixes the assignment probabilities throughout the trial with no regard to historical allocation and response information. Nevertheless, the assignment probabilities can all be equal or different across treatment arms. For a trial with K treatments, each trial participant is simply assigned with probability $1/K$ to one of the K arms under equal randomization. If a certain treatment is believed to be more beneficial, or investigators are interested in learning more about a specific drug, more patients can be randomized to that treatment arm. For instance, the allocation ratio to a new therapy versus the standard-of-care can be specified as 2 : 1 or 3 : 1.

In SAS, the **`%SimpleRandomize`** macro can be utilized to design a simple randomized trial. The input variables include **`n`**, the total sample size of the trial, and **`groupdata`**, the data set that stores the identities of the treatments and their corresponding allocation ratios.

As an illustration, we consider a three-arm trial with treatments A, B, and C. Based on the allocation ratio of 1:1:2, we can randomize 100 patients by calling the **%SimpleRandomize** macro as shown in Example Code 9.1 on page 249.

Example Code 9.1 *Simple Randomization*

```
%macro SimpleRandomize(n,groupdata, seed);
   proc iml;
      use &groupdata.;
      read all;
      call randseed(&seed);

      u=j(&n,1);
      prob=ratio/sum(ratio);
      agroup=j(&n,1);
      call randgen(u, "Uniform");
      cprob = j(nrow(group),1);
      do j=1 to nrow(group);
         cprob[j]=sum(prob[1:j]);
      end;

      do j=1 to &n;
         k=1;
         do while (u[j]>cprob[k]);
            k=k+1;
         end;
         agroup[j]=k;
      end;
      group=group[agroup];

      create SimpleRandomization var {group}; /** create data set **/
      append;
   quit;

   proc print data=SimpleRandomization;
   run;

   proc freq data=SimpleRandomization;
      tables group;
   run;
%mend SimpleRandomize;


data ThreeArm;
   input group $ ratio;
   datalines;
   A 1
   B 1
   C 2
   ;
run;

%SimpleRandomize(n=100,groupdata=ThreeArm,seed=6);
```

The macro generates a sequence of treatment assignments for 100 subjects. We can use `proc freq` to show the frequency of the treatment assignments (Table 9.2 on page 250).

Table 9.2 Output from Example Code 9.1

Group	Frequency	Percent	Cumulative Frequency	Cumulative Percent
A	19	19.00	19	19.00
B	22	22.00	41	41.00
C	59	59.00	100	100.00

9.3 Restricted Randomization

9.3.1 Permuted Block Randomization

With equal probabilities of assignment, the number of patients in each arm is supposed to be close. Nevertheless, simple randomization typically cannot guarantee a perfect balance across different arms, especially when the sample size is small. By contrast, the restricted randomization aims to achieve an equal number of subjects in each treatment arm, for which two such procedures are introduced below.

The most popular technique for restricted randomization is the so-called permuted block randomization. Considering a sequence of blocks, each block contains a prespecified number of treatment assignments, which are permuted in a random order. For illustration, in a three-arm randomized trial with treatments, A, B, and C, the possible permutation sequences using a block size of three are the following:

1. ABC
2. ACB
3. BAC
4. BCA
5. CAB
6. CBA.

At the randomization step, a block is chosen randomly, and suppose that the third block is selected, BAC; that means, the first patient in the block receives treatment B, the second receives A, and the third receives C. This procedure ensures that exactly one patient is assigned to each treatment arm within the block. Obviously, such permuted block randomization guarantees the number of patients allocated to each treatment arm to be the same. The permuted block randomization is particularly useful in multi-center trials, where it can be used to balance treatments within each study center and, thus, has benefits for understanding between-center effects.

`proc plan` can be utilized to generate the entire randomization scheme based on permuted block randomization. For example, in a two-arm trial, eight patients are enrolled for treatment assignment. With a block size of 4, there are six possible block patterns, i.e., $\binom{4}{2} = 6$. To invoke **proc plan**, we need to specify the number of blocks, the block size, and the number of treatments, as shown in Example Code 9.2 on page 251.

Example Code 9.2 *Permuted Block Randomization*

```
proc plan seed=3;
   factors Block=2 random Sequence=4 ordered / noprint;
   treatments Treatment=4;
   output out=PermutedBlock Treatment cvals=('A' 'A' 'B' 'B') random;
run;

proc sort data = PermutedBlock;
   by block sequence;
run;

proc print data = PermutedBlock;
run;
```

The output for this permuted block design represents the treatment assignments of the eight patients. The result shows that the first block selected in the trial is block 2, and the first two patients in block 2 receive treatment B and the other two receive treatment A (Table 9.3 on page 251).

Table 9.3 *Output for Example Code 9.2*

Block	Sequence	Treatment
1	1	A
1	2	B
1	3	B
1	4	A
2	1	B
2	2	B
2	3	A
2	4	A

However, a drawback of the permuted block randomization is that potential selection bias might be introduced if the practitioner is aware of the block size. By the end of each block, the treatment assigned to the last participant in the block is known as long as the previous treatment assignments have been kept track of. A natural remedy to prevent such selection bias is to randomly mix blocks of different sizes so that the block size is unpredictable as well.

9.3.2 Biased Coin Design

Another well-known restricted randomization method is the biased coin design (BCD), which aims to provide an approximated balance among the treatment arms [2]. Each step of the BCD favors the treatment that has been underrepresented in the trial thus far. For illustration, let n_1 and n_2 denote the numbers of subjects that are assigned to arm 1 and arm 2, respectively. Let p be the prespecified randomization probability for arm 1. As the trial proceeds, a new patient will be allocated to arm 1 with a probability of

$$\Pr(\text{patient assigned to arm 1}) = \begin{cases} p, & n_1 < n_2 \\ 1/2, & n_1 = n_2 \\ 1-p, & n_1 > n_2 . \end{cases}$$

There are many choices for the specification of p: Efron recommended $p = 2/3$, such that the trial can be simply conducted by tossing a biased coin [2]. Based on a constant p, the treatment allocation cannot characterize the extent of unbalance between the two groups. To accommodate the sample size information, Wei recommended the allocation probability to arm 1 as

$$p = \frac{1}{2}\left(1 - \frac{\Delta}{n}\right),$$

where $\Delta = n_1 - n_2$ and $n = n_1 + n_2$ [3]. As one step further, Antognini and Giovagnoli proposed an adjustable BCD to correct the patient distribution towards balance: the more imbalanced the two groups, the more strength is imposed to pull the samples back to balance [4].

The **%BCDrandomize** macro implements the BCD of Wei [3] to generate the treatment assignment for each new patient. Users need to input the accumulated number of patients in each group (**n1** and **n2**). At the beginning of a two-arm trial, no patient has been recruited. We use the following code to randomize the first patient with an equal probability to each arm and, by chance, the first patient is assigned to treatment B (Table 9.4 on page 253).

Example Code 9.3 *Biased Coin Design*

```
/* f(x)=1-x <- probability of assignment to A */
/* g(x)=x <- probability of assignment to B */
/* where x = (diff in num of subjects in each trt)/(total num of subjects) */

%macro BCDrandomize(n1, n2, seed);
   data Assignment;
   %let numer=%EVAL(&n1-&n2);
   %let denom=%EVAL(&n1+&n2);

   /* assign subject to B with probability x, A with prob 1-x */
   %if %SYSEVALF(&n1=0) & %SYSEVALF(&n2=0) %then %let DiffRatio = %SYSEVALF(0);
   %else %let DiffRatio = %SYSEVALF(&numer/&denom);
   %let Allocprob = %SYSEVALF(1/2-&DiffRatio/2);
   %let RandNum = %SYSFUNC(ranuni(&seed)); *uniform[0,1] random var;
   %if %SYSEVALF(&RandNum <= &Allocprob) %then %let Assign=A;
   %else %let Assign=B;
   /* create subject num var */
   %let AssignNum = %EVAL(&n1+&n2+1);
   groupA = &n1;
   groupB = &n2;
```

```
        allop = &Allocprob;
        newGroup = "&Assign";

        label groupA = "Number in arm A"
        groupB = "Number in arm B"
        allop = "Allocation probability to arm A"
        newGroup = "Next assignment";
        run;

        proc print data=Assignment label noobs;
        run;
    %mend BCDrandomize;

    %BCDrandomize(n1=0,n2=0,seed=123);
    %BCDrandomize(n1=5,n2=10,seed=123);
```

Table 9.4 *New Trial for Example Code 9.3*

Number in arm A	Number in arm B	Allocation probability to arm A	Next assignment
0	0	0.5	B

With the trial ongoing, the BCD can adaptively change the allocation ratio. Suppose that the trial has assigned 5 patients to group A and 10 patients to group B. We apply the **%BCDrandomize** macro again as in the second call of Example Code 9.3 on page 252 (Table 9.5 on page 253).

Table 9.5 *Ongoing Trial for Example Code 9.3*

Number in arm A	Number in arm B	Allocation probability to arm A	Next assignment
5	10	0.66667	A

9.4 Covariate-Adaptive Randomization

9.4.1 Stratified Randomization

Prior to randomization, there are often some baseline prognostic factors (covariates) collected, such as age, gender, and disease severity, which may have an important impact on the treatment outcomes. It is thus desirable to balance treatment allocation over these covariates so that valid and efficient treatment comparisons can be conducted.

The simplest way to balance the treatment assignment over important covariates is through stratification. As shown in Figure 9.1 on page 254, trial participants are first grouped into mutually exclusive strata based on the values of their prognostic variables, and then they are randomly allocated to each treatment within each stratum.

Figure 9.1 Illustration of Stratified Randomization

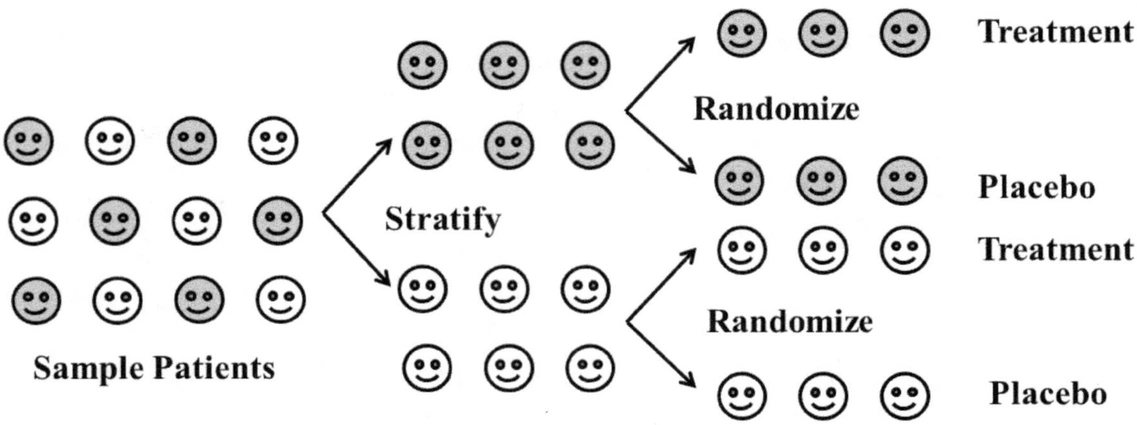

If the number of strata is small, stratified randomization can strike a balance with respect to various combinations of the covariates. However, if the number of strata is relatively large in comparison to the number of subjects, stratification can be meaningless. Because the number of strata increases multiplicatively with the number of stratification factors, some strata may become very sparse or even empty. This, in turn, may yield a considerable imbalance among treatment arms [5].

proc plan can be used to design a stratified randomization procedure. Suppose that a trial has enrolled 24 patients, and we need to stratify patients based on two prognostic factors: gender and blood pressure. The factor gender has two levels—male or female, and the blood pressure has 3 levels—high, normal, and low. In conjunction with permuted block randomization, the stratification based on the two factors results in six mutually exclusive groups. If we take the block size of 4, the output of Example Code 9.4 on page 254 produces a stratified block randomization scheme for such a trial (Table 9.6 on page 254).

Example Code 9.4 Stratified Randomization

```
proc plan seed=123;
    factors Block=1 random Gender=2 ordered Pressure=3 ordered Sequence=4
    ordered/noprint;
    treatments Treatment=4 random;
    output out=StratifiedRandomization Gender cvals=('Male' 'Female') ordered
           Pressure cvals=('High' 'Normal' 'Low') ordered
                 Treatment cvals=('A' 'A' 'B' 'B') random;
run;

proc print data = StratifiedRandomization;
run;
```

Table 9.6 Output from Example Code 9.4

Gender	Pressure	Sequence	Treatment
Male	High	1	A
Male	High	2	B
Male	High	3	A

Gender	Pressure	Sequence	Treatment
Male	High	4	B
Male	Normal	1	A
Male	Normal	2	B
Male	Normal	3	A
Male	Normal	4	B
Male	Low	1	B
Male	Low	2	B
Male	Low	3	A
Male	Low	4	A
Female	High	1	B
Female	High	2	B
Female	High	3	A
Female	High	4	A
Female	Normal	1	B
Female	Normal	2	A
Female	Normal	3	A
Female	Normal	4	B
Female	Low	1	B
Female	Low	2	B
Female	Low	3	A
Female	Low	4	A

9.4.2 Covariate-Adaptive Randomization by Minimization

When there are a large number of prognostic factors in a trial, it becomes difficult to achieve overall balance across all of the covariates. Taves [6] and Pocock and Simon [7] proposed the minimization method (also known as dynamic allocation, covariate-adaptive, or adjusted randomization) for sequential treatment assignment. During the randomization process, the allocation probability of each subject is determined by the current overall balance among the treatment groups.

In detail, let I denote the total number of prognostic factors, among which continuous factors need to be categorized into meaningful ordinal levels. In a two-arm trial, let n_{i1} be the number of subjects that are assigned to arm 1 and n_{i2} assigned to arm 2, then the difference for factor i is given by

$$g_i = |n_{i1} - n_{i2}|, \quad i = 1, \ldots, I.$$

The total imbalance is measured by a weighted sum over the marginal imbalance for each factor $G = \sum_{i=1}^{I} w_i g_i$, where w_i is a weight characterizing the importance of the ith factor. Based on previous allocations of patients, each new patient is more likely to be assigned to the treatment arm that would lead to the least overall imbalance G. Table 9.7 on page 256 shows an illustration of the minimization method, with 40 patients distributed across two prognostic factors of sex and tumor stage.

Table 9.7 Illustration of the Minimization Method

		Treatment		Imbalance	New Patient	Potential Imbalance	
Prognostic Factor	**Level**	**A**	**B**			**Assigned to A**	**Assigned to B**
Sex	Male	9	7	2	1	3	1
	Female	10	14	4		4	4
Tumor Stage	I	7	6	1	1	2	0
	II	10	13	3		3	3
	III	2	2	0		0	0
					Total	12	8

For illustration, we present an example to demonstrate how to achieve overall balance on two prognostic factors: sex and tumor stage. Assuming equal weights $w_1 = w_2 = 1$ for sex and tumor stage, suppose 40 subjects have been enrolled and the next subject entering the trial is a male patient with tumor stage I. If this new participant were assigned to arm B, the total imbalance between the two treatment groups would be minimized, in contrast to being assigned to arm A. Therefore, this subject will be assigned to arm B with a larger probability, say 0.75, in order to reduce the imbalance of treatment assignment.

The `%MinimizationRandomize` macro performs the minimization method to sequentially allocate the newly recruited subjects. To invoke the macro, users need to specify four input parameters:

1. `TreatedPatients` is the data set that contains the information of the patients who have already been assigned treatments. The first column in the data set indicates the treatment for each patient, and the remaining columns correspond to prognostic factors, whose values should be discrete integers starting from 1.
2. `FactorWeight` is the data set that specifies the weights for prognostic factors.
3. `NewPatient` is the data set that stores the covariate information of the new patient.

4. **p** is a large probability (**p** > 0.5) which is specified to reduce the imbalance of prognostic factors.

The following code utilizes the **%MinimizationRandomize** macro to allocate three newly recruited subjects: a male with tumor stage I, a male with tumor stage II and a female with tumor stage II. These subjects will be assigned to the treatment arm that leads to a smaller imbalance with probability $p = 0.75$ (Example Code 9.5 on page 257).

Example Code 9.5 *Covariate-Adaptive Allocation by Minimization*

```
data FactorWeight;
   input w;
   datalines;
1
1
;
run;

%macro MinimizationRandomize(TreatedPatients,NewPatient,FactorWeight,p,seed);
   proc iml;
      use &TreatedPatients.;
      read all into X;
      use &TreatedPatients.;
      read all var {group};
      use &NewPatient.;
      read all into Y;
      use  &FactorWeight.;
      read all;
      call randseed(&seed);

      X=X//Y;

      imA=0;
      groupA=group//'A';

      do i=1 to ncol(X);
         do j=1 to max(X[,i]);
            imA=imA+w[i]*abs(sum(groupA[loc(X[,i]=j)]='A')
            -sum(groupA[loc(X[,i]=j)]='B'));
         end;
      end;

      imB=0;
      groupB=group//'B';

      do i=1 to ncol(X);
         do j=1 to max(X[,i]);
            imB=imB+w[i]*abs(sum(groupB[loc(X[,i]=j)]='A')
            -sum(groupB[loc(X[,i]=j)]='B'));
         end;
      end;
      print imA imB;

      u=1;
      call randgen(u, "Uniform");
```

```
      if (imA<=imB & u<=&p) then
      call symput('newgroup','A');
      if (imA<=imB & u>&p) then
      call symput('newgroup','B');
      if (imA>imB & u<=&p) then
      call symput('newgroup','B');
      if (imA>imB & u>&p) then
      call symput('newgroup','A');

      NextGroup=symget("newgroup");;
      print NextGroup;
   quit;

   data &NewPatient.;
      length group $ 1;
      group=symget("newgroup");
      set &NewPatient.;
   run;

   proc print data=&TreatedPatients.;
   run;

   data &TreatedPatients.;
      set &TreatedPatients. &Newpatient.;
   run;

   proc print data=&TreatedPatients.;
   run;
%mend MinimizationRandomize;

* 1st subject: male, tumor I;
data NewPatient;
   input gender tumorstage;
   datalines;
1 1
;
run;

%MinimizationRandomize(TreatedPatients,NewPatient,FactorWeight,p=0.75,seed=6);

* 2nd subject: male, tumor II;
data NewPatient;
   input gender tumorstage;
   datalines;
1 2
;
run;

%MinimizationRandomize(TreatedPatients,NewPatient,FactorWeight,p=0.75,seed=6);

* 3rd subject: female, tumor II;
data NewPatient;
   input gender tumorstage;
   datalines;
2 2
;
```

```
run;

%MinimizationRandomize(TreatedPatients,NewPatient,FactorWeight,p=0.75,seed=6);
```

The macro produces a set of outputs. First, it provides the total imbalance, when the new patient is assigned to group A and B, respectively. Second, the macro would suggest a group for the new subject based on the minimization method. Last, the **TreatedPatients** data set is updated by including the data of the new patient. The full outputs for the above example are omitted here, while we summarize the results of randomization in Table 9.8 on page 259.

Table 9.8 *Output from Example Code 9.5*

Sub	Treatment	Sex	Tumor Stage	Imbalance (assigned to A)	Imbalance (assigned to B)
1	B	Male	1	12	8
2	A	Male	2	8	8
3	A	Female	2	6	10

Therefore, to minimize the total imbalance, the first subject should be assigned to treatment B. For the second subject, the total imbalance is the same regardless of whether this participant is assigned to treatment A or B. As a result, we can choose a treatment purely at random. Clearly, the third subject would receive treatment A so as to minimize the total imbalance.

9.4.3 Model-Based Optimal Covariate-Adaptive Randomization

To implement the minimization method, continuous covariates need to be categorized. However, it is often arbitrary to determine the number of categories and the corresponding cutoff values. As an alternative, one can develop an optimal randomization procedure such that the variance of the estimated treatment effect in the presence of covariates is minimized. Specifically, let Y_j be the outcome of the jth patient, X_j be the p-dimensional covariates (including the intercept), Z_j be the treatment indicator that takes a value of 1 if the jth patient is assigned to the treatment group, and -1 if to the control group. For continuous outcome Y_j, we assume a linear model,

$$Y_j = X_j^T\beta + \delta Z_j + \varepsilon_j,$$

where ε_j is the random error that follows a normal distribution with mean 0 and variance σ^2, β and δ are the parameters to be estimated with δ denoting the treatment effect. The variance of the estimated treatment effect is

$$\mathrm{Var}\left(\hat{\delta}\right) = \frac{\sigma^2}{n - Z^T X\left(X^T X\right)^{-1} X^T Z},$$

where X denotes the $n \times p$ matrix of covariates and Z is the $n \times 1$ vector of Z_j, $j = 1, \ldots, n$. Therefore, minimizing $\mathrm{Var}\left(\hat{\delta}\right)$ can be achieved by minimizing the loss function

$$\mathscr{L}_n = Z^T X\left(X^T X\right)^{-1} X^T Z,$$

which can be interpreted as the number of units lost due to inefficiency of treatment allocation.

Suppose that n patients have already been assigned to the two treatment groups, and the covariates X_{n+1} of the $(n + 1)$th patient have been collected. To construct a sequential randomization procedure, the treatment assignment of the $(n + 1)$th patient is chosen to minimize the loss $\mathscr{L}_{n+1}$ with a high probability. Atkinson [8] claimed that the allocation rule depends on

$$R_{n+1} = X_{n+1}^T\left(X^TX\right)^{-1}X^TZ.$$

For example, the probability that the $(n + 1)$th patient is assigned to the treatment group can be specified as

$$\Pr\left(Z_{n+1} = 1 \middle| R_{n+1}\right) = \frac{\left(1 - n^{-1}R_{n+1}\right)^{\gamma}}{\left(1 - n^{-1}R_{n+1}\right)^{\gamma} + \left(1 + n^{-1}R_{n+1}\right)^{\gamma}}$$

where $\gamma \geq 0$ is a prespecified tuning parameter to control the degree of randomness [9]. Obviously, if $\gamma = 0$, the above procedure reduces to equal randomization; if $\gamma = \infty$, it becomes a deterministic allocation rule. Typically, $\gamma = 5$ is recommended to achieve a balance between the selection bias and the loss.

To illustrate the model-based optimal CAR, we apply it to assign patients with different prognostic factors based on the macro **%ModelOptRandomize**. Users need to input the data set of the previously treated patients (**TreatedPatients**), including their covariates and treatment assignments (last column). The macro then invokes the model-based optimal CAR to assign new patients based on their prognostic factors (**NewPatient**). Consider a two-arm trial with treatments A and B, and the three important prognostic factors are gender, the standardized blood pressure, and the standardized injury severity score. Suppose that 20 patients have been enrolled, and three more subjects enter the trial sequentially with their covariates provided in Example Code 9.6 on page 260. The **%ModelOptRandomize** macro carries out the model-based optimal CAR to examine the potential treatment assignments for the three new patients. Once the model-based optimal CAR is implemented for a new patient, the **%ModelOptRandomize** macro would update the trial data set (**TreatedPatients**) by concatenating the covariates of the new participant to the design matrix (Table 9.9 on page 262).

Example Code 9.6 *Model-Based Optimal CAR*

```
data TreatedPatients;
   input Intercept Gender Pressure Severity Treatment;
   *Pressure: blood pressure;
   *Severity: Severity score;
   datalines;
1  0  1.16 -0.80  1
1  1  1.84  2.25  1
1  1  0.41 -1.38  0
1  0  0.99  1.12  1
1  1 -1.18 -0.30  0
1  1  1.47 -0.94  0
1  1 -1.16  0.24  1
1  1  1.92 -1.29  1
1  0  1.13 -0.77  0
1  1 -0.42  0.69  0
1  1 -0.17 -0.59  1
1  1 -0.73  1.22  1
```

```
1  1 -0.00 -0.59  0
1  1  1.26 -0.45  0
1  0 -0.48  2.23  1
1  1 -0.58 -2.29  0
1  1  0.06 -0.69  1
1  1 -0.09  1.10  1
1  1  0.23 -1.63  1
1  0  0.37 -2.23  0
;
run;

%macro ModelOptRandomize(TreatedPatients,NewPatient,gamma,seed);
   proc iml;
      use &TreatedPatients.;
      read all into X;
      use &NewPatient.;
      read all into Z;
      n=nrow(X);
      call randseed(&seed);

      X[,ncol(X)]=-(X[,ncol(X)]=0)+(X[,ncol(X)]=1);
      delta=X[,ncol(X)];
      X=X[,1:(ncol(X)-1)];
      L=delta`*X*inv(X`*X)*X`*delta;
      R=Z*inv(X`*X)*X`*delta/n;
      p=(1-R)**&gamma/((1-R)**&gamma+(1+R)**&gamma);

      call randgen(u, "Uniform");
      trt=u<p;
      *if trt=0 then trt=-1;
      call symputx("trt",trt);
   quit;

   data &NewPatient.;
      set &NewPatient.;
      Treatment=&trt;
      output;
   run;

   proc append base=&TreatedPatients. data=&NewPatient.;
   run;
%mend ModelOptRandomize;

data NewPatient1;
   input Intercept Gender Pressure Severity;
   datalines;
1  0   0.20   -1.98
;
run;

data NewPatient2;
   input Intercept Gender Pressure Severity;
   datalines;
1  1   -0.80   -0.30
;
run;
```

```
data NewPatient3;
   input Intercept Gender Pressure Severity;
   datalines;
1  1   0.15   2.50
;
run;

%ModelOptRandomize(TreatedPatients,NewPatient1,gamma=5,seed=6);
%ModelOptRandomize(TreatedPatients,NewPatient2,gamma=5,seed=6);
%ModelOptRandomize(TreatedPatients,NewPatient3,gamma=5,seed=6);

proc print data=TreatedPatients;
run;
```

Table 9.9 *Output from Example Code 9.6*

Obs	Gender	Pressure	Severity	Treatment
1	0	1.16	-0.80	1
2	1	1.84	2.25	1
3	1	0.41	-1.38	0
4	0	0.99	1.12	1
5	1	-1.18	-0.3	0
6	1	1.47	-0.94	0
7	1	-1.16	0.24	1
8	1	1.92	-1.29	1
9	0	1.13	-0.77	0
10	1	-0.42	0.69	0
11	1	-0.17	-0.59	1
12	1	-0.73	1.22	1
13	1	0	-0.59	0
14	1	1.26	-0.45	0
15	0	-0.48	2.23	1
16	1	-0.58	-2.29	0
17	1	0.06	-0.69	1
18	1	-0.09	1.1	1
19	1	0.23	-1.63	1
20	0	0.37	-2.23	0

Obs	Gender	Pressure	Severity	Treatment
21	0	0.20	-1.98	0
22	1	-0.80	-0.30	1
23	1	0.15	2.50	0

9.5 Response-Adaptive Randomization

9.5.1 Play-the-Winner Rule

From an ethical standpoint, clinical trials should utilize the evidence accumulated from the data to assign more patients to the superior arm, so that more patients will benefit from the better treatment. Response- or outcome-based adaptive randomization aims to achieve this goal by skewing the number of patients to a potentially better treatment group.

The play-the-winner rule attempts to allocate more patients to the potentially better treatment: staying with the winner until a failure outcome occurs and then switching to the alternative treatment [10]. This rule is often applied to the dichotomous cases, where the outcome is either a success or failure. In a study comparing two treatments A and B, the procedure is displayed in Figure 9.2 on page 263: the first patient is randomized to either treatment A or B with an equal probability. If the previous patient's response is a success, the treatment for that patient retains for the next patient; while in the case of a failure, the next patient will receive the other treatment. Success is a solid circle and failure is an open circle.

Figure 9.2 *Play-the-Winner Rule with Dichotomous Outcomes with Treatments A and B*

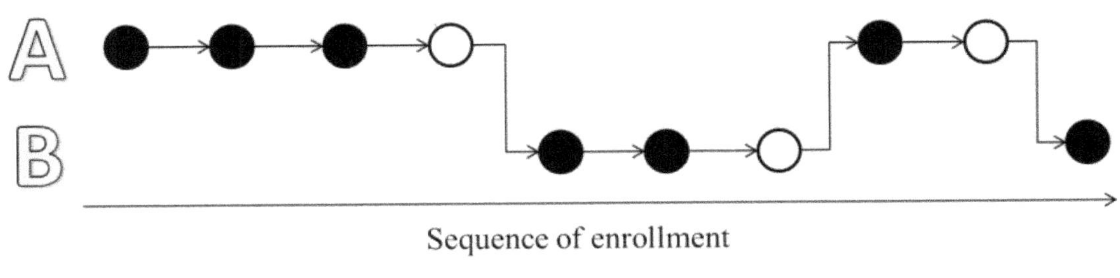

Such an alternating process continues until the total sample size is exhausted. The ratio of the numbers of subjects assigned to treatments A and B tends to $(1 - p_B)/(1 - p_A)$ as the number of patients in the trial goes to infinity, where p_A and p_B denote the response rates of treatments A and B, respectively.

9.5.2 Randomized Play-the-Winner Rule

The original play-the-winner rule as discussed above lacks randomness because each treatment assignment is fully determined by the outcome of the previous patient, regardless of the outcomes of other patients in the trial. Such a deterministic rule would increase the potential for selection bias. As a remedy, Wei and Durham introduced the randomized version of the play-the-winner rule; that is, to switch to the other treatment with a higher probability in the case of observing a failure outcome, instead of a definitive switch [11]. As a well-known example, the Michigan extracorporeal membrane oxygenator (ECMO) trial utilized such a scheme to allocate infants to either conventional therapy or the ECMO [12].

The randomized play-the-winner rule can be illustrated with an urn model (Figure 9.3 on page 264). Suppose that there are two types of balls, marked as A or B, in the urn. Starting with m balls of each type, a ball is randomly drawn with replacement to determine the treatment for a new patient. If the ball is of type A, the subject is assigned to arm A, and if the response is a success, additional α balls of type A and β balls of type B are added to the urn, with $\alpha \geq \beta \geq 0$. Therefore, the next ball to be drawn would have a higher probability of

$$\Pr(\text{Treatment A}) = \frac{\alpha + m}{\alpha + \beta + 2m} \geq 0.5,$$

to be a ball of type A, and the next patient would be more likely to be assigned to arm A. On the other hand, if the response of the subject that is assigned to arm A is a failure, additional β balls of type A and α balls of type B are added to the urn, such that the next ball to be drawn would have a lower probability of

$$\Pr(\text{Treatment A}) = \frac{\beta + m}{\alpha + \beta + 2m} \leq 0.5,$$

to be a ball of type A, and so is the probability of the next patient assigned to arm A.

Figure 9.3 *Urn Model Under Randomized Play-the-Winner Rule*

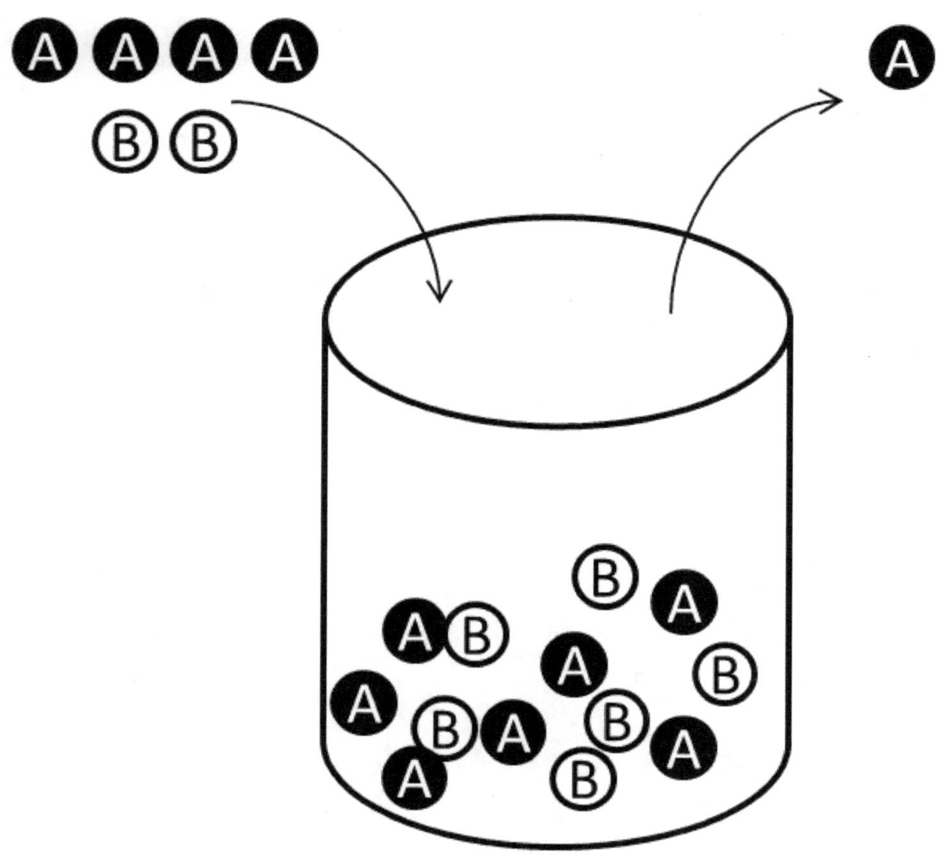

Example Code 9.7 on page 265 carries out the randomized play-the-winner rule to determine the next treatment assignment. For example, suppose that 20 patients have been assigned to treatment A and 13 assigned to treatment B. Among the treated patients, 14 from treatment A and 5 from treatment B have a favorable response. We start with an empty urn (i.e., $m = 0$), and set $\alpha = 1$ and $\beta = 0$. The **%RPWrandomize** macro can be utilized to determine the treatment group for the next patient.

Example Code 9.7 *Randomized Play-the-Winner Rule*

```
%macro RPWrandomize(n1,y1,n2,y2,m,alpha,beta,seed);
   proc iml;
      call randseed(&seed);
      /* # of balls of type A */
      n1ball=&m+&y1*&alpha+(&n2-&y2)*&alpha+&y2*&beta+(&n1-&y1)*&beta;
      /* # of balls of type B */
      n2ball=&m+&y2*&alpha+(&n1-&y1)*&alpha+&y1*&beta+(&n2-&y1)*&beta;
      /* Probability that next drawn ball is A */
      p1=n1ball/(n1ball+n2ball);
      /* Assign the next patient based on p */
      Assignment=j(1);
      call randgen(Assignment, "BERNOULLI",p1);
      if Assignment=1 then Assignment='A';
      else Assignment='B';
      print p1[colname="Allocation probability to arm A" label=""]
      Assignment[colname="Next assignment" label=""];
   quit;
%mend RPWrandomize;

%RPWrandomize(n1=20,y1=14,n2=13,y2=5,m=0,alpha=1,beta=0,seed=123);
```

Table 9.10 on page 265 shows that the calculated probability that the next patient is assigned to treatment A is 0.67, and the suggested next treatment is also treatment A.

Table 9.10 *Randomized Play-the-Winner Assignment*

Allocation Probability to Arm A	Next Assignment
0.6666667	A

9.5.3 Optimal Adaptive Randomization

Adaptive randomization can be optimized by minimizing the variance or minimizing the number of nonresponders in a trial [13-15]. As an illustration, let us consider a two-arm trial with dichotomous responses. Let p_1 and p_2 be the response rates of treatments 1 and 2, respectively. We are interested in testing H_0: $p_1 = p_2$ versus H_1: $p_1 \neq p_2$.

Neyman's allocation is obtained by minimizing the variance of the test statistic, which results in the allocation ratio between arm 1 and arm 2 as

$$r_{\text{Neyman}} = \frac{\sqrt{p_1(1-p_1)}}{\sqrt{p_2(1-p_2)}}.$$

From an ethical perspective, Rosenberger et al. [12] proposed an optimal allocation scheme that minimizes the expected number of nonresponders while fixing the variance of the test statistic, which leads to an optimal allocation ratio of

$$r_{\text{opt}} = \frac{\sqrt{p_1}}{\sqrt{p_2}}.$$

For continuous outcomes, we assume normality for patients' responses in arms 1 and 2, $Y_1 \sim \text{N}(\mu_1, \sigma_1^2)$ and $Y_2 \sim \text{N}(\mu_2, \sigma_2^2)$. We are interested in testing $H_0\colon \mu_1 = \mu_2$ versus $H_1\colon \mu_1 \neq \mu_2$.

By minimizing the variance of the estimated treatment difference, Neyman's allocation ratio is given by

$$r_{\text{Neyman}} = \frac{\sigma_1}{\sigma_2}.$$

If a smaller response is preferred, we may minimize the total expected response $n_1\mu_1 + n_2\mu_2$, subject to fixing the variance as a constant. This leads to an allocation ratio of

$$r_{\text{opt}} = \frac{\sigma_1\sqrt{\mu_2}}{\sigma_2\sqrt{\mu_1}}.$$

The SAS macros **% NeymanRandomize** and **% OptimalRandomize** generate the next treatment assignment based on the Neyman's and optimal randomization schemes. The example is the same as the one used in the randomized play-the-winner rule.

Example Code 9.8 *Neyman's and Optimal Randomization Schemes*

```
%macro NeymanRandomize(n1,y1,n2,y2,seed);
   proc iml;
      call randseed(&seed);
      /* Estimate of p1 */
      p1=&y1/&n1;
      /* Estimate of p2 */
      p2=&y2/&n2;
      /* Neyman's allocation ratio */
      r1=sqrt(p1*(1-p1)/p2/(1-p2));
      p1=r1/(1+r1);
      /* Assign the next patient based on p */
      Assignment=j(1);
      call randgen(Assignment, "BERNOULLI",p1);
      if Assignment=1 then Assignment='A';
      else Assignment='B';
      print p1[colname="Allocation probability to arm A" label=""]
      Assignment[colname="Next assignment" label=""];
   quit;
%mend NeymanRandomize;

%macro OptimalRandomize(n1,y1,n2,y2,seed);
   proc iml;
      call randseed(&seed);
      /* Estimate of p1 */
      p1=&y1/&n1;
      /* Estimate of p2 */
      p2=&y2/&n2;
      /* Neynman allocation ratio */
      r1=sqrt(p1/p2);
      p1=r1/(1+r1);
      /* Assign the next patient based on p */
      Assignment=j(1);
```

```
        call randgen(Assignment, "BERNOULLI",p1);
        if Assignment=1 then Assignment='A';
        else Assignment='B';
        print p1[colname="Allocation probability to arm A" label=""]
        Assignment[colname="Next assignment" label=""];
    quit;
%mend OptimalRandomize;

%NeymanRandomize(n1=20,y1=14,n2=13,y2=5,seed=123);
%OptimalRandomize(n1=20,y1=14,n2=13,y2=5,seed=123);
```

Based on the two randomization schemes, both the two outputs recommend treatment B for the next patient (Table 9.11 on page 267).

Table 9.11 *Neyman and Optimal Randomization Assignments*

Randomization Scheme	Allocation probability to Arm A	Next Assignment
Neyman	0.4850509	B
Optimal	0.5743003	B

There is a tradeoff between minimizing the expected number of treatment failures (nonresponses) and maximizing the power of hypothesis testing. To select a suitable randomization scheme for a clinical trial, simulation studies need to be conducted to compare several different adaptive randomization procedures. For illustration, we consider a two-arm clinical trial with binary responses. The sample size n for each pair of p_1 and p_2 is determined to yield a type I error rate of 0.05 (two-sided) and a power of 0.90 under equal allocation. We investigate the performance of four response-adaptive randomization procedures: the equal randomization, the randomized play-the-winner rule (RPW) with $\alpha = 1$, $\beta = 0$ and $m = 0$, Neyman's allocation procedure, and the optimal adaptive scheme (Opt) that minimizes the total number of nonresponders.

The SAS macro **% RARsim** (available from supplemental website) simulates 5,000 replications (**nsim =5000**) under each scenario. Tables 9.12-9.14 summarize the operating characteristics of the four adaptive randomization methods, which includes the mean of the allocation proportions to treatment 1, i.e., n_1/n (Table 9.12), the power of the hypothesis test (Table 9.13), and the expected number of treatment failures (Table 9.14). Standard deviations are given in parentheses.

Table 9.12 *Simulation Study of Response Adaptive Randomization Procedures (n1/n)*

p_1	p_2	n	Opt	Neyman	RPW	Equal
0.2	0.2	200	0.50 (0.05)	0.50 (0.05)	0.50 (0.03)	0.50 (0.04)
0.5	0.5	200	0.50 (0.04)	0.50 (0.04)	0.50 (0.03)	0.50 (0.03)
0.2	0.3	784	0.45 (0.03)	0.47 (0.02)	0.47 (0.02)	0.50 (0.02)
0.2	0.4	218	0.42 (0.05)	0.45 (0.04)	0.43 (0.04)	0.50 (0.03)
0.4	0.6	260	0.45 (0.04)	0.50 (0.03)	0.40 (0.05)	0.50 (0.03)
0.4	0.7	112	0.44 (0.06)	0.52 (0.05)	0.33 (0.09)	0.50 (0.05)

p_1	p_2	n	**Opt**	**Neyman**	**RPW**	**Equal**
0.6	0.8	218	0.46 (0.04)	0.54 (0.04)	0.34 (0.10)	0.50 (0.03)

Table 9.13 *Simulation Study of Response Adaptive Randomization Procedures (Power)*

p_1	p_2	n	**Opt**	**Neyman**	**RPW**	**Equal**
0.2	0.2	200	0.04	0.05	0.05	0.04
0.5	0.5	200	0.04	0.05	0.04	0.04
0.2	0.3	784	0.90	0.90	0.90	0.90
0.2	0.4	218	0.90	0.89	0.89	0.90
0.4	0.6	260	0.90	0.90	0.88	0.90
0.4	0.7	112	0.90	0.88	0.87	0.90
0.6	0.8	218	0.90	0.89	0.86	0.90

Table 9.14 *Simulation Study of Response Adaptive Randomization Procedures (Treatment Failures)*

p_1	p_2	n	**Opt**	**Neyman**	**RPW**	**Equal**
0.2	0.2	200	159.9 (5.6)	159.9 (5.6)	159.9 (5.7)	159.9 (5.7)
0.5	0.5	200	100.0 (7.1)	100.0 (6.9)	99.9 (7.1)	99.9 (7.1)
0.2	0.3	784	584.3 (12.5)	585.6 (11.9)	585.1 (12.3)	585.1 (12.3)
0.2	0.4	218	149.0 (6.9)	150.5 (6.6)	149.4 (7.1)	149.4 (7.1)
0.4	0.6	260	127.4 (8.0)	129.9 (7.7)	124.7 (8.7)	124.7 (8.7)
0.4	0.7	112	48.2 (5.1)	50.9 (4.9)	44.7 (6.2)	44.7 (6.2)
0.6	0.8	218	63.8 (6.5)	67.2 (6.6)	58.4 (7.9)	58.4 (7.9)

Based on the simulation result, it is clear that both the optimal adaptive design and the randomized play-the-winner rule assign more patients to the better treatment arm. However, the Neyman's allocation procedure is unethical when $p_1 + p_2 > 0.5$, because it results in more patients receiving the worse treatment. A simple remedy is to take an equal randomization instead. The randomized play-the-winner rule tends to be highly variable for large values of p_1 and p_2, and the nominal level for the power cannot be maintained. The optimal-adaptive design performs well in terms of power, compared with the Neyman allocation and the RPW rule. In addition, the optimal adaptive design is also ethical since it has a relatively low number of treatment failures.

9.5.4 Bayesian Response-Adaptive Randomization

In the aforementioned randomization methods, the allocation probability ratios only depend on the point estimates of the response probabilities. However, at the early stage of a clinical trial, the variabilities of these point estimates are typically large due to the small sample size. To address this problem, there is usually a pre-phase of equal randomization at the beginning of a trial, such that more stable allocation probabilities can be attained. On the other hand, the Bayesian approaches can naturally incorporate the estimation variability in determining the randomization probabilities.

Specifically, let p_1 and p_2, denote the response rates of the two treatments, respectively. Based on the accumulated data (D) in the trial, the posterior probability that treatment 1 has a higher response rate than treatment 2 is $\lambda = \Pr(p_1 > p_2 | D)$.

By comparing the posterior distributions p_1 and p_2, λ automatically accounts for both the point and variance estimates of the treatment response rates. Thall and Wathen [16] suggested randomizing each new patient to treatment 1 through a power transformation,

$$\pi(\lambda, \gamma) = \frac{\lambda^\gamma}{\lambda^\gamma + (1-\lambda)^\gamma},$$

where $0 \le \gamma \le 1$. If $\gamma = 0$, the randomization scheme reduces to equal randomization regardless of the value of λ. In contrast to using a constant value for γ, the power parameter γ may be allowed to depend on the accumulating sample size n, e.g., $\gamma_n = n/2N$, where N is the maximum sample size planned for the study. We apply the Bayesian adaptive randomization to the previous example by using the macro **%BayesianRandomize**. To implement the procedure, one needs to specify the following parameters:

1. **n1,y1,n2,y2** are the total sample size and number of successes for treatment A and B, respectively.

2. **alpha1,beta1,alpha2,beta2** are the hyperparameters in the beta prior distributions for the success probabilities under the two treatment groups, respectively.

3. **design** is the design parameter, **design=1** means using a constant tuning parameter. If **design=1** is utilized, it requires that you specify the value of γ. On the other hand, **design=2** allows γ to vary with the sample size, i.e., $\gamma_n = n/2N$. Users need to input the maximum sample size (**N**) if **design=2**.

We illustrate the macro by setting a constant $\gamma = 1$, as well as a varying γ in Example Code 9.9 on page 269. Results are summarized in Table 9.15 on page 270.

Example Code 9.9 *Bayesian Response Adaptive Randomization*

```
%macro BayesianRandomize(n1,y1,n2,y2,alpha1=0.5,beta1=0.5,alpha2=0.5,
beta2=0.5,Gamma=1,design=1,N=150,seed=123);
   proc iml;
      call randseed(&seed);
      /* Posterior probability that treatment A is superior to treatment B */
      /* Using MCMC approximation to compute the probability */
      posta=j(10000,1);
      postb=j(10000,1);
      call randgen(posta, "BETA",&y1+&alpha1,&n1-&y1+&beta1);
      call randgen(postb, "BETA",&y2+&alpha2,&n2-&y2+&beta2);
      lambda=sum(posta>postb)/10000;
```

```
        if &design=1 then Gamma=&Gamma;
        else Gamma=(&n1+&n2)/&N/2;

        p1=lambda##Gamma/(lambda##Gamma+(1-lambda)##Gamma);
        Assignment=j(1);
        call randgen(Assignment, "BERNOULLI",p1);
        if Assignment=1 then Assignment='A';
        else Assignment='B';
        print Gamma p1[colname="Allocation probability to arm A" label=""]
        Assignment[colname="Next assignment" label=""];
    quit;
%mend BayesianRandomize;

%BayesianRandomize(n1=20,y1=14,n2=13,y2=5,alpha1=0.5,beta1=0.5,
alpha2=0.5,beta2=0.5,design=1,Gamma=1,seed=123);
%BayesianRandomize(n1=20,y1=14,n2=13,y2=5,alpha1=0.5,beta1=0.5,
alpha2=0.5,beta2=0.5,design=2,N=150,seed=123);
```

Table 9.15 *Output from Example Code 9.9*

γ	Allocation Probability to Arm A	Next Assignment
1	0.9618	A
0.11	0.5878	B

Although RAR can help to mitigate ethical issues, it may cause an imbalance among the prognostic factors across different groups. For a more balanced design, covariate-adjusted and response-adaptive randomization procedures can be used to address concerns with both response and covariates. Under such a randomization scheme, the allocation probability is skewed to more effective treatments, and the distributions of the covariates are simultaneously adjusted toward balance [17, 18].

9.6 Summary

This chapter reviews various types of adaptive-randomization designs in clinical trials. When used appropriately, adaptive designs may improve the efficiency and reduce the cost of a trial. Also, the information from the recruited patients can be maximally utilized, and the risk to the patients can be substantially reduced.

However, in practice, randomized trials are still dominated by the conventional fixed-randomization scheme due to the following concerns:

- Patients may not be balanced on certain covariates, especially those with possible time trends.
- Hypothesis tests during interim monitoring and at the trial completion are unconventional and difficult.
- Delayed outcomes may affect the practical implementation of adaptive randomization designs.

To facilitate practical use of adaptive randomization, more automatic and frequent updating systems should be built. Necessary infrastructures and cooperation between statisticians and clinicians need to be established. Further investigation on the statistical properties of various types of randomized design is warranted [19].

References

1. Hu F & Rosenberger WF. (2006). *The Theory of Response-Adaptive Randomization in Clinical Trials*. Hoboken, New Jersey: John Wiley & Sons.
2. Efron B. (1971). Forcing a sequential experiment to be balanced. *Biometrika* 58: 403-417.
3. Wei LJ. (1978). The adaptive biased coin design for sequential experiments. *The Annals of Statistics* 6: 92-100.
4. Antognini AB & Giovagnoli A. (2004). A new biased coin design for the sequential allocation of two treatments. *Journal of the Royal Statistical Society: Series C (Applied Statistics)* 53: 651-664.
5. Therneau TM. (1993). How many stratification factors are too many to use in a randomization plan? *Controlled Clinical Trials* 14: 98-108.
6. Taves DR. (1974). Minimization: A new method of assigning patients to treatment and control groups. *Clinical Pharmacology and Therapeutics* 15: 443-453.
7. Pocock SJ & Simon R. (1975). Sequential treatment assignment with balancing for prognostic factors in the controlled clinical trial. *Biometrics* 31: 103-115.
8. Atkinson AC. (1999). Optimum biased-coin designs for sequential treatment allocation with covariate information (with discussion). *Statistics in Medicine* 18: 1741-1755.
9. Smith RL. (1984). Properties of biased coin designs in sequential clinical trials. *The Annals of Statistics* 12: 1018-1034.
10. Zelen M. (1969). Play the winner rule and the controlled clinical trial. *Journal of the American Statistical Association* 64: 131-146.
11. Wei LJ & Durham S. (1978). The randomized play-the-winner rule in medical trials. *Journal of the American Statistical Association* 73: 840-843.
12. Bartlett RH, Roloff DW, Cornell RG, Andrews AF, Dillon PW & Zwischenberger JB. (1985). Extracorporeal circulation in neonatal respiratory failure: A prospective randomized study. *Pediatrics* 76: 479-487.
13. Rosenberger WF, Stallard N, Ivanova A, Harper CN & Ricks ML. (2001). Optimal adaptive designs for binary response trials. *Biometrics* 57: 909-913.
14. Melfi VF, Page C & Geraldes M. (2001). An adaptive randomized design with application to estimation. *Canadian Journal of Statistics* 29: 107-116.
15. Hu F & Rosenberger WF. (2003). Optimality, variability, power: Evaluating response-adaptive randomization procedures for treatment comparisons. *Journal of the American Statistical Association* 98: 671-678.
16. Thall PF & Wathen JK. (2007). Practical Bayesian adaptive randomization in clinical trials. *European Journal of Cancer* 43: 859-866.
17. Ning J & Huang X. (2010). Response-adaptive randomization for clinical trials with adjustment for covariate imbalance. *Statistics in Medicine* 29: 1761-1768.

18. Yuan Y, Huang X & Liu S. (2011). A Bayesian response-adaptive covariate-balanced randomization design with application to a leukemia clinical trial. *Statistics in Medicine* 30: 1218-1229.

19. Yin G. (2012). *Clinical Trial Design: Bayesian and Frequentist Adaptive Methods*. Hoboken, New Jersey: John Wiley & Sons.

Authors

Ruitao Lin, Ph.D. Candidate, Department of Statistics and Actuarial Science, The University of Hong Kong, Hong Kong, China.

Guosheng Yin, Professor, Department of Statistics and Actuarial Science, The University of Hong Kong, Hong Kong, China.

Chapter 10
Optimal Response-Adaptive Randomization Designs in Binary Outcome Clinical Trials

---

10.1 Introduction

10.1.1 Randomized Clinical Trials

The most common goal of a randomized clinical trial (RCT) is to compare the effects of one or more experimental treatments versus control treatment (standard of care) in the target patient population. Randomization plays a fundamental role in the RCT design. By introducing a deliberate element of chance into the assignment of treatments, one increases the likelihood that important patient characteristics (known and unknown) that may affect the outcome of interest are similarly distributed across the treatment groups, and therefore, any observed treatment difference should be attributed to the treatment effects, not the effects of study patients [1]. Importantly, randomization by itself is not sufficient to achieve the goals of a RCT and it should be complemented by other techniques such as masking, allocation concealment, stratification or adjustment of randomization for covariates (when appropriate), covariate-adjusted analysis and the careful conduct of the trial [2].

When designing an RCT, it is essential to formulate the primary scientific question to be answered in the trial. This requires careful consideration of the disease, the target patient population, the choice of experimental and control treatments, and the primary outcome variable. This primary question is frequently quantified in the form of testing a hypothesis of the difference of treatment effects. The trial should have sufficient sample size to provide a reliable answer to the primary question [3]. One can also include additional research questions (that are less important but still within the scope of the trial) as secondary objectives.

Once the trial objectives are formalized, there are several important statistical considerations, including but not limited to: 1) the choice of the target allocation ratio; 2) the choice of the randomization procedure; 3) the choice of the study sample size; 4) the choice of statistical methodology for data analysis. Let us consider the first two items in more detail. Many RCTs employ equal allocation designs, such as 1:1 allocation for a two-arm study. Equal allocation is frequently recommended in practice because it often maximizes the power of statistical tests and it is also consistent with the view of clinical equipoise at the beginning of the trial [3, pg. 98]. A number of randomization procedures for implementing equal allocation are available. These include complete (simple) randomization, permuted block randomization, the maximal procedure [4], and biased coin designs [5]. On the other hand, there are a number of situations when a fixed unequal allocation may be preferred. For instance, the 2:1 allocation, where twice as many patients are assigned to the experimental treatment compared to the control, may have an ethical advantage over the 1:1 allocation if the experimental treatment turns out to be beneficial [6,7]. Unequal allocation may also be preferred for gaining more information on the safety profile of the experimental treatment, for economic efficiency, or for accounting for possible differential drop-outs or cross-overs of study patients [8]. Randomization procedures to implement fixed unequal allocation include, for example, permuted block designs and brick tunnel randomization [9].

In some trials, the choice of an allocation ratio is not straightforward. For instance, if variability of the outcome is different across the treatment arms, equal allocation may not be an optimal choice. In a two-arm trial, the allocation minimizing variance of the estimated treatment difference (Neyman allocation) is proportional to the standard deviations of the outcome in the two treatment groups. Since these standard deviations are frequently unknown at the outset, how should one go about designing a trial in this case? On the other hand, at the trial design stage there may be some prior evidence (albeit not definitive) suggesting that the experimental treatment will be an improvement over standard of care. In this case, the true equipoise no longer exists and an investigator may want to consider a design with, say, 2:1 or 3:1 allocation ratio favoring experimental treatment. However, why a ratio of 2:1 or 3:1? Such choices are based on the investigator's expectation of the treatment effect which is a judgment call. These examples of clinical trials where statistical efficiency and ethics are of central concern highlight that fixed equal or unequal allocation designs may lack flexibility. This motivates the introduction of response-adaptive randomization into the trial design.

10.1.2 Response-Adaptive Randomization

With response-adaptive randomization (RAR), treatment randomization probabilities are modified according to the history of treatment assignments and responses from patients in the trial to achieve some pre-determined experimental objective (e.g. to achieve an allocation ratio that is desirable from the standpoint of statistical efficiency and ethics), while maintaining validity and integrity of the trial results. For instance, an objective may be to reduce the number of treatment failures with no loss of statistical power [10].

RAR has a long history in the biostatistics literature [11,12]. However, its use in practice has been limited, mainly due to a negative experience with a poorly designed ECMO trial in the 1980s [13]. At the same time, in the past two decades research on RAR has advanced substantially—many new methodologies have been developed and statistical properties of various RAR designs have been established. The monograph by Hu and Rosenberger provides a modern theory of RAR in clinical trials [14]. Recent statistical research has focused on the development of optimal RAR procedures that can simultaneously address the objectives related to statistical efficiency and ethics. Optimal RAR procedures should be contrasted with heuristic RAR procedures such as the randomized play-the-winner rule [12] or Bayesian adaptive randomization [15]. The former procedures target explicitly the objectives of statistical efficiency and ethics, whereas the latter ones are primarily concerned with assigning more patients to the empirically better treatment.

It is instructive to review clinical trial scenarios where RAR can be applied with the most net benefit. Palmer and Rosenberger in [16] provide an excellent discussion of the delicate balance between individual ethics (doing what is best for every subject in the trial) and collective ethics (doing what is best for future patients who stand to benefit from the trial results). They consider two dimensions of disease characteristics—severity and prevalence—and suggest that individual ethics should definitely outweigh collective ethics when disease is severe or life threatening and when disease is rare or very rare. Indeed, when disease is (very) rare, the majority of patients with the disease will be treated within the trial and very few patients will be treated outside the trial. Also, if disease outcome is severe or life threatening, then even modest reduction in treatment failures in the trial is desirable and can be viewed as a significant contribution from an ethical standpoint. Since RAR is aligned with the principle of individual ethics, it can be an attractive research design in trials for rare diseases and trials with grave outcomes.

The ethical objective is one reason for using RAR. Another important reason is the pursuit of statistical efficiency. By applying RAR in trials with heteroscedastic outcomes, one can target allocations that lead to more accurate estimates of the treatment effects or more powerful tests compared to equal randomization [17-19]. In the draft guidance on adaptive designs, the FDA provides the following view on RAR: "...more recently the approach has been revised to suit the objective of dose-response evaluation" and it is "...particularly valuable for exploratory studies" [20]. Indeed, RAR can be used in phase II dose-ranging studies to increase allocation frequency at dose levels that carry the most information on the shape of a dose-response curve or at dose levels of special interest. One good example where these ideas were applied is the ASTIN trial, an adaptive dose-ranging study in acute ischemic stroke which evaluated 15 different dose levels and the placebo, with the goal to determine the dose producing 95% of the maximum treatment effect (ED95) [21]. The ASTIN study used Bayesian RAR design where the randomization probability to any dose level was set proportional to posterior probability that the given dose is the ED95. The dose-response curve was found to be flat and the study was terminated early for futility, thereby achieving substantial savings in the cost and patient resources.

Before discussing various RAR designs, it is instructive to state some key assumptions for RAR trials [2,22]:

- "Statement of the obvious": Better treatment will actually perform better in the trial.
- The treatment with better outcome does not cause serious toxicity.
- Study outcomes should be observable relatively quickly, and the patient inclusion rate should be relatively low to enable adaptations in the design.
- Data must be of excellent quality to enable accurate estimation and adaptation throughout the trial.
- The disease is stable over time (there is no drift in patient characteristics).
- The trial is carefully planned with extensive simulations run under different experimental scenarios.

Clearly, RAR designs are more complex experiments and require more upfront planning than designs with fixed-schedule randomization [2].

10.1.3 A Classification of Response-Adaptive Randomization Designs

10.1.3.1 RAR Urn Models

The FDA draft guidance on adaptive designs classifies RAR methods as "adaptive study designs whose properties are less well understood" [20]. Indeed, there is a limited number of trials which successfully implemented RAR and, to our knowledge, none of the RAR trials have been run in a confirmatory (phase III) setting. However, as the knowledge on statistical properties, merits, and limitations of RAR is increasing, it is likely that more trials using RAR will be performed in the future [2,23]. In this subsection we briefly discuss three major types of RAR designs: 1) RAR urn models, 2) Bayesian adaptive randomization, and 3) optimal RAR procedures. In terms of maturity levels, the first two types can be viewed as "established methods" with some examples of real-life applications, whereas the third type includes the procedures whose potential is yet to be demonstrated in practice.

Urn models provide a useful probabilistic mechanism for implementing RAR in clinical trials [24]. The most famous RAR urn model is the randomized play-the-winner rule (RPWR), developed in 1978 by Wei and Durham [12]. The method assumes a two-arm comparative trial with binary outcomes, where a patient's treatment assignment is determined by randomly drawing a ball from the urn, and the urn composition is sequentially updated based on the outcomes from previous patients in the trial such that balls representing more successful treatment are chosen more frequently. The RPWR has a heuristic appeal of assigning fewer patients to the less successful therapy—the limiting allocation proportion of study patients assigned to a given treatment is inversely proportional to the failure rate of that treatment. However, such an allocation is not optimal in terms of any statistical criterion (in particular, statistical power with this approach may be lower than with 1:1 allocation). The RPWR was used to design a pediatric trial of extracorporeal membrane oxygenation (ECMO), which compared the ECMO therapy versus the conventional therapy [13]. At the trial outset there was a strong ethical rationale for implementing a skewed allocation in favor of the ECMO arm. In the actual trial, the RPWR stopped after 12 infants were randomized (one infant was randomized to the conventional therapy and died, and 11 infants were randomized to ECMO treatment and all survived). As such, the study failed from the statistical perspective because it did not provide conclusive results about the relative merits of the two therapies. According to the modern theory of RAR, the failure of the ECMO trial can be explained by the trial's small sample size, the RPWR's high variability, and the dependence on the initial composition of the balls in the urn (initially the urn contained one ball of each type, and after several assignments the urn composition became extremely skewed in favor of the ECMO arm, leaving almost no chance for the conventional therapy to be chosen). Despite this negative experience, the ECMO trial is a good setting where RAR designs with robust statistical properties could have been used. One method that could have been beneficial in this setting is the drop-the-loser rule, an urn design with the same limiting allocation as the RPWR, but with much lower variability and higher speed of convergence to the target allocation [25]. Many other urn models with established statistical properties are available; refer to §10.5 of [22], Chapter 4 of [14], and [26] for further details.

10.1.3.2 Bayesian Adaptive Randomization

Bayesian adaptive randomization, originally proposed by Thompson in [27], is another heuristic approach to facilitate RAR. Let p_E and p_C denote the success probabilities for experimental (E) and control (C) treatments, respectively. Assume that p_E and p_C follow independent beta prior distributions, and the posteriors of p_E and p_C are updated sequentially based on accumulating patient outcome data. The current eligible patient is randomized between treatments E and C with probabilities $\lambda_E = \Pr(p_E > p_C|data)$ and $\lambda_C = 1 - \lambda_E$. In other words, the current patient is assigned with higher probability to the treatment that is viewed more successful given current data. Thall and Wathen in [15] noted that such a randomization procedure, while holding ethical promise, can be highly variable due to the random nature of λ_E, λ_C. The authors suggested stabilizing the treatment allocation probabilities as follows:

$$\lambda_E = \frac{\{\Pr(p_E > p_C|data)\}^\gamma}{\{\Pr(p_E > p_C|data)\}^\gamma + \{\Pr(p_E < p_C|data)\}^\gamma} \text{ and } \lambda_C = 1 - \lambda_E,$$

where $\gamma \in [0,1]$ is a tuning parameter ($\gamma = 0$ corresponds to 1:1 randomization and $\gamma = 1$ is the original Thompson's procedure [27]). Based on empirical evidence, Thall and Wathen recommended using in practice $\gamma = 1/2$ or $\gamma = n/(2N)$ (where n is the current sample size and N is the maximum allowable sample size) [15]. An application of this approach in a soft tissue sarcoma trial is described in [28]. Some authors described applications of Bayesian adaptive randomization in multi-arm randomized clinical trials in oncology where it was imperative to maximize individual patients' benefit from participating in the trial [29-31]. Korn and Freidlin in [32] argued that ethical benefits due to Bayesian adaptive randomization (as quantified by a reduction in the number of non-responders in the trial) are typically very modest compared to a fixed-schedule 1:1 or 2:1 randomization, and even these benefits can be outweighed by other complexities inherent to adaptive randomization (e.g. outcomes must be observed fast, patient inclusion rate must be low, and data must be periodically ublinded to modify treatment randomization probabilities). In a follow-up note, Berry in [33] acknowledged that ethical gains of Bayesian adaptive randomization are indeed somewhat limited in two-arm trials, but they can be much more pronounced in multi-objective, multi-arm trials. The potential gains of RAR should be assessed not only in terms of ethics (e.g. reduction in the number of non-responders), but also in terms of statistical efficiency criteria (e.g. enhanced estimation precision or increased power of statistical tests). In particular, phase II dose-ranging trials and randomized phase II trials evaluating different experimental therapeutics with the common control arm provide a nice setting where RAR can provide a dual benefit of placing more patients on better-performing treatment arms and an increasing amount of statistical information for the chosen experimental objectives [21,31].

10.1.3.3 Optimal Response-Adaptive Randomization

As was mentioned in Section 10.1.2, modern research on RAR has focused on the development of optimal RAR procedures for multi-objective clinical trials with two or more treatment arms and different types of primary outcomes (binary, continuous (Gaussian), and time-to-event). The idea is to determine an allocation design that is optimal for selected trial objectives and construct a RAR procedure with minimal variability that converges to the chosen optimal allocation [34]. The RAR component is required because optimal allocation typically depends on model parameters that are to be estimated using accumulating outcome data from the trial. Optimal RAR designs have firm theoretical basis, and they can frequently be more efficient and more ethical than conventional equal allocation randomization designs [14,17-19]. Under widely satisfied conditions, optimal RAR designs have similar asymptotic properties (e.g. consistency and asymptotic normality of both allocation proportions and maximum likelihood estimators) to the fixed randomization designs [35]. A recent review of proper statistical inferential procedures following optimal RAR designs can be found in [36]. It should be acknowledged that many optimal RAR designs are relatively new methods that have not yet demonstrated their potential in practice. To facilitate implementation of these designs, validated information systems (to perform interactive data entry and dynamic update of treatment randomization probabilities) must be developed. In addition, input from the health authorities (FDA, EMA) will be essential for successful implementation of optimal RAR designs in clinical trials.

10.1.4 Organization of This Chapter

The purpose of this chapter is to provide an exposition on the methodology of optimal RAR designs to a statistician or a clinical trialist who is new to this subject, and to provide some SAS code to simulate treatment allocation sequences and operating characteristics of selected RAR designs. A particular class of RAR designs (optimal RAR for two-arm binary outcome trials) is chosen because it is quite basic but, at the same time, it incorporates all of the key elements of RAR, and it is well suited for illustration purposes. The chapter is not meant to be a comprehensive study on how to choose the best RAR design for use in practice. For book-length discussions on this subject please refer to [14,37].

In Section 10.2, we review and compare several optimal allocation rules for two-arm binary outcome trials. Section 10.3 describes RAR designs that can be used to converge to the chosen optimal allocation. We also discuss theoretical aspects of optimal RAR designs - the relationship between optimality, variability and power, asymptotically best RAR procedures, and statistical inference following RAR. In Section 10.4, we discuss Monte Carlo simulation of optimal RAR designs. In Section 10.5, we discuss the issues of sample size and power for RAR trials. Section 10.6 describes some additional important considerations and practical issues for RAR trials. In Section 10.7, we illustrate utility of RAR by redesigning a real life clinical trial. Concluding remarks are given in Section 10.8.

10.2 Optimal Allocation

Consider a binary outcome clinical trial to compare an experimental treatment, E, versus a control treatment, C. Let p_E denote the probability of success on E ($q_E = 1 - p_E$) and p_C denote the probability of success on C ($q_C = 1 - p_C$). Suppose the trial has a sample size n which is fixed and predetermined. Let ρ denote the allocation proportion for the experimental treatment where $0 < \rho < 1$. This means roughly $n_E = n\rho$ patients are assigned to E and $n_C = n(1-\rho)$ patients are assigned to C. An experimental design problem is to find an optimal allocation ρ^* as a solution to some formal optimization problem. In a two-arm comparative trial, a common objective is to have sufficient power to test the primary study hypothesis. Consider testing the hypothesis $H_0: p_E = p_C$ versus $H_1: p_E \neq p_C$ using the Wald test

$$Z_W = \frac{\hat{p}_E - \hat{p}_C}{\sqrt{\frac{\hat{p}_E \hat{q}_E}{n_E} + \frac{\hat{p}_C \hat{q}_C}{n_C}}}$$

where $\hat{p}_E, \hat{q}_E, \hat{p}_C, \hat{q}_C$ are consistent estimators of the corresponding parameters. Under H_1, Z_W has asymptotically normal distribution with mean

$d = (p_E - p_C)\left\{\frac{p_E q_E}{n_E} + \frac{p_C q_C}{n_C}\right\}^{-1/2}$ and unit variance. The allocation that maximizes power for a fixed sample size n and fixed p_E, q_E, p_C, q_C is one that minimizes the value of $\left\{\frac{p_E q_E}{n\rho} + \frac{p_C q_C}{n(1-\rho)}\right\}$ for $\rho \in (0,1)$. This optimal solution is known as the *Neyman allocation* and it is given by

$$\rho_N^* = \frac{\sqrt{p_E q_E}}{\sqrt{p_E q_E} + \sqrt{p_C q_C}} \quad (10.1)$$

The Neyman allocation assigns a greater proportion of patients to a more variable treatment group. Unfortunately, when $p_E + p_C > 1$, the Neyman allocation is skewed in favor of the less successful treatment, which is inappropriate from an individual ethics perspective.

Rosenberger and co-authors in [10] considered the following question: For fixed variance of the Wald test statistic under the alternative hypothesis, which allocation minimizes the expected number of treatment failures? The optimization problem in this case is formulated as follows:

$$\begin{cases} \min\limits_{\rho \in (0,1)} n\{q_E \rho + q_C(1-\rho)\} \\ s.t. \quad \frac{p_E q_E}{n\rho} + \frac{p_C q_C}{n(1-\rho)} = const \end{cases}$$

The optimal solution is the *RSIHR allocation* named after Rosenberger, Stallard, Ivanova, Harper, and Ricks [10]:

$$\rho_{RSIHR}^* = \frac{\sqrt{p_E}}{\sqrt{p_E} + \sqrt{p_C}} \quad (10.2)$$

Unlike the Neyman allocation, RSIHR allocation always assigns a greater proportion of patients to the more successful treatment.

Now consider testing the hypothesis of equality of treatment effects using the score test based on the log-odds ratio, $\theta = \log\{p_E q_C / (p_C q_E)\}$. For testing $H_0: \theta = 0$, one computes $Z = (n_C S_E - n_E S_C)/n$ and $V = n_E n_C SF/n^3$, where S_E and S_C are the number of successes on E and C, respectively, $S = S_E + S_C$ and $F = n - S$ [38]. When n is large, Z is approximately normally distributed with mean θV and variance V. Using the large sample approximations $S \approx n\bar{p}$ and $F \approx n(1-\bar{p})$, where $\bar{p} = (n_E p_E + n_C p_C)/n$, the variance of the score statistic is approximated as

$$V \approx n\rho(1-\rho)(\rho p_E + (1-\rho)p_C)(\rho q_E + (1-\rho)q_C).$$

Magirr in [39] considered the problem of minimizing expected number of treatment failures $n\{q_E\rho + q_C(1-\rho)\}$ subject to the fixed value of V. It can be shown using simple algebra that this is equivalent to minimizing the value of $\{\rho(1-\rho)(\rho p_E + (1-\rho)p_C\}^{-1}$ for $\rho \in (0,1)$. The optimal solution is

$$\rho^*_{SCORE} = \frac{p_E - 2p_C + \sqrt{p_E^2 - p_E p_C + p_C^2}}{3(p_E - p_C)}, \quad p_E \neq p_C. \quad (10.3)$$

If $p_E = p_C$, the optimal solution is $\rho^*_{SCORE} = 1/2$. This allocation rule will be referred to as *score allocation.* It can be shown that for any $p_E, p_C \in (0,1)$ one has $1/3 \le \rho^*_{SCORE} \le 2/3$. Furthermore, $\rho^*_{SCORE} > 1/2$ for $p_E > p_C$ and $\rho^*_{SCORE} < 1/2$ for $p_E < p_C$, which implies that a greater proportion of patients are assigned to the more successful treatment.

Baldi Antognini and Giovagnoli [40] considered the following compound criterion combining ethical and inferential objectives:

$$\Phi_\omega(\rho) = \omega\left\{\frac{\Psi_E(\rho)}{\Psi_E^*}\right\} + \left(1-\omega\right)\left\{\frac{\Psi_I(\rho)}{\Psi_I^*}\right\}.$$

Here $\omega \in (0,1)$ is a user-defined weight that determines a tradeoff between ethics and inference, $\Psi_E(\rho) = q_E\rho + q_C(1-\rho)$ is the expected proportion of treatment failures, $\Psi_E^* = \min(q_E, q_C)$, $\Psi_I(\rho) = \{p_E q_E/\rho + p_C q_C/(1-\rho)\}$ is the variance of the estimated treatment difference, and $\Psi_I^* = \{\sqrt{p_E q_E} + \sqrt{p_C q_C}\}^2$ is the minimum value of $\Psi_I(\rho)$ for $\rho \in (0,1)$. The motivation for using standardized criteria of ethics and inference is to bring them to a comparable scale. The optimal allocation ρ^*_ω minimizing $\Phi_\omega(\rho)$ is the unique solution in (0,1) of the equation

$$\frac{\omega}{1-\omega}\frac{p_E - p_C}{\min(q_E, q_C)}\left\{\frac{\sqrt{p_C q_C}}{\sqrt{p_E q_E}} + 1\right\}^2 = \frac{\left\{\frac{p_C q_C}{p_E q_E} - 1\right\}(\rho^*_\omega)^2 + 2\rho^*_\omega - 1}{\{\rho^*_\omega(1-\rho^*_\omega)\}^2}. \quad (10.4)$$

Baldi Antognini and Giovagnoli in [40] explored different choices of the weight ω. In our presentation, we set $\omega = 1/2$ (equal interest in ethics and inference), and this allocation rule will be referred to as *compound optimal allocation.* There are other useful optimal allocation rules for two-arm binary outcome trials which we omit here due to a limited space. The interested reader is referred to [41-44].

Figure 10.1 shows the values of the four optimal allocation proportions (1)–(4) for a range of scenarios when $p_C = 0.4$ and $0.2 \le p_E \le 0.9$. The RSIHR allocation (2), score allocation (3), and compound optimal allocation (4) are always skewed in favor of the more successful treatment, whereas the Neyman allocation (1) can be skewed in favor of the inferior treatment. When treatment effects are the same $(p_E = p_C = 0.4)$, all four rules reduce to equal allocation.

Figure 10.1 *Allocation Proportion to Treatment E for Four Optimal Allocation Rules*

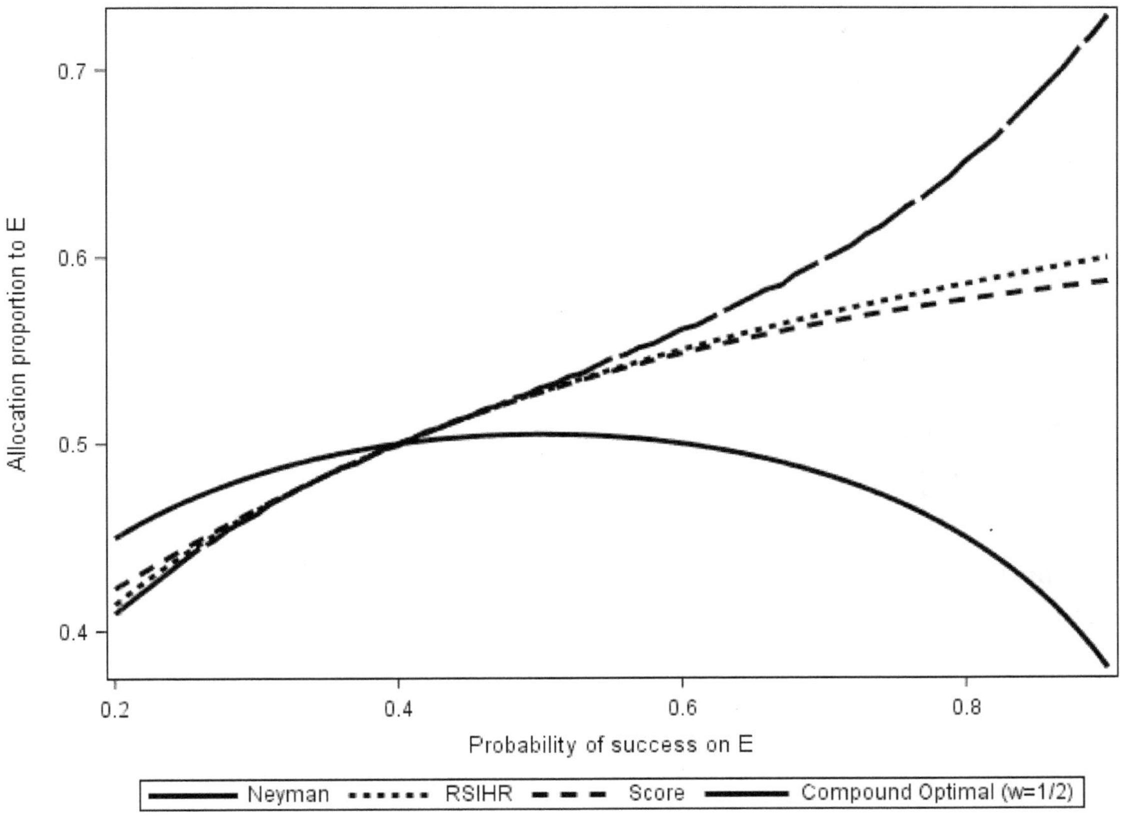

Table 10.1 (generated by program `ch10.2.sas` in the supplemental material) presents the values of power of the Wald test and total expected treatment failures for several scenarios of a trial with $n = 100$ patients. Six rules are compared: 1:1 allocation, 2:1 allocation, and four optimal allocation rules (1)–(4). In terms of power, the four optimal allocation rules are almost identical to 1:1 allocation; however, 2:1 allocation has 1% to 8% lower power compared to the other rules. The RSIHR (2), score (3), and compound optimal (4) allocation rules result in modest but consistent reductions in the expected number of treatment failures compared to 1:1 allocation. These numbers are 1 to 3 fewer failures when the absolute difference between treatment success probabilities is 0.2 to 0.3, and it can be 3 to 6 fewer failures when difference between success probabilities is 0.4. The 2:1 allocation yields the lowest number of failures when $p_E > p_C$ and the highest number of failures when $p_E < p_C$.

Table 10.1 *Power (Expected Number of Failures) for Six Allocation Rules for n=100 Subjects*

p_E	p_C	**1:1**	**2:1**	**Neyman**	**RSIHR**	**Score**	**Compound optimal** ($\omega = 1/2$)
0.2	0.4	0.61 (70)	0.53 (73)	0.61 (69)	0.61 (68)	0.61 (68)	0.61 (68)
0.5	0.4	0.17 (55)	0.16 (53)	0.17 (55)	0.17 (55)	0.17 (55)	0.17 (55)

p_E	p_C	**1:1**	**2:1**	**Neyman**	**RSIHR**	**Score**	**Compound optimal** ($\omega = 1/2$)
0.6	0.4	0.53 (50)	0.49 (47)	0.53 (50)	0.53 (49)	0.53 (49)	0.53 (49)
0.7	0.4	0.89 (45)	0.84 (40)	0.89 (46)	0.88 (43)	0.88 (43)	0.87 (42)
0.8	0.4	0.99 (40)	0.98 (33)	0.99 (42)	0.99 (37)	0.99 (37)	0.99 (34)

10.3 Response-Adaptive Randomization for Implementing Optimal Allocation

10.3.1 Preliminaries

Optimal allocation rules discussed in Section 10.2 depend on treatment success probabilities p_E and p_C. For the time being let us assume that p_E and p_C are known. Furthermore, suppose that all n eligible patients are available for the trial at once. Then, if we want to implement, say, RSIHR allocation (2), we would have to split the n patients into two groups of sizes n_E and n_C, where

$$n_E = n\frac{\sqrt{p_E}}{\sqrt{p_E}+\sqrt{p_C}} \text{ and } n_C = n - n_E$$

(n_E and n_C can be rounded up to integers if necessary).

However, there are several potential issues with this approach. First, it is infeasible to have all n patients at once. Most clinical trial take years to run and eligible patients are recruited over time. Second, in practice p_E and p_C are unknown, and in fact the trial is run to estimate p_E and p_C. Third, study patients cannot be simply "split" into two treatment groups—an investigator may be subjective when deciding on treatment assignments and may introduce bias into the design.

RAR can be used to target the desired optimal allocation. The idea of RAR is to use accumulating data (outcomes) from patients in the trial to estimate p_E and p_C and modify treatment randomization probabilities for the current patient such that the design converges to the desired target allocation. By convergence of the design we mean that the sample treatment allocation proportions converge to the corresponding target allocation proportions. RAR requires that primary outcome data are unmasked periodically or sequentially for the purpose of estimating p_E and p_C and updating treatment randomization probabilities. In practice, RAR trials must be conducted by a centralized randomization unit, and the roles and responsibilities of the study personnel involved in data collection, data cleaning, data analysis, and generation of treatment assignments must be clearly defined in the trial protocol [2,45].

We now describe the basic setup for RAR. The trial starts with randomizing $2m_0$ patients (m_0 is some small positive integer) equally between E and C using some restricted randomization procedure, such as the permuted block design. This is done to ascertain some initial data to estimate p_E and p_C. We make an assumption that *each patient's outcome is available immediately after randomization.* While this is quite a restrictive assumption because in practice some time must pass before a patient's response is observable, it serves as a useful starting point for developing RAR theory [14]. Consider a point in the trial when $m \geq 2m_0$ patients have been treated and the $(m + 1)$st patient is ready to be randomized into the trial. The treatment assignment for the $(m + 1)$st patient will depend on the data accrued thus far. For $j = 1, \ldots, m$, let $\delta_j = 1$ (or 0) if the jth patient's treatment is E (or C) and let $Y_j = 1$ (or 0) if the jth patient's outcome is success (or failure). Note that $p_E = \Pr(Y_j = 1 | \delta_j = 1)$ and $p_C = \Pr(Y_j = 1 | \delta_j = 0)$ for $j = 1, \ldots, m$. Given $\mathbf{\Delta}_m = (\delta_1, \ldots, \delta_m)$ and $\mathbf{Y}_m = (Y_1, \ldots, Y_m)$, the treatment assignment for the $(m + 1)$st patient will have to be determined.

Hu and Rosenberger in [14] define a RAR procedure as one for which randomization probability to treatment E for the $(m + 1)$st patient is determined as

$$\phi_{m+1, E} = \Pr(\delta_{m+1} = 1 | \mathbf{\Delta}_m, \mathbf{Y}_m), \; m > 2m_0. \quad (10.5)$$

Therefore, the randomization probability to treatment E is $\phi_{m+1, C} = 1 - \phi_{m+1, E}$. Note that the quantity in (10.5) is random because it depends on $\mathbf{\Delta}_m$ and $\mathbf{Y}_m$ which are random vectors. Based on $\mathbf{\Delta}_m$ and $\mathbf{Y}_m$, let $N_E(m) = \sum_{j=1}^{m} \delta_j$ and $N_C(m) = \sum_{j=1}^{m} (1 - \delta_j)$ denote the number of patients assigned to E and C, and let $S_E(m) = \sum_{j=1}^{m} \delta_j Y_j$ and $S_C(m) = \sum_{j=1}^{m} (1 - \delta_j) Y_j$ denote the number of successes on E and C. The success probabilities p_E and p_C are estimated as follows:

$$\widehat{p}_{Em} = \frac{S_E(m)}{N_E(m)} \text{ and } \widehat{p}_{Cm} = \frac{S_C(m)}{N_C(m)}. \quad (10.6)$$

It should be noticed that $\widehat{p}_{Em}$ and $\widehat{p}_{Cm}$ in (10.6) are not usual estimators of binomial proportions because with RAR treatment assignments $\delta_1, \ldots, \delta_m$ are correlated and the denominators $N_E(m)$ and $N_C(m)$ are random variables. Martingale theory is used to establish asymptotic properties of the estimators in this case [14].

In Sections 10.3.2, 10.3.3, and 10.3.4 we discuss several approaches to facilitate optimal RAR procedures. All these procedures possess the following important asymptotic properties:

1. The maximum likelihood estimators $\widehat{p}_{Em}$ and $\widehat{p}_{Cm}$ in (10.6) are strongly consistent for p_E and p_C; they are asymptotically uncorrelated and have an asymptotically bivariate normal distribution.
2. The sample treatment allocation proportion $N_E(m)/m$ is strongly consistent for the target allocation ρ and has an asymptotically normal distribution with a known structure for the asymptotic variance.

Therefore, standard asymptotic estimators and tests can be used for statistical inference following optimal RAR procedures [35,36].

10.3.2 Sequential Maximum Likelihood Estimation Design

With the *sequential maximum likelihood estimation* (SMLE) design, treatment randomization probabilities are set equal to the current estimates of the target allocation proportions [22,46]. In particular, Rosenberger and co-authors in [10] proposed the following SMLE procedure targeting the RSIHR allocation (10.2):

$$\phi_{m+1,\,E} = \frac{\sqrt{\widehat{p}_{Em}}}{\sqrt{\widehat{p}_{Em}} + \sqrt{\widehat{p}_{Cm}}} \quad (10.7)$$

They proved strong consistency and asymptotic normality of both estimators and the sample allocation proportions with the procedure (10.7) and showed that the Wald test $Z_W = \left(\widehat{p}_{Em} - \widehat{p}_{Cm}\right)\left\{\frac{\widehat{p}_{Em}\widehat{q}_{Em}}{N_E(m)} + \frac{\widehat{p}_{Cm}\widehat{q}_{Cm}}{N_C(m)}\right\}^{-1/2}$ is asymptotically standard normal under $H_0: p_E = p_C$. They also showed via simulation that the procedure (10.7) can lead to a modest reduction in treatment failures with minimal or no loss in power compared to equal randomization designs. A limitation of the SMLE design is that it can be quite variable, which can have a negative impact on power. More elaborate RAR procedures are described in Sections 10.3.3 and 10.3.4.

10.3.3 Doubly Adaptive Biased Coin Design

The Doubly Adaptive Biased Coin Design (DBCD) is a class of RAR procedures that can target any allocation proportion ρ provided that some mild regularity conditions are met [47,48]. The key ingredient of DBCD is the allocation function $g(x, \rho)$, defined on $[0,1] \times [0,1]$. Hu and Zhang [48] proposed the following allocation function:

$$g(x,\rho) = \begin{cases} \dfrac{\rho\left\{\frac{\rho}{x}\right\}^{\gamma}}{\rho\left\{\frac{\rho}{x}\right\}^{\gamma} + (1-\rho)\left\{\frac{1-\rho}{1-x}\right\}^{\gamma}}, & 0 < x < 1; \\ 1 - x, & x = 0,1\,. \end{cases} \quad (10.8)$$

The user-defined parameter $\gamma \geq 0$ controls the degree of randomness ($\gamma = 0$ is most random and $\gamma \to \infty$ is almost a deterministic procedure). The role of γ will become clear momentarily.

Suppose that the target allocation has been chosen as $\rho = \rho\left(p_E, p_C\right)$. After m patients, the target allocation is estimated as $\widehat{\rho}_m = \rho\left(\widehat{p}_{Em}, \widehat{p}_{Cm}\right)$. The DBCD assigns the $(m + 1)$st patient to E with probability

$$\phi_{m+1,\,E} = g\left(\frac{N_E(m)}{m}, \widehat{\rho}_m\right),$$

where $g(x, \rho)$ is as in (10.8). If $\gamma = 0$, the DBCD is equivalent to $\phi_{m+1,\,E} = \widehat{\rho}_m$, the SMLE design.

Hu and Zhang in [48] proved that under the condition that $\rho = \rho\left(p_E, p_C\right)$ is continuous in its arguments and is twice continuously differentiable in a small neighborhood of the true value of $\left(p_E, p_C\right)$, both the sample treatment proportions and the estimators are strongly consistent and asymptotically normal. In particular, $N_E(m)/m$ has an asymptotically normal distribution with mean ρ and asymptotic variance

$$\sigma_\gamma^2 = \frac{\rho(1-\rho)}{1+2\gamma} + \frac{2(1+\gamma)}{1+2\gamma}\left\{\left(\frac{\partial\rho}{\partial p_E}\right)^2\frac{p_E q_E}{\rho} + \left(\frac{\partial\rho}{\partial p_C}\right)^2\frac{p_C q_C}{1-\rho}\right\}.$$

A small value of σ_γ^2 is desirable from the standpoint of statistical power. Clearly, σ_γ^2 is decreasing in γ. When $\gamma = 0$, σ_γ^2 is largest. When $\gamma \to \infty$, σ_γ^2 is smallest, but the procedure is almost deterministic. Rosenberger and Hu in [35] recommended using $\gamma = 2$ as a tradeoff between power and randomness.

Let us describe the DBCD procedure with $\gamma = 2$ targeting the RSIHR allocation (10.2). After m patients, the target is estimated as $\hat{\rho}_m = \sqrt{\hat{p}_{Em}}/(\sqrt{\hat{p}_{Em}} + \sqrt{\hat{p}_{Cm}})$. Then the $(m+1)$st patient is randomized to E with probability

$$\phi_{m+1,\,E} = \frac{\hat{\rho}_m \left\{ \frac{\hat{\rho}_m}{N_E(m)/m} \right\}^2}{\hat{\rho}_m \left\{ \frac{\hat{\rho}_m}{N_E(m)/m} \right\}^2 + \left(1 - \hat{\rho}_m\right)\left\{ \frac{1 - \hat{\rho}_m}{N_C(m)/m} \right\}^2}.$$

10.3.4 Efficient Randomized-Adaptive Design

Hu and co-authors in [50] considered the following question: Can a RAR procedure be found that preserves allocation randomness, and can target any pre-specified allocation and has minimal variability? They proposed a class of efficient randomized-adaptive designs (ERADE) for which the $(m+1)$st patient is randomized to E with probability

$$\phi_{m+1,\,E} = \begin{cases} \delta\hat{\rho}_m, & N_E(m)/m > \hat{\rho}_m; \\ \hat{\rho}_m, & N_E(m)/m = \hat{\rho}_m; \\ 1 - \delta(1 - \hat{\rho}_m), & N_E(m)/m < \hat{\rho}_m, \end{cases}$$

where $0 \le \delta \le 1$is a user-defined parameter that controls the degree of randomness ($\delta = 0$ is most deterministic between and $\delta = 1$ is most random). Hu and co-authors recommended setting δ between 0.4 and 0.7 [50]. ERADE is an extension of the biased-coin design [5] which is used to target equal allocation.

The theoretical properties of ERADE are similar to those of DBCD: both sample proportions and estimators are strongly consistent and asymptotically normal. However, a fundamental difference between the two designs is that the allocation function for ERADE is discrete, whereas for DBCD it is continuous in ρ. This means that ERADE is less variable than DBCD. In fact, ERADE is equivalent to DBCD with $\gamma \to \infty$ and it is an asymptotically best RAR procedure [51]. The sample proportion $N_E(m)/m$ for ERADE is asymptotically normal with mean ρ and asymptotic variance $\left(\frac{\partial \rho}{\partial p_E}\right)^2 \frac{p_E q_E}{\rho} + \left(\frac{\partial \rho}{\partial p_C}\right)^2 \frac{p_C q_C}{1-\rho}$, which is the lower bound on the variance of a RAR procedure targeting allocation ρ.

10.3.5 Theoretical Comparison of Various RAR Designs

Hu and Rosenberger in [34] derived a relationship between optimality, variability and power that can be used to facilitate a comparison among various RAR designs. They considered a second-order Taylor series expansion of a non-centrality parameter of the chi-square test following RAR, and showed that three important factors that have an impact on power of the test are the allocation target for a fixed design, the speed of convergence to the target, and the variability of the sample allocation proportion. For RAR procedures with the same allocation target, only variability of the sample proportions can be compared. A procedure with small variability is desirable. Hu and co-authors in [51] defined an asymptotically best RAR procedure as one that attains the smallest possible asymptotic variance of $N_E(m)/m$. A version of Theorem 1 of [51] for binary outcome trials can be formulated as follows:

Theorem 1 Consider a two-arm binary outcome trial using an RAR procedure with target allocation $\rho = \rho(p_E, p_C)$. Suppose the following regular conditions hold:

1. $p_E, p_C \in (0,1)$
2. $N_E(n)/n \rightarrow \rho \in (0,1)$ almost surely
3. $\sqrt{n}\left(N_E(n)/n - \rho\right) \rightarrow N\left(0, \sigma^2\right)$ in distribution, where $\sigma^2 > 0$.

Then we have $\sigma^2 \geq B(p_E, p_C) = \left(\frac{\partial \rho}{\partial p_E}\right)^2 \frac{p_E q_E}{\rho} + \left(\frac{\partial \rho}{\partial p_C}\right)^2 \frac{p_C q_C}{1-\rho}$. The quantity $B(p_E, p_C)$ is called the lower bound for the variance of RAR procedures with allocation target ρ. A RAR procedure that attains the lower bound is called an asymptotically best RAR procedure.

For illustration, let us consider three RAR designs targeting the RSIHR allocation $\rho = \rho^*_{RSIHR}$: 1) SMLE procedure (Section 10.3.2), 2) DBCD with $\gamma = 2$ (Section 10.3.3), and 3) ERADE (Section 10.3.4). Clearly, $\rho = \rho^*_{RSIHR}$ is a twice continuously differentiable function of (p_E, p_C) with $\frac{\partial \rho}{\partial p_E} = \frac{\rho(1-\rho)}{2p_E}$ and $\frac{\partial \rho}{\partial p_C} = -\frac{\rho(1-\rho)}{2p_C}$. One can easily show that the lower bound for the variance of $N_E(m)/m$ (the asymptotic variance of ERADE) is

$$\sigma^2_{ERADE} = B(p_E, p_C) = \frac{1}{4\left(\sqrt{p_E} + \sqrt{p_C}\right)^3}\left\{\frac{p_C q_E}{\sqrt{p_E}} + \frac{p_E q_C}{\sqrt{p_C}}\right\}. \quad (10.9)$$

The asymptotic variance of DBCD(γ) (Section 10.3.3) is

$$\sigma^2_{DBCD(\gamma)} = \frac{\sqrt{p_E p_C}}{(1+2\gamma)\left(\sqrt{p_E} + \sqrt{p_C}\right)^2} + \frac{2(1+\gamma)}{1+2\gamma}\sigma^2_{ERADE}. \quad (10.10)$$

The asymptotic variance of the SMLE procedure, σ^2_{SMLE}, is obtained by calculating $\sigma^2_{DBCD(\gamma)}$ with $\gamma = 0$. Clearly, $\sigma^2_{SMLE} > \sigma^2_{DBCD(\gamma=2)} > \sigma^2_{ERADE}$.

Figure 10.2 is a plot of asymptotic variance $N_E(m)/m$ of three RAR designs (SMLE, DBCD(γ), and ERADE) for a range of scenarios when $p_C = 0.4$ and $0.2 \leq p_E \leq 0.9$. Interestingly, the variance is monotone decreasing as p_E is increasing from 0.2 to 0.9. For SMLE the variance is decreasing from 0.6 to 0.38; for DBCD($\gamma = 2$) it is decreasing from 0.26 to 0.12; and for ERADE it is decreasing from 0.18 to 0.06. For a completely randomized design (CRD) targeting 1:1 allocation (a non-adaptive procedure for which every allocation is made independently with probability 1/2), the variance is constant, 0.25, for any values of p_C and p_E. As such, in the considered scenarios both DBCD ($\gamma = 2$) and ERADE are overall less variable than CRD.

Figure 10.2 *Asymptotic Variance of the Sample Proportion for Three RAR Designs*

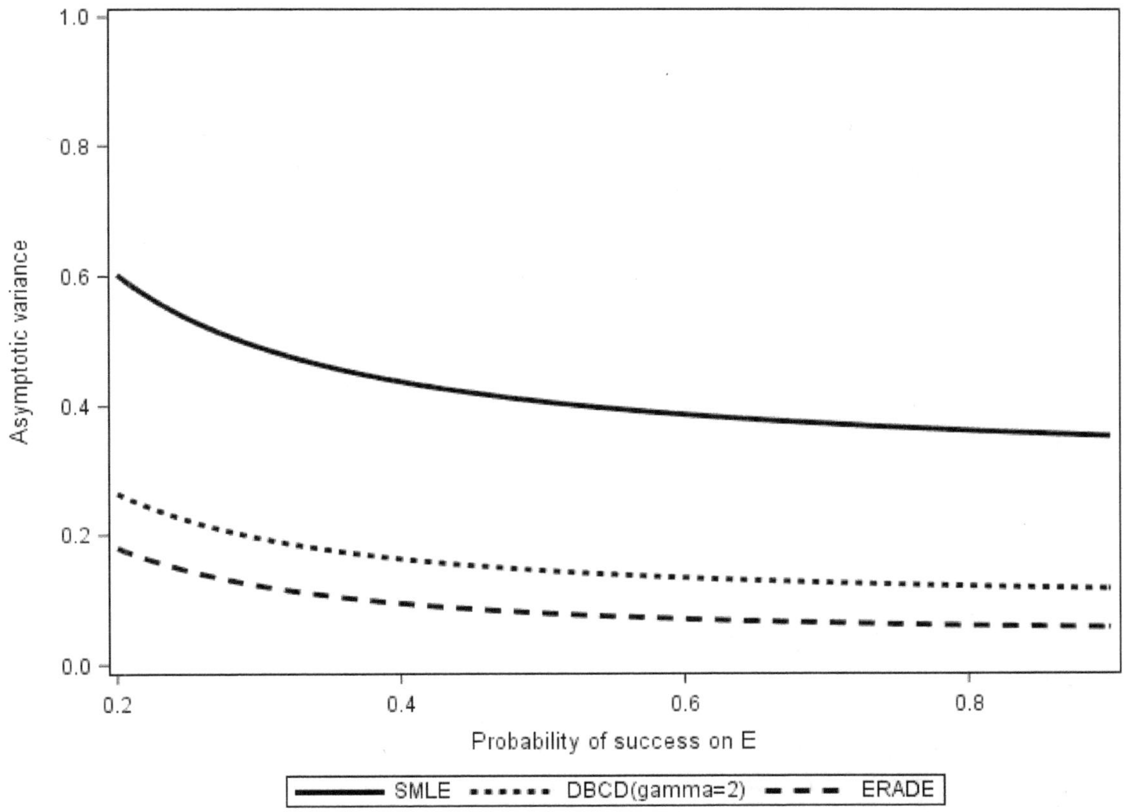

10.4 Simulation of Optimal Response-Adaptive Randomization Procedures

10.4.1 Simulating a Single RAR Sequence

If the target allocation ratio is pre-specified (e.g. 1:1 or 2:1), a treatment randomization sequence can be pre-generated before any subject is enrolled into a trial. In contrast, a RAR sequence cannot be pre-generated because treatment randomization probabilities are adaptively modified throughout the trial based on cumulative patient outcome data.

Standard computer packages such as SAS an R have built-in random number generators that can be used to simulate RAR designs under certain assumptions on outcomes from patients in the trial. We start with a simulation of a single randomization sequence. Program **`ch10.4.1.sas`** in the supplemental material generates a sequence of treatment assignments for a trial with $n = 40$ patients using the DBCD($\gamma = 2$) procedure (Section 10.3.3) targeting the RSIHR allocation (10.2). We assume that the true success probabilities for the treatments are $p_E = 0.7$ and $p_C = 0.4$, and therefore, $\rho = \sqrt{0.7}/(\sqrt{0.7} + \sqrt{0.4}) = 0.57$. The first $2m_0$ patients are randomized between E and C using equal randomization (in Program **`ch10.4.1.sas`**, we set $2m_0 = 10$). Specifically, randomization probability to E for the first 10 patients is set equal to

$$\phi_{1,E} = \frac{1}{2}; \qquad \phi_{m+1,E} = \frac{5 - N_E(m)}{10 - m}, \; m = 1, \ldots 9$$

where $N_E(m)$ is the number of treatment E assignments among the m patients. The response-adaptive part starts from the 11th patient. The randomization probability for the $(m + 1)$th patient ($m = 10, \ldots, 39$) is determined as follows. Assuming that all outcome data from previous m patients are available, obtain $N_E(m)$, $N_C(m)$, $S_E(m)$, $S_C(m)$, and estimate treatment success probabilities as $\widehat{p}_{k,m} = \left(S_k(m) + 0.5\right)/\left(N_k(m) + 1\right)$. Note that $\widehat{p}_{k,m}$ are Bayesian estimates under a noninformative prior, to avoid estimated success probabilities equal to zero or one. The estimated target allocation is updated as $\widehat{\rho}_m = \sqrt{\widehat{p}_{E,m}}/\left(\sqrt{\widehat{p}_{E,m}} + \sqrt{\widehat{p}_{C,m}}\right)$, and the randomization probability to E for the $(m + 1)$st patient is set equal to

$$\phi_{m+1,E} = \frac{\widehat{\rho}_m\left\{\frac{\widehat{\rho}_m}{N_E(m)/m}\right\}^2}{\widehat{\rho}_m\left\{\frac{\widehat{\rho}_m}{N_E(m)/m}\right\}^2 + \left(1 - \widehat{\rho}_m\right)\left\{\frac{1 - \widehat{\rho}_m}{N_C(m))/m}\right\}^2}, \; m = 10, \ldots, 39.$$

For the $(m + 1)$st patient, a uniform random number $U_{m+1} \in [0,1]$ is generated, and the following rule is applied:

If $U_{m+1} \le \phi_{m+1,E}$, assign treatment E; else if $U_{m+1} > \phi_{m+1,E}$, assign treatment C.

Table 10.2 shows the changes in randomization probabilities as the trial progresses. The first column is the patient number. Columns 2 and 3 represent current treatment numbers for E and C. Columns 4 and 5 represent the current numbers of successes on E and C. Columns 6 and 7 display current estimates of success probabilities for E and C, and column 8 displays the current estimate of the target allocation. As noted above, the treatment assignments for the first 10 patients are not response-adaptive and, therefore, the values in columns 4–8 are not populated in this case (NA). Column 9 is the randomization probability for the current patient. Column 10 is the treatment assignment (1 if treatment is E, and 0 if treatment is C). The last column is the outcome of the patient (1 if success, and 0 if failure).

Table 10.2 *Simulation of a Single Sequence of DBCD*

Patient	$N_{E,m-1}$	$N_{C,m-1}$	$S_{E,m-1}$	$S_{C,m-1}$	$\widehat{p}_{E,m-1}$	$\widehat{p}_{C,m-1}$	$\widehat{\rho}_{m-1}$	$\phi_{m,E}$	δ_m	Y_m
1	0	0	NA	NA	NA	NA	NA	0.50	0	0
2	0	1	NA	NA	NA	NA	NA	0.56	1	1
3	1	1	NA	NA	NA	NA	NA	0.50	1	1
4	2	1	NA	NA	NA	NA	NA	0.43	0	1
5	2	2	NA	NA	NA	NA	NA	0.50	1	0
6	3	2	NA	NA	NA	NA	NA	0.40	1	1
7	4	2	NA	NA	NA	NA	NA	0.25	0	0
8	4	3	NA	NA	NA	NA	NA	0.33	0	0
9	4	4	NA	NA	NA	NA	NA	0.50	1	1

Patient	$N_{E,m-1}$	$N_{C,m-1}$	$S_{E,m-1}$	$S_{C,m-1}$	$\widehat{p}_{E,m-1}$	$\widehat{p}_{C,m-1}$	$\widehat{\rho}_{m-1}$	$\phi_{m,E}$	δ_m	Y_m
10	5	4	NA	NA	NA	NA	NA	0.00	0	0
11	5	5	4	1	0.75	0.25	0.63	0.88	1	0
12	6	5	4	1	0.64	0.25	0.62	0.80	1	1
13	7	5	5	1	0.69	0.25	0.62	0.77	0	0
14	7	6	5	1	0.69	0.21	0.64	0.85	1	1
15	8	6	6	1	0.72	0.21	0.65	0.83	1	0
16	9	6	6	1	0.65	0.21	0.64	0.76	1	1
17	10	6	7	1	0.68	0.21	0.64	0.74	1	0
18	11	6	7	1	0.63	0.21	0.63	0.67	0	0
19	11	7	7	1	0.63	0.19	0.65	0.76	1	1
20	12	7	8	1	0.65	0.19	0.65	0.74	0	0
21	12	8	8	1	0.65	0.17	0.66	0.81	1	0
22	13	8	8	1	0.61	0.17	0.66	0.77	0	1
23	13	9	8	2	0.61	0.25	0.61	0.69	0	1
24	13	10	8	3	0.61	0.32	0.58	0.65	1	1
25	14	10	9	3	0.63	0.32	0.59	0.63	1	1
26	15	10	10	3	0.66	0.32	0.59	0.61	0	0
27	15	11	10	3	0.66	0.29	0.60	0.68	1	1
28	16	11	11	3	0.68	0.29	0.60	0.67	1	1
29	17	11	12	3	0.69	0.29	0.61	0.65	0	1
30	17	12	12	4	0.69	0.35	0.59	0.62	1	0
31	18	12	12	4	0.66	0.35	0.58	0.58	0	1
32	18	13	12	5	0.66	0.39	0.56	0.57	1	0
33	19	13	12	5	0.63	0.39	0.56	0.52	0	1
34	19	14	12	6	0.63	0.43	0.55	0.52	1	1
35	20	14	13	6	0.64	0.43	0.55	0.50	0	0
36	20	15	13	6	0.64	0.41	0.56	0.56	1	0
37	21	15	13	6	0.61	0.41	0.55	0.52	1	0

Patient	$N_{E,m-1}$	$N_{C,m-1}$	$S_{E,m-1}$	$S_{C,m-1}$	$\hat{p}_{E,m-1}$	$\hat{p}_{C,m-1}$	$\hat{\rho}_{m-1}$	$\phi_{m,E}$	δ_m	Y_m
38	22	15	13	6	0.59	0.41	0.55	0.48	1	1
39	23	15	14	6	0.60	0.41	0.55	0.47	0	1
40	23	16	14	7	0.60	0.44	0.54	0.47	0	0

Consider the 20th patient, for example. Based on the data from the first 19 patients, the treatment numbers are 12 for E and 7 for C, the number of successes are 8 for E and 1 for C, the estimated success probabilities are 0.65 for E and 0.19 for C, the estimated target allocation is 0.65, and the randomization probability for E is 0.74. The treatment assignment turns out to be $E\left(\delta_{20}=0\right)$, and the patient's outcome is a failure $\left(Y_{20}=0\right)$. For the last (40th) patient, the last four columns are as follows: estimated target allocation is 0.54, the randomization probability for E is 0.47, the treatment assignment is $E\left(\delta_{40}=0\right)$, and the patient's outcome is failure $\left(Y_{40}=0\right)$. For this generated sequence, the allocation proportion for E after 40 patients is 23/40=0.575, which is quite close to the target allocation of 0.57.

10.4.2 Operating Characteristics of RAR designs via Monte Carlo Simulation

By simulating a RAR trial (say, 10,000 times) one can generate empirical distributions of important design characteristics, such as treatment allocation proportion, number of treatment failures, etc. This can enable a comparison of various randomization designs under different experimental scenarios. Supplemental program `ch10.4.2.sas` can be used to simulate operating characteristics of five types of randomization procedures:

I. Completely Randomized Design (CRD)

II. Permuted Block Design (PBD)

III. SMLE procedure

IV. DBCD($\gamma=2$) procedure

V. ERADE procedure.

For procedure I, every patient is randomized between E and C with probability 1/2. For procedure II, treatment assignments are made at random in blocks of size $2m_0$ (where m_0 is a pre-specified positive integer) such that treatment balance is achieved after every cohort of $2m_0$ patients. For procedures III, IV, and V, first $2m_0$ patients are randomized between E and C using permuted block randomization, and the remaining patients are randomized between E and C according to a RAR algorithm with RSIHR target allocation $\rho=\rho^*_{RSIHR}=\frac{\sqrt{p_E}}{\sqrt{p_E}+\sqrt{p_C}}$.

The design characteristics include the following:

- Allocation proportion $N_E(n)/n$;
- Number of trial subjects assigned to superior treatment: $N_E(n)1\{p_E\geq p_C\}+N_C(n)1\{p_E<p_C\}$;
- Total number of failures in the trial: $F(n)=F_E(n)+F_C(n)$, where $F_k(n)$ is the number of failures on treatment $k=E,C$;

- Estimated treatment difference $\widehat{\Delta}(n) = \widehat{p}_{En} - \widehat{p}_{Cn}$;
- Empirical (average) power of the Wald test (with 2-sided $\alpha = 0.05$).

Supplemental program **ch10.4.2.sas** was run to simulate the operating characteristics of the five designs I – V for a scenario when $p_E = 0.7$ and $p_C = 0.4$, based on 10,000 simulations. The trial sample size was set $n = 120$ which corresponds to ~92% power of the Wald test for the equal allocation design. The target allocation is 0.5 for designs I and II and it is 0.57 for designs III, IV, and V.

Figure 10.3 shows simulated distributions of the allocation proportion. For design I (CRD), the distribution is centered around 0.5 but variability is nontrivial (the range for the allocation proportion is 0.33 to 0.68). For design II (PBD), the treatment sample sizes are always perfectly balanced; therefore, the allocation is constant at 0.5. The RAR designs III (SMLE), IV (DBCD with $\gamma = 2$) and V (ERADE) have approximately normal distributions that are centered around target allocation 0.57. Consistent with theory, ERADE has the lowest variability and SMLE has the highest variability among the three RAR designs.

Figure 10.3 *Distributions of the Simulated Allocation Proportion for Five Designs*

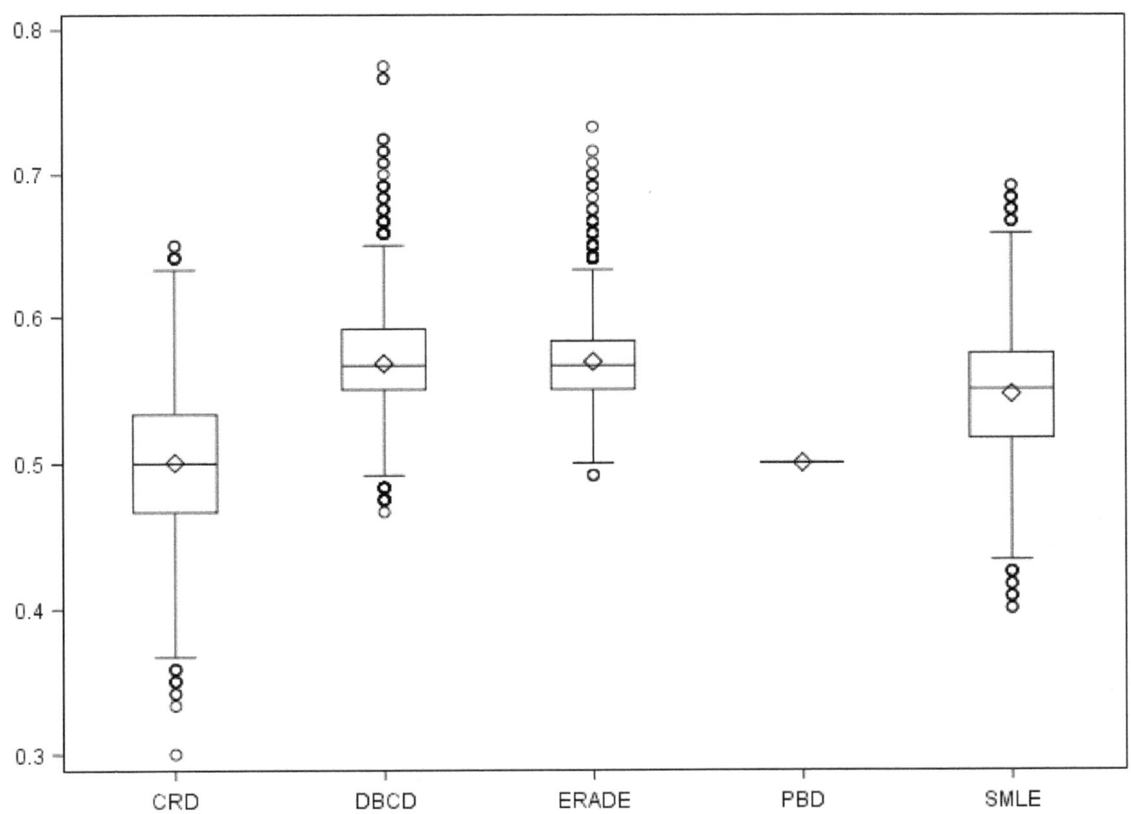

Table 10.3 shows selected summary statistics from the simulation. Since in our example $p_E = 0.7$ and $p_C = 0.4$, treatment E is superior. The average number of treatment E assignments is 66 for SMLE, 68 for DBCD and ERADE, and it is 60 for balanced designs I and II (note the different ranges of this characteristic among the five designs). In regards to the total number of treatment failures, RAR designs yield 2–3 fewer failures on average compared to the balanced designs. All five designs result in unbiased

estimates and have similar mean squared errors (MSEs) of the treatment difference. The empirical power of the Wald test for the designs is 0.92-0.93.

Overall, in this example, RAR designs provide some reduction in treatment failures that are almost identical in terms of quality of estimation and power to balanced randomization designs. While in our simulation we considered the Wald test, other tests can be considered as well. Gu and Lee in [52] performed a comprehensive simulation study to explore the properties of nine different test statistics in two-arm binary outcome RAR trials. They found that for small trials ($n = 30$), the Cook's correction to the chi-square test and Williams' correction to the log-likelihood ratio test have the best performance.

Table 10.3 *Summary Statistics of Simulated Allocation Proportion for Five Designs*

	PBD	**CRD**	**SMLE**	**DBCD** ($\gamma = 2$)	**ERADE**
Target allocation proportion for E	0.50	0.50	0.57	0.57	0.57
Number on E - Mean (SD)	60.0 (0)	60.1 (6)	65.6 (5)	68.1 (4)	68.3 (3)
Number on E - Min-Max	60-60	36-78	46-83	56-88	57-87
Treatment Failures - Mean (SD)	54.0 (5)	53.9 (5)	52.3 (5)	51.5 (5)	51.5 (5)
Treatment Failures - Min-Max	33-72	33-75	33-73	32-71	33-70
Estimated Treatment Difference - Mean (SD)	0.30 (0)	0.30 (0)	0.30 (0)	0.30 (0)	0.30 (0)
Estimated Treatment Difference - MSE	0.0074	0.0077	0.0078	0.0078	0.0079
Average Power of the Wald Test	0.93	0.92	0.92	0.92	0.92

10.5 Power and Sample Size for Response-Adaptive Randomization

For a randomized design with a fixed predetermined allocation ρ (e.g. $\rho = 1/2$ or $\rho = 2/3$), both the total sample size n and the treatment group sizes $n_E = n\rho$ and $n_C = n(1-\rho)$ are fixed quantities, appropriately chosen to achieve the desired power of a test. For a RAR trial, the total sample size n is fixed, but the treatment group sizes

$N_E(n)$ and $N_C(n)$ are random. Therefore, when planning a RAR trial, some special considerations are required for sample size and power.

Hu and Rosenberger in [14] presented an approach to determine an appropriate sample size for a RAR design with target allocation $\rho(p_E, p_C)$. Consider testing a one-sided hypothesis $H_0: p_E = p_C$ versus $H_a: p_E > p_C$. For a given significance level α, H_0 is rejected if the test statistic

$$\frac{\widehat{p}_{En} - \widehat{p}_{Cn}}{\sqrt{\frac{\widehat{p}_{En}\widehat{q}_{En}}{N_E(n)} + \frac{\widehat{p}_{Cn}\widehat{q}_{Cn}}{N_C(n)}}} > z_{1-\alpha},$$

where $z_{1-\alpha}$ is the $100(1-\alpha)$th quantile of the standard normal distribution. Under the assumptions that $N_k(n) \to \infty$ almost surely, $\widehat{p}_{kn}\widehat{q}_{kn} \to p_k q_k$ in probability, and $\sqrt{n}(\widehat{p}_{kn} - p_k) \to N(0, p_k q_k)$ in distribution for $k = E, C$ (which hold true for RAR procedures considered in Sections 10.3.2, 10.3.3, and 10.3.4), the power function can be approximated as

$$P(p_E, p_C, N_E(n), N_C(n)) \approx \Pr\left\{\frac{\widehat{p}_{En} - \widehat{p}_{Cn}}{\sqrt{\frac{p_E q_E}{N_E(n)} + \frac{p_C q_C}{N_C(n)}}} > z_{1-\alpha}\right\} = \Phi\left(\frac{p_E - p_C}{\sqrt{\frac{p_E q_E}{N_E(n)} + \frac{p_C q_C}{N_C(n)}}} - z_{1-\alpha}\right),$$

(10.11)

where Φ is the cumulative distribution function of the standard normal distribution.

Importantly, quantity (10.11) is a random variable because $N_E(n)$ and $N_C(n)$ are random. Under further asymptotic assumptions (that are met for RAR procedures considered thus far):

- $N_E(n)/n \to \rho \in (0,1)$ almost surely and
- $\sqrt{n}(N_E(n)/n - \rho) \to N(0, \sigma^2)$ in distribution for some $\sigma^2 > 0$,

one can obtain a second-order Taylor's approximation to the power function of a RAR design [14]. It is shown that the power of a RAR design with target allocation ρ is mainly determined by the power of a fixed allocation design with allocation ρ and the values of $(N_E(n)/n - \rho)$ and $(N_E(n)/n - \rho)^2$ (the expected value of the latter term is the variance of the allocation proportion). Therefore, one can facilitate the planning of a sample size for RAR designs based on asymptotic approximations.

Three types of sample size can be distinguished: 1) sample size to achieve power $1-\beta$ for a fixed allocation design (type I sample size), 2) sample size to achieve power $1-\beta$ on average (type II sample size), and 3) sample size to achieve power $1-\beta$ with probability $1-\xi$ (for some small positive ξ) (type III sample size) [14].

Let us consider a type I sample size. For a fixed allocation, the treatment group sample sizes are $N_E(n) = n\rho$ and $N_C(n) = n(1-\rho)$, and the sample size to achieve power $1-\beta$ is obtained from solving $\Phi\left(\frac{p_E - p_C}{\sqrt{\frac{p_E q_E}{n\rho} + \frac{p_C q_C}{n(1-\rho)}}} - z_{1-\alpha}\right) = 1 - \beta$. The solution is

$$n_I = \left(\frac{p_E q_E}{\rho} + \frac{p_C q_C}{1-\rho}\right)\frac{\left(z_{1-\alpha} + z_{1-\beta}\right)^2}{\left(p_E - p_C\right)^2} \quad (10.12)$$

(if necessary, n_I in (10.12) can be rounded to the next largest integer).

To determine type II sample size (n_{II}), we should consider the average power function. By our assumption, $\sqrt{n}\left(\frac{N_E(n)}{n} - \rho\right) \to N\left(0, \sigma^2\right)$; therefore, $N_E(n) \approx \rho n + \sigma\sqrt{n}Z$ and $N_C(n) \approx (1-\rho)n - \sigma\sqrt{n}Z$, where Z is a standard normal random variable. The average power function is then approximated as

$$EP\left(p_E, p_C, N_E(n), N_C(n)\right) \approx \int_{-\infty}^{\infty} \Phi\left(\frac{p_E - p_C}{\sqrt{\frac{p_E q_E}{\rho n + \sigma\sqrt{n}x} + \frac{p_C q_C}{(1-\rho)n - \sigma\sqrt{n}x}}} - z_{1-\alpha}\right)\phi(x)\, dx,$$

(10.13)

where $\phi(x) = (2\pi)^{-1/2}\exp\left(-x^2/2\right)$. To achieve power $1-\beta$ on average, we find the smallest positive integer n_{II} for which $EP\left(p_E, p_C, N_E(n_{II}), N_C(n_{II})\right) \geq 1-\beta$.

In practice every clinical trial is run only once, and it is important to ensure that with high probability the statistical test has adequate power. The type III sample size (n_{III}) for a RAR design to achieve fixed power $1-\beta$ with probability $1-\xi$ is the smallest positive integer that satisfies the $\Pr\left(P\left(p_E, p_C, N_E(n_{III}), N_C(n_{III})\right) \geq 1-\beta\right) \geq 1-\xi$. In [14], the authors show that n_{III} can be found (approximately) as the smallest positive integer that satisfies the following two conditions:

$$\frac{p_E q_E}{\rho n_{III} - z_{1-\xi/2}\sigma\sqrt{n_{III}}} + \frac{p_C q_C}{(1-\rho)n_{III} + z_{1-\xi/2}\sigma\sqrt{n_{III}}} < \left(\frac{p_E - p_C}{z_{1-\alpha} + z_{1-\beta}}\right)^2, \quad (10.14)$$

and

$$\frac{p_E q_E}{\rho n_{III} + z_{1-\xi/2}\sigma\sqrt{n_{III}}} + \frac{p_C q_C}{(1-\rho)n_{III} - z_{1-\xi/2}\sigma\sqrt{n_{III}}} < \left(\frac{p_E - p_C}{z_{1-\alpha} + z_{1-\beta}}\right)^2. \quad (10.15)$$

In (10.14) and (10.15), σ is an asymptotic standard deviation of $N_E(n)/n$.

Supplemental program **ch10.5.sas** can be used to determine the three types of sample size for CRD targeting equal allocation $\rho = 1/2$ and ERADE targeting RSIHR allocation $\rho = \frac{\sqrt{p_E}}{\sqrt{p_E} + \sqrt{p_C}}$ for a 1-sided test with $\alpha = 0.025$, desired level of power $1-\beta = 0.90$, and desired probability $1-\xi = 0.95$ to achieve 90% power.

Table 10.4 shows the requisite sample sizes for four experimental scenarios of (p_E, p_C). The fourth, fifth, and sixth columns in Table 10.4 show type I, type II, and type III sample sizes, respectively. For each type of the sample size, the ERADE design requires 2-3 more patients than CRD to achieve the same level of power. The type II sample size is typically 1 more patient than the type I sample size. This means that, on average, RAR designs have nearly the same power as the fixed allocation designs (which is consistent with the theory in [14] suggesting that the average power loss for RAR designs is of order n^{-1}). The type III sample size is typically 4-7 more patients than the type I sample size. Overall, these results suggest that CRD and ERADE do not lose too much power due to randomization compared to the corresponding fixed allocation designs.

Table 10.4 Three Types of Sample Size for Two Randomization Designs

(p_E, p_C)	Design	Target allocation	n_I	n_{II}	n_{III}
(0.5, 0.4)	CRD	0.50	1030	1031	1035
	ERADE	0.53	1032	1033	1037
(0.6, 0.4)	CRD	0.50	253	254	257
	ERADE	0.55	255	256	260
(0.7, 0.4)	CRD	0.50	106	107	111
	ERADE	0.57	109	109	113
(0.8, 0.4)	CRD	0.50	53	54	60
	ERADE	0.59	56	57	61

10.6 Additional Considerations

10.6.1 More Than Two Treatments and Non-Binary Outcomes

Many RCTs involve more than two treatment arms. For instance, in a phase II dose ranging study, the treatment arms may be a placebo and/or an active control and several doses of an investigational drug. The study objectives may include estimation of various treatment contrasts and testing hypotheses of equality of treatment effects. Frequently, the optimal allocation ratio is unequal across treatment arms [53]. As noted in [33], "… the adaptive randomization light shines brightest in complicated multi-arm settings," and indeed, optimal RAR designs are expected to provide more substantial gains over equal randomization in trials with more than two treatment arms (e.g. by placing more patients at the "most informative" dose levels). A general framework for finding optimal allocation designs to minimize a weighted sum of treatment sample sizes subject to constraints on power in a multi-arm setting was proposed by Tymofyeyev and co-authors in the context of a binary outcome trial [17]. Subsequently, their approach was extended to multi-arm, multi-objective clinical trials with normal and time-to-event outcomes [18,19,54,55]. For trials where the primary objectives involve estimation of multiple treatment contrasts, one can use the D_A-optimal allocation [56]. For implementing optimal allocation in a multi-arm trial, one can use the DBCD procedure [48] or an immigrated urn model [26]. Both the DBCD and the immigrated urn model are RAR designs that yield consistent and asymptotically normal estimators and sample allocation proportions under widely satisfied conditions.

10.6.2 Delayed Response

One assumption for developing the theory of RAR is that each patient's outcome is instantaneous. In practice, patient outcomes are measured at certain time points after the treatment has been administered. If the recruitment period is long enough and the outcomes are observed relatively quickly after randomization, RAR can still be applied successfully. This was justified theoretically in [57,58]. Simulation studies show that when approximately 60% or more of the patient outcome data are observed during the recruitment phase and used for purposes of adaptation, the large-sample properties of RAR designs are unaffected by delayed response [18,59]. However, if a delay in observing response is significant, convergence to the target allocation can be slowed down, which can diminish the advantages of RAR.

10.6.3 Misclassified Response

RAR requires access to accumulating primary outcome data from patients in the trial. These data must be of excellent quality to enable accurate estimation and adaptation throughout the trial. In some trials, binary responses may be misclassified and this may introduce bias into the design. Li and Wang in [60] considered a problem of finding optimal allocation for RAR designs where responses are subject to misclassification. While their approach can be useful for mitigating certain biases, efforts should always be made to ensure a high quality assessment of data in RAR trials.

10.6.4 Time Trends

In some clinical trials there may be systematic trends in unknown prognostic factors over time. For instance, the earliest enrolled patients may have a worse prognosis than the patients enrolled later due to changing aspects in the disease, standards of care, and other factors. One of the major criticisms of RAR is that it can lead to biased estimates and an inflated probability of type I error in the presence of time trends [35]. Several approaches to mitigate these issues have been proposed in the literature. The authors of [61,62] suggested applying RAR in blocks such that randomization probabilities are held constant within each block of patients but change adaptively between blocks. The subsequent data analysis through regression modeling should also adjust for the blocking factor. Simon and Simon in [63] developed randomization tests to analyze data following RAR trials. Their approach ensures control of the type I error rate in the presence of time trends. Hu and Roseberger in [64] proposed applying weighted likelihood techniques to reduce bias and mean squared error introduced by time trends. Finally, if covariates that cause heterogeneity are known in advance, one can consider using covariate-adjusted, response-adaptive randomization designs [14,65].

10.7 Examples

10.7.1 Redesigning a Real Clinical Trial

In this section we give an example of a published clinical trial where an optimal RAR design could be useful. Connor and co-authors in [66] reported the results of a randomized, double-blind, placebo-controlled trial of the efficacy and safety of zidovudine (AZT) in reducing the risk of maternal-infant transmission of the human immunodeficiency virus (HIV) type 1. In this trial, 477 pregnant women were enrolled and randomized equally between AZT $(n_E = 239)$ and a placebo $(n_C = 238)$. In the study, 409 women gave birth to 415 live-born infants. The estimated proportions of uninfected infants at 18 months were 0.917 for the AZT group and 0.745 for the placebo group; that is, the AZT treatment regimen reduced the risk of maternal-infant HIV transmission by approximately two thirds compared to a placebo. An optimal RAR design would assign the AZT treatment more often, thereby achieving a more ethical trial design.

We consider a redesign of this trial by simulation. Four competing randomization procedures will be compared:

1. Completely Randomized Design (CRD): Every patient is randomized between the treatment groups with a probability 1/2. (While such a design would not be used in practice, it is included here to enable a comparison of variability with two RAR designs.)
2. Permuted Block Design (PBD): Randomization is applied in blocks of size 4 such that treatment numbers are equalized after every four patients.
3. RSIHR Design: The target allocation $\rho = \sqrt{p_E}/(\sqrt{p_E} + \sqrt{p_C})$ is implemented using ERADE (Section 10.3.4) with $\delta = 0.5$.
4. Compound Optimality Design: The target allocation (obtained as the unique solution to equation (10.4) with $\omega = 0.5$) is implemented by using the ERADE procedure (Section 10.3.4) with $\delta = 0.5$.

The true success probabilities are assumed to be $p_E = 0.917$ (AZT) and $p_C = 0.745$ (placebo), implying $p_E - p_C = 0.172$. With these numbers, the target allocation proportion (unknown to the investigator at the outset) to the AZT treatment is 0.525 for the RSIHR design and 0.607 for the compound optimality design. We use the total sample size $n = 477$ to match the real trial setup in [66]. In the simulation of two RAR designs, the first four patients are assigned to the AZT or placebo using the PBD with block size 4; afterwards, the allocation is performed using the ERADE procedure with the corresponding target allocation. In our simulation, we assume that each patient's outcome is observed before the next patient is enrolled in the study, and treatment randomization probabilities are updated sequentially using RAR algorithms. In practice, the outcome data from some patients may not be available yet at the time of the current patient's entry (i.e. responses are delayed), in which case one would use just the data accrued thus far to update parameter estimates and randomization probabilities. However, this scenario is not explored here.

Table 10.5 (supplemental program `ch10.7.1.sas`) shows the simulated operating characteristics of the four designs. All four designs achieved their target allocation and are very similar in terms of quality of estimation. The RSIHR design is less variable, and the compound optimal design is more variable than the CRD (empirical standard deviation of the allocation proportion for RSIHR, compound optimal, and CRD is 0.006, 0.033, and 0.023, respectively). On average, the RSIHR design assigns 12 more patients to the AZT treatment, and the compound optimal design assigns 53 more patients to the AZT treatment compared to the balanced randomization designs (CRD and PBD). Also, on average, the RSIHR design results in 2 fewer treatment failures, and the compound optimal design results in 8 fewer treatment failures than the balanced designs. Therefore, in this example, the ethical gains of the RSIHR design are rather modest, whereas the compound optimal design provides the best balance between individual and collective ethics.

Table 10.5 *Redesign of the AZT Trial Using Four Randomization Procedures*

	PBD	CRD	RSIHR	Compound Optimality
Allocation proportion for E - Mean (SD)	0.500 (0.001)	0.500 (0.023)	0.526 (0.006)	0.610 (0.033)

	PBD	CRD	RSIHR	Compound Optimality
Number on E - Mean (SD)	238.49 (0.50)	238.46 (11.05)	250.89 (2.65)	291.16 (15.72)
Number on E - Min-Max	238-239	199-279	241-261	245-348
Treatment Failures - Mean (SD)	80.66 (8.01)	80.75 (8.22)	78.53 (7.67)	71.62 (8.09)
Treatment Failures - Min-Max	51-115	52-114	52-109	45-101
Parameter Estimate (p_E) - Mean (SD)	0.9168 (0.0177)	0.9170 (0.0179)	0.9170 (0.0174)	0.9164 (0.0162)
Parameter Estimate (p_E) - MSE	0.0003	0.0003	0.0003	0.0003
Parameter Estimate (p_C)- Mean (SD)	0.7449 (0.0284)	0.7445 (0.0284)	0.7444 (0.0289)	0.7429 (0.0322)
Parameter Estimate (p_C)- MSE	0.0008	0.0008	0.0008	0.0010
Estimated Treatment Difference - Mean (SD)	0.1719 (0.0334)	0.1725 (0.0334)	0.1726 (0.0335)	0.1735 (0.0363)
Estimated Treatment Difference - MSE	0.0011	0.0011	0.0011	0.0013

10.7.2 Implementing DBCD

10.7.2.1 Three Cohort Design

Here we describe two examples that can be modified by the reader in order to implement RAR designs in practice. Sample results are provided in the supplemental materials.

Supplemental program `ch10.7.2.sas` illustrates a practical implementation of the DBCD ($\gamma = 2$) for a three cohort design. In this example, 60 patients are randomized into the trial. The first cohort of 20 patients is randomized to either E or C using PBD with block size 4, with responses generated from a Bernoulli distribution with a probability of 0.4 or 0.2, respectively. The second cohort (20 patients) is randomized to either E or C using the DBCD ($\gamma = 2$), given the data from Cohort 1. Responses are generated from a Bernoulli distribution with probability of 0.4 or 0.2 for E or C, respectively. The last cohort is randomized to E or C using the DBCD ($\gamma = 2$) given data from Cohorts 1 and 2.

10.7.2.2 Two Cohort Sequential Design

Supplemental program `ch10.7.2.sas` also illustrates a two cohort sequential design using DBCD ($\gamma = 2$). A total of 60 patients will be randomized into the trial. The first cohort (20 patients) is randomized to E or C using PBD with block size 4, with responses generated from a Bernoulli distribution with a probability of 0.4 or 0.2, respectively. After this cohort is complete, further allocation is sequential: every patient is randomized to E or C using DBCD ($\gamma = 2$), given the data from all previous patients and assuming responses are instantaneous. Patient responses are generated from a Bernoulli distribution with probability of 0.4 or 0.2 for E or C, respectively.

10.8 Summary

In this chapter we gave an exposition on optimal RAR designs for clinical trials with binary outcomes. These designs use accumulating data from patients in the trial to modify treatment randomization probabilities to achieve an allocation that is optimal for some pre-specified experimental objective(s). A common objective is to minimize the number of treatment failures in the study subject to a constraint on power of a statistical test. Optimal RAR designs can result in a modest reduction in treatment failures in the trial, while maintaining important statistical properties such as power and estimation efficiency. Therefore, such designs can be attractive in clinical trials where outcomes are grave and even a modest reduction in treatment failures is viewed as highly desirable from the individual ethics perspective. The advantages of optimal RAR designs over balanced randomization designs are more pronounced when the treatment difference is large; however, when the treatment effects are the same, RAR reduces to equal allocation randomization. Optimal RAR designs have well-established asymptotic properties: under widely satisfied conditions, both estimators and sample allocation proportions are strongly consistent and follow asymptotically normal distributions. Therefore, standard asymptotic inference procedures can be applied for data analysis following RAR trials.

The main objective of this chapter is to provide an exposition to the methodology of optimal RAR designs, but not to give a comprehensive guidance on how to choose the "best" design for use in practice. Our discussion focused primarily on two-arm binary outcome trials. Some authors indicate that for two-arm binary outcome trials "adaptive randomization is inferior to 1:1 randomization" in terms of benefit to future patients, and it offers "modest to no benefit" to the patients in the trial [32]. In [67], the maximum possible ethical gain of the RSIHR allocation (as measured by the percentage of reduction in the expected number of nonresponders) was quantified. Such a reduction is found to be, in general, quite small (typically 3% or less compared to 1:1 randomization). This finding is also confirmed by our simulation study (cf. Section 10.7). Note that the papers [32,67] examined only two specific types of RAR procedures (Bayesian adaptive randomization using Thall and Wathen's approach [15], and the RAR design targeting RSIHR allocation [10]). However, the scope of optimal RAR designs is much broader—it also includes other types of optimal allocation (e.g. compound optimality design—Design IV in Section 10.7), and multi-arm RAR trials, and trials with binary, count, continuous, and time-to-event outcomes [14]. In more general settings, RAR can provide more substantial improvements, both in terms of statistical efficiency and ethics, over equal allocation randomization [17-19,31]. One important topic that we have not discussed in this chapter is a combination of RAR with group-sequential designs which allow stopping the trial early for futility (if there is lack of treatment effect) or efficacy (if treatment effect is pronounced). Some authors theoretically showed advantages of group-sequential RAR designs [68-71].

It is important to note that RAR designs are operationally more complex and require more upfront planning than designs with fixed randomization schedules. RAR is applicable in trials where the recruitment period is relatively long and the outcomes can be observed quickly; the data must be of high quality to mitigate the potential for bias throughout the trial conduct. See [2,22,45] for further considerations on implementing

RAR designs in practice. In conclusion, if used judiciously, optimal RAR designs can be useful in randomized comparative clinical trials with objectives primarily related to statistical efficiency and ethics.

References

1. Altman DG & Bland JM. (1999). Treatment allocation in controlled trials: why randomize? *British Medical Journal* 318: 1209.
2. Sverdlov O & Rosenberger WF. (2013). Randomization in clinical trials: can we eliminate bias? *Clinical Investigation* 3: 37-47.
3. Friedman LM, Furberg CD & DeMets DL. (2010). *Fundamentals of Clinical Trials, Fourth Edition.* New York: Springer.
4. Berger VW, Ivanova A & Knoll MD. (2003). Minimizing predictability while retaining balance through the use of less restrictive randomization procedures. *Statistics in Medicine* 22: 3017-3028.
5. Efron B. (1971). Forcing a sequential experiment to be balanced. *Biometrika* 58: 403-417.
6. Pocock SJ. (1979). Allocation of patients to treatment in clinical trials. *Biometrics* 35: 183-197.
7. Sposto R & Krailo MD. (1987). Use of unequal allocation in survival trials. *Statistics in Medicine* 6: 119-125.
8. Dumville JC, Hahn S, Miles JNV & Torgerson DJ. (2006). The use of unequal randomisation ratios in clinical trials: a review. *Contemporary Clinical Trials* 27: 1-12.
9. Kuznetsova O & Tymofyeyev Y. (2011). Brick tunnel randomization for unequal allocation to two or more treatment groups. *Statistics in Medicine* 30: 812-824.
10. Rosenberger WF, Stallard N, Ivanova A, Harper CN & Ricks ML. (2001). Optimal adaptive designs for binary response trials. *Biometrics* 57: 909-913.
11. Zelen M. (1969). Play the winner rule and the controlled clinical trial. *Journal of the American Statistical Association* 64: 131-146.
12. Wei LJ & Durham S. (1978). The randomized play-the-winner rule in medical trials. *Journal of the American Statistical Association* 73: 840-843.
13. Bartlett RH, Rolloff DW, Cornell RG, Andrews AF, Dillon PW & Zwischenberger JB. (1985). Extracorporeal circulation in neonatal respiratory failure: a prospective randomized trial. *Pediatrics* 76: 479-487.
14. Hu F & Rosenberger WF. (2006). *The Theory of Response-Adaptive Randomization in Clinical Trials.* New York: Wiley.
15. Thall PF & Wathen JK. (2007). Practical Bayesian adaptive randomisation in clinical trials. *European Journal of Cancer* 43: 859-866.
16. Palmer CR & Rosenberger WF. (1999). Ethics and practice: Alternative designs for phase III randomized clinical trials. *Controlled Clinical Trials* 20: 172-186.
17. Tymofyeyev Y, Rosenberger WF & Hu F. (2007). Implementing optimal allocation in sequential binary response experiments. *Journal of the American Statistical Association* 102:224-234.

18. Sverdlov O, Tymofyeyev Y & Wong WK. (2011). Optimal response-adaptive randomized designs for multi-armed survival trials. *Statistics in Medicine* 30: 2890 2910.

19. Sverdlov O, Ryeznik Y & Wong WK. (2014). Efficient and ethical response-adaptive randomization designs for multi-arm clinical trials with Weibull time-to-event outcomes. *Journal of Biopharmaceutical Statistics* 24: 732-754.

20. US Food and Drug Administration. (2010). Guidance for industry: Adaptive design clinical trials for drugs and biologics (draft). Available at: http://www.fda.gov/downloads/DrugsGuidanceComplianceRegulatoryInformation/Guidances/UCM201790.pdf (http://www.fda.gov/downloads/DrugsGuidanceComplianceRegulatoryInformation/Guidances/UCM201790.pdf).

21. Krams M, Lees KR, Hacke W, Grieve AP, Orgogozo JM & Ford GA. (2003). Acute Stroke Therapy by Inhibition of Neutrophils (ASTIN): an adaptive dose-response study of UK 279,276 in acute ischemic stroke. *Stroke* 34: 2543-2548.

22. Rosenberger WF & Lachin J. (2002). *Randomization in Clinical Trials: Theory and Practice*. New York: Wiley.

23. McEntegart D. (2008). Book review of *The Theory of Response-Adaptive Randomization in Clinical Trials* by Hu F & Rosenberger WF. *Pharmaceutical Statistics* 7: 72-73.

24. Rosenberger WF. (2002). Randomized urn models and sequential design (with discussion). *Sequential Analysis* 21: 1-28 (discussion: 29-41).

25. Ivanova A. (2003). A play-the-winner-type urn design with reduced variability. *Metrika* 58: 1-13.

26. Zhang LX, Hu F, Cheung SH & Chan WS. (2011). Immigrated urn models—theoretical properties and applications. *The Annals of Statistics* 39: 643-671.

27. Thompson WR. (1933). On the likelihood that one unknown probability exceeds another in view of the evidence of the two samples. *Biometrika* 25: 275-294.

28. Thall PF & Wathen JK. (2005). Covariate-adjusted adaptive randomization in a sarcoma trial with multi-stage treatments. *Statistics in Medicine* 24: 1947-1964.

29. Giles FJ, Kantarjan HM, Cortes JE, Garcia-Manero G, Verstovsek S, Faderl S, Thomas DA, Ferrajoli A, O'Brien S, Wathen JK, Xiao LC, Berry DA & Estey EH. (2003). Adaptive randomized study of Idarubicin and Cytarabine versus Troxacitabine and Cytarabine versus Troxacitabine and Idarubicin in untreated patients 50 years or older with adverse karyotype acute myeloid leukemia. *Journal of Clinical Oncology* 21: 1722-1727.

30. Cheung YK, Inoue LYT, Wathen JK & Thall PF. (2006). Continuous Bayesian adaptive randomization based on event times with covariates. *Statistics in Medicine* 25: 55-70.

31. Trippa L, Lee EQ, Wen PY, Batchelor TT, Cloughesy T, Parmigiani G & Alexander BM. (2012). Bayesian adaptive randomized trial design for patients with recurrent glioblastoma. *Journal of Clinical Oncology* 30: 3258-3263.

32. Korn EL, Freidlin B. (2011). Outcome-adaptive randomization: is it useful? *Journal of Clinical Oncology* 29: 771-776.

33. Berry DA. (2011). Adaptive clinical trials: the promise and the caution. *Journal of Clinical Oncology* 29: 606-609.

34. Hu F & Rosenberger WF. (2003). Optimality, variability, power: Evaluating response-adaptive randomization procedures for treatment comparisons. *Journal of the American Statistical Association* 98: 671-678.

35. Rosenberger WF, Sverdlov O & Hu F. (2012). Adaptive randomization for clinical trials. *Journal of Biopharmaceutical Statistics* 22: 719-736.

36. Yi Y & Wang X. (2015). Statistical inference following response-adaptive randomization. In Sverdlov O, ed. *Modern Adaptive Randomized Clinical Trials: Statistical and Practical Aspects*. Boca Raton, Florida: CRC Press.

37. Atkinson A & Biswas A. (2014). *Randomised Response-Adaptive Designs in Clinical Trials*. Boca Raton, Florida: CRC Press.

38. Whitehead J. (1997). *The Design and Analysis of Sequential Clinical Trials, Second Edition*. New York: Wiley.

39. Magirr D. (2011). Block response-adaptive randomization in clinical trials with binary endpoints. *Pharmaceutical Statistics* 10: 341-346.

40. Baldi Antognini A & Giovagnoli A. (2010). Compound optimal allocation for individual and collective ethics in binary clinical trials. *Biometrika* 97: 935-946.

41. Brittain E & Schlesselman JJ. (1982). Optimal allocation for the comparison of proportions. *Biometrics* 38: 1003-1009.

42. Zhang L & Biswas A. (2007). Optimal failure-success response-adaptive designs for binary responses. *Drug Information Journal* 41: 709-718.

43. Azriel D, Mandel M & Rinott Y. (2012). Optimal allocation to maximize the power of two-sample tests for binary response. *Biometrika* 99: 101-113.

44. Yi Y & Yuan Y. (2013). An optimal allocation for response-adaptive designs. *Journal of Applied Statistics* 40: 1996-2008.

45. Gallo P. (2006). Operational challenges in adaptive design implementation. *Pharmaceutical Statistics* 5: 119-124.

46. Melfi VF, Page C & Geraldes M. (2001). An adaptive randomized design with application to estimation. *The Canadian Journal of Statistics* 29: 107-116.

47. Eiseley JR. (1971). The doubly adaptive biased coin design for sequential clinical trials. *Journal of Statistical Planning and Inference* 38: 249-261.

48. Hu F & Zhang LX. (2004). Asymptotic properties of doubly adaptive biased coin designs for multitreatment clinical trials. *The Annals of Statistics* 32: 268-301.

49. Rosenberger WF & Hu F. (2004). Maximizing power and minimizing treatment failures in clinical trials. *Clinical Trials* 1: 141-147.

50. Hu F, Zhang LX & He X. (2009). Efficient randomized-adaptive designs. *The Annals of Statistics* 37: 2543-2560.

51. Hu F, Rosenberger WF & Zhang LX. (2006). Asymptotically best response-adaptive randomization procedures. *Journal of Statistical Planning and Inference* 136: 1911-1922.

52. Gu X & Lee JJ. (2010). A simulation study for comparing testing statistics in response-adaptive randomization. *BMC Medical Research Methodology* 10: 48.

53. Sverdlov O & Rosenberger WF. (2013). On recent advances in optimal allocation designs in clinical trials. *Journal of Statistical Theory and Practice* 7: 753-773.

54. Zhu H & Hu F. (2009). Implementing optimal allocation for sequential continuous responses with multiple treatments. *Journal of Statistical Planning and Inference* 139: 2420-2430.

55. Gwise T, Zhou J & Hu F. (2011). An optimal response adaptive biased coin design with k heteroscedastic treatments. *Journal of Statistical Planning and Inference* 141: 235-242.

56. Wong WK & Zhu W. (2008). Optimal treatment allocation rules under a variance heterogeneity model. *Statistics in Medicine* 27: 2850-2864.

57. Hu F, Zhang LX, Cheung SH & Chan WS. (2008). Doubly adaptive biased coin designs with delayed responses. *The Canadian Journal of Statistics* 36: 541-559.

58. Zhang LX, Chan WS, Cheung SH & Hu F. (2007). A generalized drop-the-loser rule for clinical trials with delayed responses. *Statistica Sinica* 17: 387-409.

59. Zhang L & Rosenberger WF. (2007). Response-adaptive randomization for survival trials: the parametric approach. *Applied Statistics* 56: 153-165.

60. Li X & Wang X. (2013). Response-adaptive designs with misclassified responses. *Communications in Statistics—Theory and Methods* 42: 2071-2083.

61. Karrison T, Huo D & Chappell R. (2003). Group sequential, response-adaptive designs for randomized clinical trials. *Controlled Clinical Trials* 24: 506-522.

62. Chappell R & Karrison T. (2007). Letter to the editor. *Statistics in Medicine* 26: 3046-3052.

63. Simon R & Simon N. (2011). Using randomization tests to preserve type I error with response adaptive and covariate adaptive randomization. *Statistics and Probability Letters* 81: 767-772.

64. Hu F & Rosenberger WF. (2000). Analysis of time trends in adaptive designs with application to a neurophysiology experiment. *Statistics in Medicine* 19: 2067-2075.

65. Rosenberger WF & Sverdlov O. (2008). Handling covariates in the design of clinical trials. *Statistical Science* 23: 404-419.

66. Connor EM, Sperling RS, Gelber R, Kiselev P, Scott G, O'Sullivan MJ, VanDyke R, Bey M, Shearer W, Jacobson RL, Jimenez E, O'Neill E, Bazin B, Delfraissy JF, Culnane M, Coombs R, Elkins M, Moye J, Stratton P & Balsley J for the Pediatric AIDS clinical trials group protocol 076 study group. (1994). Reduction of maternal-infant transmission of human immunodeficiency virus type 1 with zidovudine treatment. *The New England Journal of Medicine* 331: 1173-1180.

67. Yuan Y & Yin G. (2011). On the usefulness of outcome-adaptive randomization. *Journal of Clinical Oncology* 29: e390-e392.

68. Zhu H & Hu F. (2010). Sequential monitoring of response-adaptive randomized clinical trials. *The Annals of Statistics* 38: 2218-2241.

69. Zhu H & Hu F. (2012). Interim analysis of clinical trials based on urn models. *Canadian Journal of Statistics* 40: 550-568.

70. Lai TL & Liao OYW. (2012). Efficient adaptive randomization and stopping rules in multiarm clinical trials for testing a new treatment. *Sequential Analysis* 31: 441-457.

71. Chambaz A & van der Laan MJ. (2014). Inference in targeted group-sequential covariate-adjusted randomized clinical trials. *Scandinavian Journal of Statistics* 41: 104-140.

Authors

Oleksandr Sverdlov, Associate Director of Biostatistics, EMD Serono, Inc., a subsidiary of Merck KgaA, Rockland, MA, USA.

Zorayr Manukyan, Director of Biostatistics, Biotherapeutic Research Unit, Pfizer Inc., Cambridge, MA, USA.

Gaurav Sharma, Statistician, The EMMES Corporation, Rockville, MD, USA.

Chapter 11
Population Enrichment Designs

11.1 Introduction

11.1.1 Background

Traditional clinical development of an experimental therapy utilizes the "one-size-fits-all" approach by testing the regimen in an unselected or untargeted patient population with a specific disease. The assumption is that response in the population with the disease is homogeneous. With the advent of molecularly targeted therapies, genetic engineering such as DNA sequencing and mRNA transcript profiling now makes a finer taxonomy of disease possible, which enables the development of precise diagnostic, prognostic, and therapeutic paradigms for specific subsets of patients, i.e. personalized medicine. Therefore, these targeted therapies may benefit only a subset of the entire population and may not benefit or even harm the rest of the population. On the other hand, proteomic and genetic biomarkers have the potential to provide substantial added value to the current medical practice. For instance, in oncology, some biomarkers provide the possibility to integrate an accurate predictor of efficacy with a specific mechanism-based therapy using the genetic makeup of the tumor and the genotype of each individual patient to guide the selection of cancer treatment (Table 11.1 on page 306).

As a result of these new opportunities and challenges, the traditional paradigm of drug development not taking into account response heterogeneity may be suboptimal. To embark on the mission of personalized medicine, innovative statistical designs beyond the interaction test of a traditional fixed design are becoming increasingly attractive, which allow assessment of treatment effects due to phenotypic or genomic heterogeneity of patients. Furthermore, focused clinical trials using a biomarker strategy may result in smaller study sizes, higher probability of trial success, enhancement of the benefit-risk relationship, and potentially mitigating ever-escalating development costs.

In 2012, the FDA released a draft guidance on enrichment strategies for clinical trials to support approval of human drugs and biological products. In their guidance, the term enrichment is defined as "*the prospective use of any patient characteristic to select a study population in which detection of a drug effect (if one is in fact present) is more likely than it would be in an unselected population.*" Further, enrichment strategies fall into three broad categories (excerpts from the guidance):

1. *Strategies to decrease heterogeneity – These include selecting patients with baseline measurements in a narrow range (decreased inter-patient variability) and excluding patients whose disease or symptoms improve spontaneously or whose measurements are highly variable (decreased intra-patient variability). The decreased variability provided by these strategies increases study power.*

2. *Prognostic enrichment strategies – choosing patients with a greater likelihood of having a disease-related endpoint event (for event-driven studies) or a substantial worsening in condition (for continuous measurement endpoints). These strategies will increase the absolute effect difference between groups but will not alter relative effect.*

3. *Predictive enrichment strategies – choosing patients more likely to respond to the drug treatment than other patients with the condition being treated. Such selection can lead to a larger effect size (both absolute and relative) and permit use of a smaller study population. Selection of patients could be based on a specific aspect of a patient's physiology or a disease characteristic that is related in some manner to the study drug's mechanism, or it could be empiric (e.g., the patient has previously appeared to respond to a drug in the same class).*

In this chapter, we give an overview of population enrichment designs that are growing in the statistical literature, with a focus on designs of predictive enrichment strategies so as to increase the power and efficiency to detect an effective therapy with regard to a predictive biomarker in a clinical trial. A predictive biomarker is a type of biomarker that identifies patients who are likely to benefit from a particular treatment, in contrast to a prognostic biomarker which is associated with only the disease outcome. The focus of this chapter is on the efficacy endpoint of interest; design issues with respect to predictive biomarkers on safety will not be discussed.

Table 11.1 *Some Oncology Drugs Approved in the US for Patient Populations by Molecular Targets*

Compound/Target	**Indication (prevalence target)**
Crizotinib (Xalkori®)/ EML4-ALK-translocation	Non-small cell lung cancer with EML4-ALK-translocation (4-7%)
Ceritinib (Zykadia®)/ EML4-ALK-translocation	Non-small cell lung cancer with EML4-ALK-translocation (4-7%)
Vemurafenib (Zelboraf®)/ *BRAF* mutation	Advanced melanoma with mutant *BRAF* (30-40%)

Compound/Target	Indication (prevalence target)
Trastuzumab (Herceptin®); Lapatinib (Tykerb®)/ Her2	Her2 expressing breast cancer (25%); Her2 expressing metastatic gastric cancer (20-30%)
Her2 expressing metastatic gastric cancer (20-30%)	ER(+) breast cancer (60-70%)
Aromatase inhibitors (letrozole, exemestane)	CD20(+) B-cell lymphomas (90%+)
Rituximab (Rituxan®)/ CD20	Advanced Head/neck cancer (~100%); EGFR(+) metastatic colorectal cancer (60-80%); KRAS^{WT} metastatic colorectal cancer (60%)

11.1.2 Issues to Consider

There are a number of issues (Table 11.2 on page 307) that one needs to consider before designing a trial with a predictive biomarker component. It's an important step as we are armed with alternative design options in a rapidly growing literature.

First, we need to evaluate the strength of preclinical evidence for a potential predictive biomarker. If there is compelling preliminary evidence that the experimental therapy does not provide benefit to all the patients, and the benefit is restricted to a subset of patients expressing a molecular or genetic value, an enrichment strategy may be adopted. Otherwise, an unselected or all-comers strategy may be wise so that there is no missed opportunity for drug development, patients, and the marketplace. The second issue is whether the prevalence (percentage) of the biomarker positive group is high, moderate or low. If the prevalence is high, population enrichment may be redundant and a traditional design could render the greatest commercial value and market reach. Likewise, an all-comers design may not be feasible for a low-prevalence situation. Thirdly, the accuracy of the measurements that are used to identify the enrichment population and the sensitivity and specificity of the enrichment criterion in distinguishing responders and non-responders are also critical issues. An accurate, reproducible, and adequately validated assay is essential for establishing desired therapeutic activity and clinical validation of the biomarker (usually realized by a companion diagnostic kit from a central lab to identify the patients) in a prospective manner. In addition, the feasibility and timing to obtain a biopsy (de-novo or archived) or serum sample at baseline prior to randomization determines whether the biomarker can be prospectively validated.

Table 11.2 *Issues to Consider in Selecting a Design with Predictive Biomarker Component*

Strength of preclinical evidence for a marker	Whether we should use an enrichment/targeted strategy (e.g. crizotinib in ALK+ non-small cell lung cancer) or an unselected/all-comers strategy (e.g. cetuximab and panitumumab in wild-type KRAS colorectal cancer)
Prevalence of the marker	Percentage of the population having the biomarker positive (such as mutation or aberration) status
Reproducibility and validity of assays	Whether the assay is accurate, reliable, and has been analytically validated (local or central lab)
Feasibility and timing of assessments for the biomarker status	Whether the biomarker can be prospectively validated or retrospectively validated

We will further discuss these issues in this chapter when reviewing the existing methods of population enrichment designs.

11.2 Classical Designs

11.2.1 Retrospective Design

Classical population enrichment designs fall into two categories: retrospective enrichment design and prospective enrichment design.

Retrospective enrichment design is a traditional all-comers design with retrospective validation of a biomarker, usually not available or assessable at the beginning of the trial, thereby making prospective testing unfeasible. Retrospective validation is conducted after the completion of the study and may involve previously conducted trials in the same patient population. As stated by Mandrekar and Sargent [1] when conducted appropriately, this design can aid in bringing forward effective treatments to marker-defined patient populations in a timely manner that might otherwise be impossible due to ethical and logistical (i.e. large trial and long time to complete) considerations. For such retrospective analysis to be valid and to minimize bias, Mandrekar and Sargent [1] summarized a list of essential elements that are critical to retrospective validation studies.

1. Data from a well-conducted randomized controlled trial
2. Availability of samples on a large majority of patients to avoid selection bias
3. Prospectively stated hypothesis, analysis techniques, and patient population
4. Predefined and standardized assay and scoring system
5. Upfront sample size and power justification

Take the development of EGFR-inhibitors cetuximab and panitumumab in metastatic colorectal cancer (CRC) as an example. Cetuximab and panitumumab were initially marketed for the indication of EGFR+ CRC, which represents 65% of advanced colorectal cancer patients. Based on retrospective analysis of previously conducted randomized phase III and II trials [2-4], it has been demonstrated that cetuximab significantly improves the overall survival for patients with wild-type *KRAS* (a protein that in humans is encoded by the *KRAS* gene), with no survival benefit in patients harboring *KRAS*-mutant status. As a result, in July 2009, the FDA approved cetuximab for treatment of *KRAS*-wild type colon cancer. Similarly, in a prospectively specified analysis of data from a previous randomized phase III trial of panitumumab versus best supportive care [5], the hazard ratio for progression-free survival (PFS) comparing panitumumab with best supportive care in the *KRAS* wild type and mutant subgroups was 0.45 and 0.99, respectively, with a statistically significant treatment by *KRAS* status interaction ($p<0.0001$). Given the lack of activity in the *KRAS*-mutant group, the label was changed to include wild-type patients only in 2009.

11.2.2 Prospective Design

11.2.2.1 Enrichment/Targeted Design

Although retrospective evaluation of predictive biomarkers could save resources and time, and make effective treatments available to patients in a much expedited timeframe, it may introduce serious bias due to the nature of retrospective selection of patient subgroups and lack of controlled validation of biomarkers. Hence, prospectively designed trials are still the gold standard in the clinical development of targeted therapies and predictive biomarkers.

Enrichment design is also referred to as biomarker-enrichment design or gene-enrichment design. All patients in the trial may not generally benefit from the study treatment under consideration. The goal of the enrichment designs is to study the clinical benefit in a subgroup of the patient population defined by a specific biomarker status. In this design, the patients are screened for the presence or absence of a biomarker(s) profile. After extensive screening, only patients with the presence of a certain biomarker characteristic or profile are enrolled in the clinical trial [6-7]. In principle, this design essentially consists of an additional criterion for patient inclusion in the trial (Figure 11.1 on page 309).

Figure 11.1 *Enrichment Design*

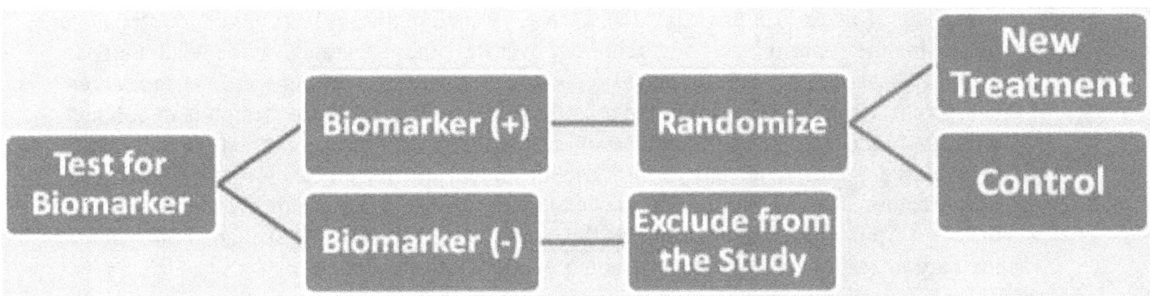

A recent example for the enrichment design was of mutated *BRAF*-kinase [8]. Almost 50% of melanomas have an activating ^{V600E} *BRAF* mutation. This leads to the hypothesis that inhibition of mutated *BRAF* kinase will have meaningful clinical benefit. Hence, only patients who tested positive for ^{V600E} *BRAF* mutation were enrolled in the study. Patients were randomized to an inhibitor of mutated *BRAF*-kinase or control treatment. As hypothesized, the large treatment benefit was observed in the pre-specified subgroup. Another example for enriched design was used in the HER2 trial where patients with HER2+ breast cancer [9]. During the conduct of the study, it is important to have rapid turnaround times for the assay results in order to enroll patients faster. In addition, the assay testing should be consistent between different labs. For example: a high discordance was found between the local and central testing for HER2 status. Hence, the Herceptin therapy may have benefitted a potentially larger group than defined as HER2+ by central testing.

The following considerations should be taken into account in this design – 1) a smaller sample size is usually required but the screening may still take the same amount of time (or even longer as explained below) as with an all-comers designs given the extensive pre-screen testing that will be conducted before enrollment; 2) the marketing label will be restricted; 3) there may still be a potential subset of patients who may benefit with the new treatment; 4) restricted enrollment does not provide data to establish that treatment is ineffective in biomarker negative patients; 5) a low prevalence of the marker may be challenging operationally and financially. Operationally, the biggest challenge is in recruitment, and financially it may not be commercially attractive.

The efficiency of this design is a function of the percent of biomarker positive patients who are likely to benefit by the target treatment, and the reliability and reproducibility of the assay also plays a pivotal role. This design is appropriate when the mechanistic behavior of drug is known and there is compelling preliminary evidence of a benefit to a subset population.

The rest of Section 11.2.2 focuses on the all-comers/unselected design and its variations. These designs differ from each other by the primary hypothesis test, randomization, and multiplicity approaches, which, in turn, affect the operating characteristics of the design, including sample size, power and type I error rate.

11.2.2.2 Marker by Treatment Interaction Design

Marker by Treatment Interaction Design is also called biomarker-stratified design [7]. This design is chosen when there is no preliminary evidence to strongly favor restricting the trial to patients with a specific biomarker profile that would necessitate a biomarker-enrichment design. This design is prospective and leads to a definitive marker validation strategy. In such cases, marker by treatment or stratified design is more informative than biomarker-enrichment design. In this design, the patients are tested for biomarker status and then randomized separately according to their positive or negative status of the marker [6]. Thus, the randomization is done using marker status as the stratification factor; however, only the patients with a valid measurable marker results are randomized. Patients in each marker group are then randomized to two separate treatments (Figure 11.2 on page 310). Two separate hypotheses tests are conducted to determine the superiority of one treatment over the other separately within each marker group. The sample size is calculated separately to power the testing within each marker sub-group. Another variation to the hypothesis test within the same design is to conduct a formal marker by treatment interaction test to see if the treatment effect varies within each marker status subgroup. In this case, the study is powered based on the magnitude of interaction. This design can be viewed as two stand-alone trials; however, it is different from a large clinical trial by the calculation of the sample size and restriction of the randomization to only patients with a valid marker result [1].

Figure 11.2 *Marker by Treatment Interaction Design*

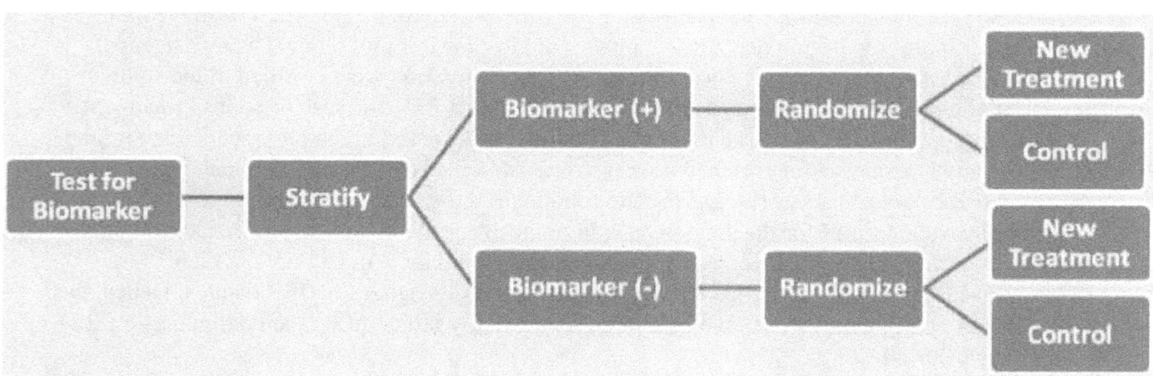

11.2.2.3 Sequential Testing Strategy Design

In principle, sequential testing designs can be considered as a special case of the classical randomized clinical trial for all comers or unselected patients.

Test Overall Difference Followed by Subgroup

Simon and Wang [10] proposed an analysis strategy where the overall hypothesis is tested to see if there is a difference in the response in new treatment versus the control group. If there is no difference and the response is not significant at a pre-specified significance level (for example 0.01), then the new treatment is compared to the control group in the biomarker status positive patients. The second comparison uses a threshold of significance, which is the proportion of the traditional 0.05 not utilized by the initial test. This approach is useful when the new treatment is believed to be effective in a wider population, and the subset analysis is supplementary and used as a fallback option.

For example, if the trial is planned for having 90% power for detecting a uniform 33% reduction in overall hazard using a two-sided significance level of .03, then the overall analysis will take place when there are 297 events. If the test is positive in 25% of patients and the test is not prognostic, then at the time of the analysis there will be approximately 75 events among the test positive patients. If the overall test of treatment effect is not significant, then the subset test will have 75% power for detecting a 50% reduction in hazard at a two-sided .02 significance level. By delaying the treatment evaluation in the test positive patients, 80% power can be achieved when there are 84 events and 90% power can be achieved when there are 109 events in the test positive subset.

Song and Chi [11] later proposed a modification of the above method. Their method takes into account the correlation between the test statistics of the hypotheses of the overall population and the biomarker positive population.

Test Subgroup Followed by the Overall Population

Bauer [12] investigated the multiple testing in the sequential sampling. Here the hypothesis for the treatment is first tested in the biomarker positive status patients and then tested in the overall population. This strategy is appropriate when there is a preliminary biological basis to believe that the biomarker status positive patients will benefit more from the new drug and there is sufficient marker prevalence to appropriately power the trial. In this closed testing procedure, the final type I error rate is always preserved. The approach of first testing in the subgroup defined by marker status has been implemented in the ongoing US-based phase III trial testing cetuximab, in addition to infusional fluorouracil, leucovorin, and oxaliplatin as adjuvant therapy in stage III colon cancer [13]. While the trial has now been amended to accrue only patients with *KRAS*–wild-type tumors, approximately 800 patients with *KRAS* mutant tumors have already been enrolled. In this trial, the primary analysis would be conducted at the 0.05 level in the patients with wildtype *KRAS*. A sample size of 1,035 patients with wild-type KRAS per arm would result in 515 total events, providing 90% power to detect a hazard ratio of 0.75 for this comparison using a two-sided, log-rank test at a significance level of 0.05. If this subset analysis is statistically significant at P =0.05, then the efficacy of the regimen in the entire population will also be tested at level 0.05, as this is a closed testing procedure. This comparison using all 2,910 patients will have 90% power to detect a hazard ratio of 0.79 comparing the two treatment arms, based on a total of 735 events.

11.2.2.4 Biomarker-Analysis Design

Biomarker-analysis design [14] essentially has two elements. The first element is a randomized trial with the presence or absence of the biomarker examined in all participants followed by the identification of a promising subgroup. This is done by using a plot of treatment benefit versus various cut-points or intervals of the biomarker. It is critical in this design that the specimen be at least collected at the randomization even if it is not examined, though it is preferred that it is examined at randomization. Collection of the specimens a priori can mitigate the risk of non-compliance with the treatment due to the incoming knowledge of the marker data [15]. As the data trickles in, the investigators need to assess the risk and benefit especially from an ethical perspective of concealing the new information.

This design can assist in understanding the following hypothesis test: (a) Targeted Treatment versus Standard of Care in the overall population; (b) Targeted Treatment versus Standard of Care in the biomarker positive population; (c) Targeted Treatment versus Standard of Care in the biomarker negative population; (d) marker-based treatment selection versus targeted therapy and (e) marker-based treatment selection versus standard of care. With multiple hypotheses that can be tested for (a) to (e), the significance levels and confidence intervals need to be adjusted according to the type and the number of hypotheses under consideration.

The biomarker subgroup selection using the cut-points can be done using plots. Various plots have been proposed in the literature which assists in better visualization and understanding of the cut-points and intervals. Some of these plots present confidence intervals that adjust for multiplicity. The following are some of the commonly used plots:

1. Marker-by-treatment predictiveness curves [16] - the risk of the response is plotted separately under targeted therapy and standard-of-care treatments for subjects with a marker in the interval.
2. Selection impact curve [17] - benefit of marker-based treatment selection is plotted directly as a function of marker cut-points.
3. Tail-oriented subgroup plot [18] - The estimated benefit of targeted therapy against the standard of care is plotted among subjects with a marker level greater than a cut-point as a function of different clinically meaningful cut-points. Hence, the tail of the distribution is specified when the estimated benefit is plotted for a marker level above a certain cut point.
4. Sliding-window subgroup plot [19] - The estimated benefit of targeted therapy against the standard of care is plotted among subjects with a marker level within an interval as a function of marker level. Hence, the sliding window is specified when the estimated benefit is plotted for a marker level within a certain interval.

The tail-oriented subgroup plot and sliding window plots [20] give confidence intervals that account for multiple testing of several cut-points or intervals.

Baker and Kramer [21] proposed a special case of biomarker analysis design for rare events. In this design, all subjects are randomized to either the targeted therapy or the control. The specimens are collected but not examined at the time of randomization. Subjects are randomly selected at the end of the trial to test for the presence or absence of the marker. The probability of random selection is ascertained based on the positive outcome of interest. King et al. [22] proposed testing for the marker only for the subjects with a positive outcome of interest. This type of design can be referred to as biomarker-nested case-control design.

11.2.2.5 Marker-Based Strategy Design

In this design, patients are randomly assigned to treatment dependent or independent of the marker status (Figure 11.3 on page 313). All patients randomized to the non-biomarker based arm receive the control treatment. In the biomarker based arm, the patients receive the targeted or experimental therapy if the marker is positive and they receive the control treatment if the marker is negative [6-7]. The outcome of all of the patients in the marker based subgroup is compared to that of all patients in the non-marker based sub-group to investigate the predictive value of the marker. One downside of this design is that patients treated with the same regimen are included on both the marker-based and the non–marker-based subgroup, resulting in a substantial redundancy, which leads to many patients receiving the same treatment regimes in both subgroups. Hence, this design can reduce the treatment effect especially if the prevalence of the marker is high requiring a large sample size. This is illustrated in the following example, in the ERCC1 trial [23] and presented in [6] about 57% of the biomarker-based strategy arm patients were assigned to the same regimen of cisplatin+docetaxel as done in the standard of care arm. Thus, the comparison weakens the between-arm treatment effect difference and reduces the statistical power to reject null hypotheses. This can lead to either getting incomplete information or it may miss a valuable biomarker in addition to delaying the evaluation of the biomarker due to the increased sample size required to achieve a desired power. One other disadvantage of this design is the inability to examine the effect of targeted therapy in patients in the negative marker status group as none of these patients receive it. Even if the patients in the negative marker status group respond to the targeted therapy, this cannot be assessed. The treatment difference between the new treatment and the control treatment can be diluted by marker-based treatment selection and sometimes it can be a poor choice as compared to the randomized design.

A modified version of this design has been proposed where the negative marker status group undergo randomization and receive the targeted therapy or the control. Thus, the modified design allows assessment of the targeted therapy in both the biomarker positive and the negative subgroup. It helps to assess whether the efficacy of the marker positive patients to therapy is because of the marker status being positive or due to an improved treatment regardless of the marker status. The assessment can also be done retrospectively if the classification of the marker needs to be revisited.

Figure 11.3 *Marker-Based Strategy Design*

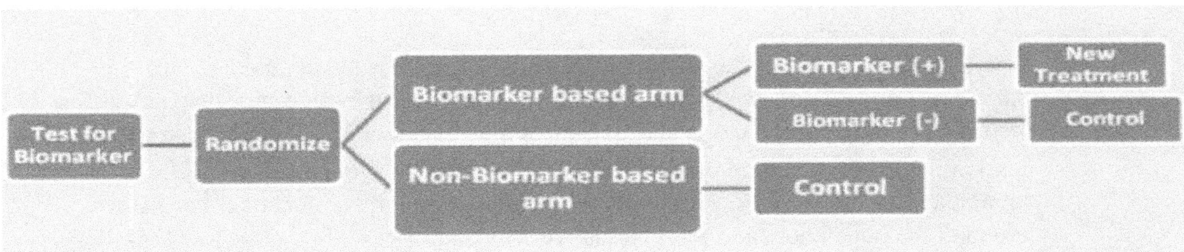

11.2.2.6 Hybrid Design

Hybrid designs should be considered when there is strong evidence from pre-clinical or prior studies that there is efficacy of some treatment(s) on the marker-based sub-group [1]. This makes it almost impossible, due to ethical reasons, to randomize patients with a particular marker to other treatment options. It is very similar to the enrichment designs, and all patients are examined for marker status and are randomly assigned to treatment or assigned to standard-of-care treatment for patients with positive biomarker values. However, only a marker-positive subgroup of patients are randomly assigned to treatments, whereas patients in the marker-negative group are assigned to a control or standard-of-care treatment (Figure 11.4 on page 313). The study is powered to detect treatment difference only in the marker-positive group. Samples are collected from all of the subjects to help testing for additional markers in the future.

Figure 11.4 *Hybrid Design*

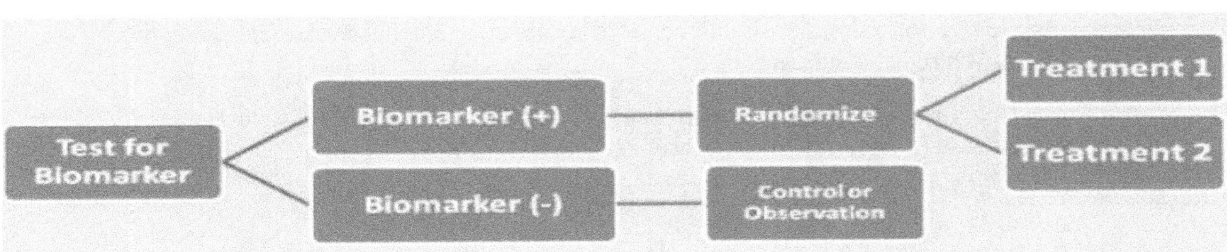

It should be noted that except for the enrichment/targeted design, all classical designs covered are all-comers designs so that all patients, regardless of their biomarker status, are enrolled in the study.

11.3 Efficiency of Classical Enrichment Designs

Simon and Maitournam [24] and Maitournam and Simon [25] considered a phase III randomized trial setting to evaluate molecular targeted treatment using a binary endpoint or continuous endpoint. The evaluations were done under the assumption that the assay was predictive of a subset of patients who benefited from the targeted therapy. They compared the all-comers design where all the patients are allowed to participate in the trial with the enrichment design with restricted subset population. They compared the operating characteristics based on average screened and randomized sample size.

For a binary endpoint, the relative efficiency of the targeted design versus the untargeted design can be expressed as

$$\frac{n}{n^T} = \left[\frac{\delta_1}{\gamma\delta_0 + (1-\gamma)\delta_1}\right]^2 f,$$

where $2n^T$ and $2n$ denote the number of patients that are needed to randomize in the enrichment and all-comers design, respectively, to achieve the same statistical power for testing the null hypothesis. δ_1 and δ_0 represent the effect size (e.g. difference in response rate) of the treatment group versus the control group in the biomarker positive and biomarker negative groups. γ accounts for the proportion of the biomarker negative group of the population, and f is the relative efficiency factor often close to 1 [24]. For the calculation of relative efficiency in light of the number of screened patients, simply multiply the equation above by $(1-\gamma)$.

For a continuous endpoint, the relative efficiency of the targeted design versus the untargeted design can be expressed in the form

$$\frac{n}{n^T} = \frac{1 + \frac{\gamma(1-\gamma)}{2\sigma^2}\left[(\mu_1-\mu_0)^2 + (\mu_{1T}-\mu_{0T})^2\right]}{\left[1-\gamma\left(1-\frac{\mu_{0T}-\mu_0}{\mu_{1T}-\mu_1}\right)\right]^2}$$

where μ_0 and μ_1 denote the mean responses for control patients in marker negative and positive groups, respectively, μ_{0T} and μ_{1T} denote the mean responses for treatment patients in marker negative and positive groups, respectively, and assume a constant variance σ^2 within each treatment group and subset. Similarly, for relative efficiency of the number of screened patients, simply multiply the equation by $(1-\gamma)$. The above results are valid only asymptotically. Alternatively, Maitournam and Simon [25] derived sample size formulas that should be more accurate for small sample sizes using the Mann–Whitney Wilcoxon test.

Macros (**`% simnorm`** and **`% simgamma`**) are developed for calculating the required sample size for a certain power based on formula (6) in [25].

$$\text{Power} \approx 1 - \Psi\left\{\frac{0.5n^2 + z_{1-\alpha/2}\sqrt{\frac{(2n+1)n^2}{12}} - 0.5 - n^2 p_1}{\sqrt{Var(W_{xy})}}\right\},$$

where $Var(W_{xy})$ is the variance of the Mann-Whitney statistic given by

$Var\left(W_{xy}\right) = n^2\left\{p_1\left(1 - p_1\right) + \left(n - 1\right)\left(p_2 + p_3 - 2p_1^2\right\}\right.$, where $p_1 = \Pr(X < Y)$ is the probability that a control outcome X is less than a treatment outcome Y, and $p_2 = \Pr\left(X < Y_1, X < Y_2\right)$ is the probability that a control outcome is simultaneously less than two independent treatment outcomes, and $p_3 = \Pr\left(X_1 < Y, X_2 < Y\right)$ is the probability that a treatment outcome is simultaneously greater than two independent control outcomes. Ψ denotes the cumulative distribution function for the standard normal distribution. Please refer to **efficiency_tct.sas** in the supplemental material of the book.

The **% MSpower** macro (Example Code 11.1) computes the smallest sample size that provides a specified power $1 - \beta$ for rejecting the null hypothesis using formula (6) in [25]. The parameters to be specified for **% MSpower** are

1. **beta**: type II error rate

2. **alpha**: type I error rate

3. **p1**: probability that a control outcome is less than a treatment outcome

4. **p2**: probability that a control outcome is simultaneously less than two independent treatment outcomes

5. **p3**: probability that a treatment outcome is simultaneously greater than two independent control outcomes.

Example Code 11.1 *MSPower Macro for Computing Required Sample Size*

```
%macro MSpower(beta, p1, p2, p3, alpha);
   data result;
      delta=1-(&alpha/2);
      za=quantile('Normal', delta);
      p1=&p1; p2=&p2; p3=&p3;alpha=&alpha;
      do i= 1 to 10000;
         nsize=i;
         denum=(i**2)*( p1*(1-p1) + (i-1)*(p2 + p3 - 2*(p1**2)) );
         den=sqrt(denum);
         a=(0.5* (i**2) + za*sqrt((i**2)*(2*i + 1)/12) - 0.5 - (i**2)*p1)/den;
         beta= CDF('Normal', a);
         power=1-beta;
         output;
         if beta<=&beta then i=10001;
      end;
   run;

   data result2;
      set result end =_end;
      end=_end;
      if end;
      if beta>&beta then do;
        warning=1;
        nsize2=">10000";
      end;
      else do;
        nsize2=compress(nsize);
      end;
      label nsize2='sample size';
    run;

   proc format;
```

```
      value wa 1='required sample size greater than 10000';
    run;

    proc print noobs label;
      var nsize2 p1 p2 p3 alpha beta power warning;
      format warning wa.;
    run;
%mend MSpower;

%MSpower(0.2, 0.7, 0.6, 0.4, 0.05);
```

The results of the macro call are shown in Table 11.3 on page 316. This indicates the smallest sample size that provides 80% power for rejecting the null hypothesis is 23 patients per treatment arm. The actual power by a total sample size of 46 patients is 82%.

Table 11.3 *Output from Example Code 11.1*

Sample Size	p1	p2	p3	alpha	beta	power
23	0.7	0.6	0.4	0.05	0.17842	0.82158

The parameters **p1**, **p2,** and **p3** could be computed using the Monte-Carlo method. If the treatment outcomes follow a Normal distribution (Example Code 11.2), the **% simnorm** macro computes the smallest sample size that provides a specified power $1-\beta$ for rejecting the null hypothesis using formula (6) in [25]. The parameters to be specified are:

1. **seed1**, **seed2**: randomization seeds used for generating random numbers
2. **mux**, **muy**: mean of treatment outcomes for the control and experimental groups
3. **stdx**, **stdy**: standard deviation of treatment outcomes for the control and experimental groups
4. **beta**: type II error rate
5. **alpha**: type I error rate
6. **simN**: number of iterations for Monte-Carlo simulation.

Example Code 11.2 *SimNorm Macro for Computing Required Sample Size*

```
%macro simnorm(seed1, seed2, mux, muy, stdx, stdy, beta, simN=10000, alpha=0.05);
   data x;
      call streaminit(&seed1);
      do i=1 to &simN;
         x=rand('normal', &mux, &stdx);
         output;
      end;
   run;

   data y;
      call streaminit(&seed2);
      do i=1 to &simN;
         y=rand('normal', &muy, &stdy);
         output;
      end;
   run;
```

```
data one;
   merge x y;
   if x<y then flag=1;
   else flag=0;
run;

proc means noprint data=one;
   var flag;
   output out=p1 mean=p1;
run;

data _null_;
   set p1;
   call symput('p1', compress(trim(p1)));
run;

data _null_;
   sy1=&seed2 +1;
   call streaminit(sy1);
   y1=rand('normal', &muy, &stdy);
   output;
   call symput('y1', compress(trim(y1)));
run;

data _null_;
   sy2=&seed2 +2;
   call streaminit(sy2);
   y2=rand('normal', &muy, &stdy);
   output;
   call symput('y2', compress(trim(y2)));
run;

data x;
   set x;
   if x<&y1 and x<&y2 then flag=1;
   else flag=0;
run;

proc means noprint data=x;
   var flag;
   output out=p2 mean=p2;
run;

data _null_;
   set p2;
   call symput('p2', compress(trim(p2)));
run;

data _null_;
   sx1=&seed1 +1;
   call streaminit(sx1);
   x1=rand('normal', &mux, &stdx);
   output;
   call symput('x1', compress(trim(x1)));
run;
```

```
      data _null_;
         sx2=&seed1 +2;
         call streaminit(sx2);
         x2=rand('normal', &mux, &stdx);
         output;
         call symput('x2', compress(trim(x2)));
      run;

      data y;
         set y;
         if y>&x1 and y>x2 then flag=1;
         else flag=0;
      run;

      proc means noprint data=y;
         var flag;
         output out=p3 mean=p3;
      run;

      data _null_;
         set p3;
         call symput('p3', compress(trim(p3)));
      run;

      title 'Normal Distribution';
      %MSpower(&beta., &p1., &p2., &p3., &alpha.);
   %mend simnorm;

   %simnorm(seed1=1, seed2=100, mux=5, muy=8, stdx=2, stdy=1.5,
   beta=0.2, simN=10000, alpha=0.05);
```

The results of **% simnorm** are shown in Table 11.4 on page 318. This indicates that, if the treatment outcomes from the control group follow a Normal distribution with mean 5, the standard deviation is 2; and if the treatment outcomes from the experimental group follow a Normal distribution with mean 8 and a standard deviation of 1.5, then estimates for **p1**, **p2**, and **p3** are 0.8837, 0.9126 and 0.9985, respectively using Monte-Carlo simulation, and the smallest sample size that provides 80% power for rejecting the null hypothesis is 12 per treatment. The actual power that leads with a total sample size of 24 is 82%.

Table 11.4 *Output from Example Code 11.2*

Sample Size	p1	p2	p3	alpha	beta	power
12	0.8837	0.9126	0.9985	0.05	0.18012	0.81988

Alternatively, if the treatment outcomes follow a Gamma distribution (Example Code 11.3 on page 319), **% simgamma** computes the smallest sample size that provides a specified power $1-\beta$ for rejecting the null hypothesis using formula (6) in [25]. The parameters to be specified are:

1. **seed1**, **seed2**: randomization seeds used for generating random numbers
2. **mux**, **muy**: mean of treatment outcomes for the control and experimental groups

3. **stdx**, **stdy**: standard deviation of treatment outcomes for the control and experimental groups

4. **beta**: type II error rate

5. **alpha**: type I error rate

6. **simN**: number of iterations for Monte-Carlo simulation.

Example Code 11.3 *SimGamma Macro for Computing Required Sample Size*

```
%macro simgamma(seed1, seed2, mux, muy, stdx, stdy, beta, simN=10000, alpha=0.05);
   data temp;
      ax=round((&mux**2)/(&stdx**2), 0.0001);
      bx=round(&mux/(&stdx**2), 0.0001);
      ay=round((&muy**2)/(&stdy**2), 0.0001);
      by=round(&muy/(&stdy**2), 0.0001);
   run;

   data _null_;
      set temp;
      call symput('ax', compress(trim(ax)));
      call symput('bx', compress(trim(bx)));
      call symput('ay', compress(trim(ay)));
      call symput('by', compress(trim(by)));

   run;

   data x;
      set temp;
      call streaminit(&seed1);
      do i=1 to &simN;
         x=rand('gamma', ax);
         x=x/bx;
         output;
      end;
   run;

   data y;
      set temp;
      call streaminit(&seed2);
      do i=1 to &simN;
         y=rand('gamma', ay);
         y=y/by;
         output;
      end;
   run;

   data one;
      merge x y;
      if x<y then flag=1;
      else flag=0;
   run;

   proc means noprint data=one;
      var flag;
      output out=p1 mean=p1;
   run;
```

```
data _null_;
   set p1;
   call symput('p1', compress(trim(p1)));
run;

data _null_;
   sy1=&seed2 +1;
   call streaminit(sy1);
   y1=rand('gamma', &ay);
   y1=y1/&by;
   output;
   call symput('y1', compress(trim(y1)));
run;

data _null_;
   sy2=&seed2 +2;
   call streaminit(sy2);
   y2=rand('gamma', &ay);
   y1=y1/&by;
   output;
   call symput('y2', compress(trim(y2)));
run;

data x;
   set x;
   if x<&y1 and x<&y2 then flag=1;
   else flag=0;
run;

proc means noprint data=x;
   var flag;
   output out=p2 mean=p2;
run;

data _null_;
   set p2;
   call symput('p2', compress(trim(p2)));
run;

data _null_;
   sx1=&seed1 +1;
   call streaminit(sx1);
   x1=rand('gamma', &ax);
   x1=x1/&bx;
   output;
   call symput('x1', compress(trim(x1)));
run;

data _null_;
   sx2=&seed1 +2;
   call streaminit(sx2);
   x2=rand('gamma', &ax);
   x2=x2/&bx;
   output;
   call symput('x2', compress(trim(x2)));
```

```
      run;

      data y;
         set y;
         if y>&x1 and y>x2 then flag=1;
         else flag=0;
      run;

      proc means noprint data=y;
         var flag;
         output out=p3 mean=p3;
      run;

      data _null_;
         set p3;
         call symput('p3', compress(trim(p3)));
      run;

      title 'Gamma Distribution';
      %MSpower(&beta., &p1., &p2., &p3., &alpha.);
   %mend simgamma;

   %simgamma(1, 100, 25, 35,5, 5, 0.2, simN=10000, alpha=0.05);
```

The results of `% simgamma` are shown in Table 11.5 on page 321. The results indicate that, if the treatment outcomes from the control group follow a Gamma distribution with a mean of 25, a standard deviation of 5 (the shape and scale parameters can be calculated accordingly); and if the treatment outcomes from the experimental group follow a Gamma distribution with a mean of 35 and a standard deviation of 5, then estimates for `p1`, `p2`, `p3` are 0.9207, 0.9935, and 1, respectively using a Monte-Carlo simulation, and the smallest sample size that provides 80% power for rejecting the null hypothesis is 9 per treatment. The actual power with a total sample size of 18 is 81%.

Table 11.5 *Output from Example Code 11.3*

Sample Size	p1	p2	p3	alpha	beta	power
9	0.9207	0.9935	1	0.05	0.19013	0.80987

When the assay is not 100% perfect to dichotomize patients to biomarker positive and negative groups, the relative efficiency formulas can be generalized to account for errors, and such errors apply only to the enrichment design, in a negative way. Let λ_{sens} denote the sensitivity of the assay for diagnosing marker+ patients and let λ_{spec} denote the corresponding specificity, then the treatment effect for the enrichment study is diluted by

$$\frac{\lambda_{sens}(1-\gamma)}{(1-\lambda_{spec})\gamma+\lambda_{sens}(1-\gamma)}.$$

If $2n^T$ denotes the number of patients randomized to the targeted trial, then $(1-\lambda_{spec})\gamma+\lambda_{sens}(1-\gamma)$ is the expected number of screened patients to enroll $2n^T$ randomized patients.

The assay specificity is critical in determining the efficiency of targeted clinical trials with regard to the required number of randomized patients, while the assay sensitivity played a vital role with regards to the required number of screened patients. The most relevant assay is the one that identifies patients who are more responsive to the new treatment than the control. It is especially important when the control is active.

Maitournam and Simon [25] did extensive simulations assessing the relative efficiency of the enrichment design versus the all-comers design and conclude:

- When the treatment effect is limited to marker+ patients and the specificity of the assay is close to 1, the enrichment design is generally much more efficient than the all-comers design with regard to both the number of randomized and number of screened patients. The efficiency decreases as the specificity of the assay degrades.
- If the treatment effect for the marker- patients is half as large as for the marker+ patients, the enrichment design requires more patients to be screened than the unselected design even if the assay is perfect. The increased number of screened patients for the enrichment design depends critically on the sensitivity of the assay. Under these conditions, there is no substantial advantage of the enrichment design in terms of the number of randomized patients unless the assay has specificity close to 1 – if that is the case, the selection of the preferred design will depend on other considerations such as relative costs of screening versus randomizing, safety and tolerability profile, and commercial value of a broader labeling indication.

11.4 Adaptive Enrichment Designs

11.4.1 Introduction

It has been well recognized and documented that increased spending in pharmaceutical and biotech research does not reflect an increase of the success rate of clinical development. Woodcock [26] outlined some of the reasons for the declining success rate of pharmaceutical development namely (i) high bar for proving drug benefits due to diminished margin for improvement, (ii) increased costs and complexity potentially decreasing the ability to bring many candidates forward into the clinic, (iii) genomics and related disciplines are not yet fully developed, (iv) chronic diseases are harder for the study sponsor to choose easy targets for investigation and investment. The United States Food and Drug Administration (FDA) hosted a "*Critical Path Initiative*" to identify key scientific challenges underlying the medical product pipeline problems and then released a *Critical Path Opportunities List* in 2006 that encouraged advancement of innovative clinical trial designs, especially learning from prior experience and ongoing accumulated data. The innovation implies the use of adaptive design methods and the potential use of a Bayesian approach. Chow et al. [27] define "*Adaptive design as a design that allows adaptations to trial and/or statistical procedures of the trial after its initiation without undermining the validity and integrity of the trial*". The PhRMA Working Group paper by Gallo et al. [28] refers to "*An adaptive design as a clinical trial design that uses accumulating data to decide on how to modify aspects of the study as it continues, without undermining the validity and integrity of the trial.*" In the past decade, the application of adaptive design methods in clinical trials has become very popular due to its flexibility and efficiency. This efficiency is at times gained at a cost of increased complexity, logistical challenges especially for adequate drug supply, and other operational issues. In most cases, intensive planning must be undertaken to carefully define go/no-go criteria, which is likely to delay the start of the trial. The sponsor should have the adequately trained resources to implement and execute adaptive designs. All eventualities should be considered including the risk and benefits in case the trial is terminated at the interim analysis. Given the continuous evolution of the electronic era with several improvements in computing, data collection and access and dynamic drug supply, the frequent use of this design is not a distant dream anymore. Some of the commonly used prospective pre-specified adaptations are (i) Group sequential design, (ii) sample size re-estimation design, (iii) adaptive dose-finding design, (iv) drop-the-loser design, (v) adaptive randomization design, (vi) adaptive treatment-switching design, (vii) hypothesis-adaptive design, (viii) an adaptive seamless trial design, and (ix) a multiple-adaptive design. Here we will primarily discuss adaptive designs related to biomarker selection and enrichment.

11.4.2 Frequentist Methods

11.4.2.1 Adaptive Signature Design

The classical designs discussed earlier involve only one biomarker and it is assumed that this biomarker positive set can be determined a prori. The adaptive signature design [29] is a design proposed to select the subgroup using a large number of potential biomarkers. This design is appropriate when both the potential biomarkers and the cut off are unknown; however, there is some evidence that the targeted therapy may work in some of the shortlisted biomarkers. The method was proposed initially using a combination of genetic markers and, hence, is also called the adaptive "gene" signature design. Recent developments in Genomic technologies (especially Pharmacogenetics) have the potential of identifying subgroups of patients who are likely to benefit from a certain targeted therapy. The design and implementation of studies with a large number of gene signatures are challenging. In this design there are three elements: (a) trial powered to detect the overall treatment effect at the end of the trial; (b) identification of the subgroup of patients who are likely to benefit from the targeted therapy at the first stage of the trial; (c) statistical hypothesis test to detect the treatment difference based on the subgroup of patients who are randomized in the latter half of the trial. These elements are pre-specified prospectively. Appropriate tests are conducted to account for multiplicity in order to control for type I error rate. The initial null hypothesis to test the benefit of the targeted therapy against the control is conducted in the overall population. This test is conducted at a slightly lower significance level than the overall alpha of 0.05 (example: 0.04 or 0.03). If the initial null hypothesis is rejected at the lower significance level, then the targeted therapy is declared superior than the control treatment for the overall population. The hypothesis testing and analysis is complete at this stage. If the first hypothesis is not rejected, then the signature component of the design is used to select a potentially promising biomarker subgroup.

It is done by the following steps: The study population is split into a training or developmental sub-sample and a validation sub-sample of patients. The training sub-sample is used to develop a model to predict the treatment difference between targeted therapy and control as a function of baseline covariates. This model is also called the benefit function, which is used to validate the results from the validation sub-sample. The benefit function used with this design is the minimum odds ratio [29] for the treatment marker interaction with a pre-specified number of biomarkers and the significance level. The risk difference is another benefit function that has been used which is the difference between the targeted therapy and the control in the probability of response as a function of baseline variables [20, 30-31]. The prediction is done for each subject in this sample and a predicted score is calculated to classify the subject as sensitive or non-sensitive. The subgroup is selected using a pre-specified cut-off for this predicted score. The second hypothesis test is conducted in this subgroup to see the benefit of the targeted therapy against the control. This test is conducted at a much lower significance (example: 0.01 or 0.02).

Generally, as the proportion of the sensitive patients increases, so does the difference in the objective response rates of the experimental arm and the control arm. Therefore, for prevalence above a certain threshold, the power of the overall effect test will dominate the power of the sensitive subset test. The adaptive signature design preserves the ability to detect the overall effect in this case. However, its advantage over the traditional design (testing for overall effect with broad eligibility) is reduced. The formulas that can assist the investigators in assessing the power relation between the sensitive subset test and the overall test are presented in [25].

The **%power** macro is developed for calculating power based on formula (1.1) in [25]. When calculating the power of the overall test, the following parameters need to be specified:

1. **pe**: the expected probability of response for a patient receiving the experimental treatment

2. **pc**: the expected probability of response for a patient receiving the control treatment

3. **alpha**: one-sided significance level

4. **N**: total sample size.

Likewise, the power of the subset test can be calculated using the macro by specifying these parameters in the sensitivity subset.

For example, if the expected probability of response for a patient receiving the experimental treatment is 0.5, and the expected probability of response for a patient receiving the control treatment is 0.2, assume that the one-sided significance level is 0.05 and the total sample size is 100, then the power of the overall test is calculated by Example Code 11.4 on page 324. In this example, the power is 94.3%.

Example Code 11.4 *Power for Adaptive Signature Design*

```
%macro power(pe, pc, alpha, N);
    data result;
        pe=&pe;
        pc=&pc;
        alpha=&alpha;
        N=&N;
        b=1-&alpha;
        pbar=(pe+pc)/2;
        za=quantile('Normal', b);
        num=(pe-pc)-za*sqrt(pbar*(1-pbar)*4/N);
        den=sqrt(pe*(1-pe)*2/N+pc*(1-pc)*2/N);
        a=num/den;
        power=CDF('Normal', a);
    run;

    proc print noobs;
        var pe pc N alpha power;
    run;
%mend power;
%power(0.5, 0.2, 0.05, 100);
```

The advantage of this design is its ability to de-risk losing the label of the broader population in pivotal trials. According to Freidlin and Simon [29], this design may be ideal to use for phase II clinical trials for developing an assay or signatures for patients who respond better to targeted therapies. One drawback of this design is that only half of the patients are used for development or validation. If prevalence of the subgroup of biomarker sensitive patients is low then this design will require a large number of patients to be screened. This may not be economically feasible, and it will be operationally challenging and will extend the enrollment period. The other drawback is that with a larger number of sub-groups that lead to high dimensional data, a large sample size may be needed to adequately power the trial.

11.4.2.2 Biomarker-Adaptive Threshold Design

In this design [32], the test for overall treatment effect is combined with the development and validation of a cutpoint for a pre-specified biomarker-based subgroup believed to be most sensitive to the targeted treatment. The statistical hypothesis test is carried out by splitting the overall type I error rate α. First, compare the treatment response on the overall population at α1 and, if not significant, then perform the second test at $\alpha - \alpha_1$.

For example, if the null hypotheses of no benefit (a) is rejected at a desired significance level of, say 0.04, then the testing is stopped or else the testing is carried out to test the hypothesis in (b) at 0.01 to control an overall α below the 0.05 level. A simplified cutoff model proposed by Altman et al. [33] is used to develop the proposed procedure. The overall patient population is then divided into two groups: biomarker-based (sensitive) and non-biomarker-based (non-sensitive). This categorization may result in some loss of information, but the proposed testing procedure is robust to departures from the simplified cut-off model. A permutation resampling approach is used for selection of the optimal cutpoint to avoid multiplicity problems [34].

An approach to sample size planning for clinical trials when the treatment effect is restricted to a subpopulation is presented in Appendix B in [32]. Assume that in a trial with time-to-event outcomes, the required number of observed events for the overall test to detect the target treatment effect (at significance level α) with power $1 - \beta$ could be calculated by the **%events** macro in Example Code 11.5 on page 325.

Example Code 11.5 *Number of Events for Biomarker-Adaptive Threshold Design*

```
%macro events(delta, alpha, beta, pi);
    data result;
        alpha=&alpha;
        power=1-&beta;
        delta=&delta;
        pi=&pi;
        za=quantile('Normal', 1-&alpha);
        zb=quantile('Normal', 1-&beta);
        logd=log(&delta);
        D=4*((za+zb)/logd)**2;
        Ds=D/(pi**2);

        label delta='hazard ratio';
        label pi="treatment effect fraction";
        label Ds='events required';
    run;

    proc print noobs label;
        var alpha power delta pi Ds;
    run;
%mend events;
%events(2, 0.05, 0.2, 0.8);
```

The parameters to be specified in the **%events** macro are:

1. **delta**: ratio of the hazard of the experimental arm over that in the control arm

2. **alpha**: significance level (one-sided type I error rate)

3. **beta**: false-negative rate (type II error rate)

4. **pi**: fraction of the population where treatment effect **delta** is limited; if the treatment effect applies to the entire study population, **pi**=1.

For example, if the hazard ratio is 0.5, the treatment effect is limited to 80% of the overall population, then the number of observed events required for a 80% power study (at a one-sided significance level of 0.05) is 80.4261, which would round up to 81 events (Example Code 11.5 on page 325).

Biomarker development and validation is usually very expensive and time consuming. Often times a reliable biomarker is not available even during the late phase of the clinical trial, namely pivotal trials. If a treatment effect is not detected in the overall population but an increased response is observed in the subgroup, an additional pivotal trial is required for regulatory approval; thus, further increasing the cost and time in the developmental process. This scenario is illustrated in the following example. Ravaud et al. [35] presented a randomized study in renal cell cancer patients who express either EGFR/ErbB2. The experimental arm was Lapatinib, an EGFR/ErbB2 tyrosine kinase inhibitor. The overall survival rate showed no statistical difference (p=0.29 with median 43.1 weeks in standard of care versus 46.9 weeks in Lapatinib). Among the subgroup of patients with over expression of EGFR in their tumors, the overall survival rate was statistically significant (p=0.02 with median 37.9 weeks in standard of care versus 46 weeks in Lapatinib). Since these findings were a result of the secondary subgroup analyses, another confirmatory trial is needed for regulatory approval of Lapatinib treatment in patients with tumors with over expression of EGFR. In the scenarios outlined above, this design and statistical testing procedure can combine the formal hypothesis test for overall population with the uncertainty in the effect in the biomarker defined subset. There is a substantial gain in efficiency providing statistically rigorous phase III evaluation of new therapies. The procedure preserves the overall type I error rate, in addition to giving the flexibility to detect a treatment effect in the overall broad population and at the same time providing a valid statistical valid test if the targeted therapy is beneficial to only a biomarker-based subset. This sequential and structured approach is carried out within a single randomized clinical trial, thereby negating the need for a new pivotal trial. This design is appropriate when the marker is known but the threshold or the cutpoint for the defining a positive or negative biomarker based subgroup is unknown. It incorporates a statistically valid hypothesis for identification, development, and validation of a cutpoint for a pre-specified biomarker.

11.4.2.3 Cross-Validated Adaptive Signature Design

This design which is an extension of the adaptive signature design was proposed to optimize the efficiency of both the development and validation components of the adaptive signature design [36]. This design enables complete cross-validation of the entire sample available in the study. This procedure preserves the overall study-wise type I error rate and increases the statistical power to detect a clinically meaningful treatment difference in the subgroup of patients who benefit from the targeted therapy.

Similar to the adaptive signature design, the initial null hypothesis to test the benefit of the targeted therapy against the control is conducted in the overall population, which is conducted at a slightly lower significance level α_1 than the overall α. If this hypothesis is rejected, then the targeted therapy is declared superior to the control treatment for the overall population and analysis is completed. If the first hypothesis is not rejected; then the signature component of the design is used select a potentially promising biomarker subgroup, also known as the sensitive subset. The sensitive subset is determined by developing the classifier using the full population. It is done by the following steps:

The study population is split into k subsamples.

Macros are developed for the cross-validated adaptive signature design and included in **`cvasd.sas`** in the supplemental material. Three data sets need to be specified in order to use the macros.

1. **`OutcomeInput`**, which is a data set containing subject information for treatment and treatment outcome. The format of the data set should follow Table 11.6 on page 327.

Table 11.6 Example for OutcomeInput Data Set

subjid	treatment	response
1	0	1
2	0	1
3	1	1
4	1	1

2. **GeneInput**, which is a data set that contains subject gene information for developing a potential biomarker. A subject is then categorized as either a sensitive subject or non-sensitive subject based on the biomarker value. The format of the data set should follow the below example in Table 11.7 on page 327.

Table 11.7 Example for GeneInput Data Set

Subj ID	gene 1	gene 2	gene 3	gene 4	gene 5	gene 6	gene 7	gene 8	gene 9	gene 10
1	0.359	0.490	1.085	0.174	-1.471	-0.207	-0.375	-0.565	-0.843	-0.388
2	1.371	1.570	1.541	-0.141	0.121	0.555	0.094	-0.002	-0.093	0.443
3	0.809	0.362	1.279	-0.134	-0.678	-0.216	0.183	-0.363	0.875	-0.027
4	1.960	0.513	0.508	-0.529	-0.191	0.293	0.153	0.113	0.249	-0.166

3. **TPInput**, a data set containing specified tuning parameter candidates that will be used in the design. The format of this data set should follow the example in Table 11.8 on page 327.

Table 11.8 Example for TPInput Data Set

eta	OS_R	gene_G
0.2	0.8	1
0.25	1.5	1

The **%decision** macro tests the benefit of the targeted therapy against the control in the overall population at a specified significance level α_1 (α_1 is usually slightly lower than the overall α). It decides if it is necessary to move to the signature component of the design (Example Code 11.6 on page 327).

Example Code 11.6 *Decision Macro Call*

```
libname perm "directory of sample data";

%macro Decision(outcome, gene, par, alpha1, seed);
   %global seedit;
```

```
    %let seedit = &seed;

    data outcome;
       set &outcome;
    run;

    data gene;
       set &gene;
    run;

    data par;
       set &par;
    run;

    proc freq data=Outcome;
    table response*treatment/chisq;
    output out=chisqtest chisq;
    run;

    data _null_;
    set  chisqtest;
    call symput ("chisq_pvalue",P_PCHI);
    run;
    /*If the chi-squre test is significant based on prespecified*/
    /*alpha1, then print result and abort*/
    /*Otherwise, need to move on to CVASD stage*/
    %if  &chisq_pvalue <&alpha1 %then %do;
    title "Chi-square Test SIGNIFICANT";
    proc print data=chisqtest;
    run;
    %abort;
    %end;
 %mend Decision;

 %Decision(perm.adsl, perm.adgene, perm.par, 0.04,12345);
```

The output (not shown) has a chi-square p-value of 0.7877. Because the test is not significant at the specified α_1 level, the signature component of the design will be implemented to select a potentially promising biomarker subgroup, also known as the sensitive subset.

The **% Resubstitution** macro (see supplemental material) calculates the resubstitution estimators of the treatment effect in the future subjects that are classified as sensitive by the final signature. To save computation time, the set of tuning parameters is selected by doing *k*-fold cross-validation on the first CV subset.

An example of implementing the developed macros for cross-validated, adaptive signature design in identifying the resubstitution estimators of predictive treatment effect for sensitive subjects is shown in Example Code 11.7 on page 328.

Example Code 11.7 *Resubstitution Estimators*

```
libname perm "directory of sample data";
%Decision(perm.adsl, perm.adgene, perm.par, 0.04,12345);
%Resubstitution(10, 5);
```

Results indicate a chi-square p-value of 0.7877 for testing the treatment response difference in the entire study population (similar to the output of Example Code 11.6). For the resubstitution estimators, the tuning parameters **eta**=0.2, **OS_R**=0.8 and

gene_G=1 are selected from the pre-specified list of tuning parameters from **perm.par**. Finally, 113 out of 124 patients are classified as sensitive, with response rates of 53% and 47% in the control and experimental groups, respectively.

The **% CVest** macro (see supplemental material) calculates the CV estimators of the treatment effect in the future subjects that are classified as sensitive by the final signature. The best set of tuning parameters is selected from the entire study population.

An example of implementing the developed macros for cross-validated, adaptive signature design in identifying the resubstitution estimators of predictive treatment effect for sensitive subjects is shown in Example Code 11.8 on page 329.

Example Code 11.8 *CV Estimators*

```
libname perm "directory of sample data";
%Decision(perm.adsl, perm.adgene, perm.par, 0.04, 12345);
%CVest(10, 5);
```

Results indicate a chi-square p-value of 0.7877 for testing the treatment response difference in the entire study population (similar to the output of Example Code 11.6 on page 327). For the CV estimators, the tuning parameters **eta**=0.25, **OS_R**=1.5 and **gene_G**=1 are selected from the pre-specified list of tuning parameters from **perm.par**. Finally, 41 out of 124 patients are classified as sensitive, with response rates of 33% and 67% in the control and experimental groups, respectively.

The cross-validation approach can considerably enhance the performance of the adaptive signature design [29] because it permits the maximization of information contributing to the development of the diagnostic signature, particularly useful in the high-dimensional data setting where the sample size or signal to noise ratio is limited. Cross-validation also maximizes the size of the sensitive patient subset used to test (validate) the signature. Molinaro et al. [37] have shown that cross-validation can provide a similar level of validity while being more efficient than the split-sample approach. One drawback is the fact that the selected gene set may not be stable when portions of the cases are omitted. Freidlin et al. [6] argued that it does not mean that the classification is unstable or that the classifier developed on the full data set will not predict accurately for independent data. In high-dimensional genetic profiling, good genomic signatures are generally not unique predictive biomarkers. However, they are usually correlated. As a result, successfully capturing the predictive genetic information is more important.

11.4.2.4 Adaptive Seamless Phase II/III Design

A seamless design combines objectives traditionally addressed in separate trials into a single trial. This type of design eliminates the time that would have occurred between the trials had they been conducted separately and may provide additional efficiencies in terms of the total number of patients or long-term follow-up.

An adaptive seamless design is the combination of trials and analysis where the final analysis uses data from patients before and after the adaptation. Though this design seems very promising, the statistical methodology for such designs must take into consideration potential biases and account for statistical issues due to multiplicity, multiple looks at the data (interim analysis), and the combination of data from independent stages. In previous years several adaptive seamless design methods have been proposed in the literature.

One of the commonly used methods is the adaptive p-value combination method and its variations [38-42]. Using these methods, many mid-trial design modifications including population selection are possible without compromising the family-wise type I error rate. The p-value based combination methods for seamless designs have been restricted to a single endpoint. Another approach that has been proposed [43] uses the multivariate normal method which is a modification to the group sequential computation. Stallard and

Todd later extended their work to incorporate a change of endpoint. Royston et al [44] proposed an approach along the same lines but include related survival outcomes in the design. These approaches make some assumptions about the joint distributions of test statistics in the interim and the final stage, and between subgroup populations and, hence, can get complicated when used for the population selection.

In the FDA guidance on adaptive designs, seamless phase II/III designs are considered as a type of design "not well-understood" due to both statistical and operational issues. In addition, seamless designs mix exploratory studies with "adequate and well controlled studies." As a result, the FDA requires that the sponsor conduct extensive simulations and communicate with the health authority as early as possible if such a design is proposed.

11.4.2.5 Flexible Adaptive Seamless (Enrichment) Design

In this design, the trial is carried out in two stages: In Stage I, all the subjects are recruited into the trial. On the basis of interim data, it is decided to either continue the study in all subjects or only the biomarker-based subgroup population. Based on the results from the interim analysis, the Stage II test would be conducted either on the full population, only the subgroup population or both the full and subgroup as a co-primary population. This is the setting of the design proposals by [45-49].

For example, Jenkins et al. [48] proposed an adaptive seamless phase II/III design with a subpopulation selection that can be more flexible. It allows the trial to select the appropriate subgroup at the interim analysis or continue in all patients with both the subgroup and the full population as co-primary populations. With this method, a combination of test statistics for the final endpoint from each stage is used for hypothesis testing. The decision to extend to the second stage is based on an intermediate or surrogate endpoint correlated to the final endpoint. This method is presented in the context of oncology using the progression free survival (PFS) and overall survival (OS) as interim and final endpoints, though it can be extended to other indications. In this design, having a co-primary endpoint recognizes the uncertainty at the interim look on the best possible endpoint and population. The additional flexibility is in the fact that the testing can be still done on the overall population, subgroup population, or the co-primary endpoint at the final analysis and also stopping the trial at the interim analysis for futility. This mitigates the risk of dropping a promising subgroup early in the trial which could be detrimental both from an ethical and commercial perspective. The proposed design uses PFS as the intermediate endpoint and overall survival as the confirmatory endpoint, though PFS has been accepted as a confirmatory endpoint in many cancer types. The design can be viewed as a special case or extension of the existing seamless design methods which combines the population and endpoints of both the stages in support of the licensing claims. This is done by combining the test statistic testing a clinically meaningful hypothesis and the two endpoints are combined without any additional bias. Suppose we have a randomized, two parallel arm trial. We partition the trial into a learning stage and a confirmatory stage like any seamless phase II/III trial. After collecting enough data (~50%) on the intermediate outcome (say PFS) on the first stage subjects, an interim analysis is conducted where both the overall population (O_P) and the pre-specified subgroup population (S_P) is examined for efficacy in the new treatment. The initial subgroup should be clearly defined and should be the only subgroup to be examined for efficacy. There is a null and alternative hypothesis associated with each of the populations (O_P and S_P). The null hypotheses ($H_0^{O_P}$ and $H_0^{S_P}$) of no difference between the experimental treatment and the control are for the final endpoint (overall survival in this case), while the alternate hypotheses ($H_1^{O_P}$ and $H_1^{S_P}$) indicate that there is increased efficacy in the new treatment compared to the control. At the interim look, there can be five possible decisions that can be made: (1) stop the trial for overwhelming efficacy in the O_P; (2) continue the trial in O_P, if the efficacy is moderate in both O_P and S_P; (3) continue the trial if the efficacy is slightly better in S_P than O_P with the co-primary subgroup hypothesis at the end of the trial; (4) enrich to include only S_P at the final analysis if the efficacy in the subgroup is much better than the O_P; (5) stop the trial for futility if the treatment is not going any better than the control. Each of the possible pre-specified decisions will differ in the sample size and in the follow-up post-interim analysis. The patients who start in the first stage will remain in the study and will be monitored for their long term (final) endpoint.

Wang et al. [45] proposed a similar design but only for a single normally distributed endpoint. We present the **% subpower** macro for design formulations.

The **% subpower** macro (Example Code 11.9 on page 331) calculates the subset power given:

1. **f**: the sample size ratio
2. **alpha_a**: the significance level for testing the overall population
3. **beta_a**: type II error of the overall trial
4. **es_ratio**: effect size ratio, **es_ratio = delta_g +/delta**
5. **alpha_g**: the significance level for testing the subgroup population.

Example Code 11.9 *Subset Power Macro*

```
%macro subpower(f,alpha_a, beta_a, es_ratio, alpha_g);
    data result;
        f=&f;
        alpha_a=&alpha_a;
        beta_a=&beta_a;
        es_ratio=&es_ratio;
        za=quantile('Normal', 1-&alpha_a);
        zb=quantile('Normal', 1-&beta_a);
        zag=quantile('Normal', 1-&alpha_g);
        d=sqrt(&f)*es_ratio*(za+zb)-zag;
        sub_power=CDF('Normal', d);
        label es_ratio="effect size ratio";
        label f="sample size ratio";
    run;

    proc print noobs label;
        var f alpha_a beta_a es_ratio sub_power;
    run;
%mend subpower;

%subpower(0.5, 0.04, 0.2, 2, 0.01)
```

For example, assuming 50% prevalence of a biomarker-based group, an alpha split of 0.04 versus 0.01 between the overall population and the subgroup, 80% power for the overall population, effect size ratio of 2, the power to detect treatment effect in the biomarker based population is 91%.

With multiple looks and subgroups there are several multiplicity methods [38, 42, 50] that can be employed to control the family-wise error rate at a nominal level, i.e., the probability of rejecting at least one true null hypothesis. A closed testing procedure is used to control multiplicity where all the possible intersection hypotheses ($H_0^{O_P}$, $H_0^{S_P}$ and

$H_0^{O_P S_P}$) is considered for rejecting any initial hypothesis (H_0^i). The stage-wise p-values for testing $H_0^{O_P}$ and $H_0^{S_P}$ are denoted by $p_i^{O_P}$ and $p_i^{S_P}$ for each stage $i \in \{1,2\}$, while $p_i^{O_P S_P}$ is a function of $p_i^{O_P}$ and $p_i^{S_P}$ for accounting for multiplicity and can be calculated using the Hochberg correction [51] or the Dunnett methods [52]. The final analysis is done on the overall population (O_P) using the inverse normal p-value combination test [53-54]. For each stage weights w_1 and w_2, where $w_1^2+w_2^2 = 1$, are specified to combine the p-values. The null hypothesis at the final analysis is rejected if $C(p_1, p_2) = w_1\Phi^{-1}(1 - p_1) + w_2\Phi^{-1}(1 - p_2) \geq c$.

11.4.3 Bayesian Methods

11.4.3.1 Bayesian Adaptive Randomization (BAR) Enrichment Design

An important feature of an adaptive clinical trial is to continually update the design by using the accumulated information from interim data, which fits naturally into the Bayesian paradigm. The Bayesian approach was actually developed specifically to deal with new data as data come in by updating prior beliefs to provide direct probability statements about the treatment effect. Moreover, in contrast to frequentist adaptive designs that require the type I error rate to be controlled, Bayesian inference is not affected by the number or timing of the interim analyses [55], allowing multiple analyses of the accumulating study data that update the probabilities under investigation. As a result, Bayesian designs are appealing to adaptive enrichment designs where adaptations in enrollment, randomization ratio, and subgroup selection are carried out based upon emerging data, particularly in exploratory studies to screen biomarkers.

In contrast to the equal (or fixed ratio) randomization approach in a frequentist design, this type of Bayesian design [56-57] implements an adaptive randomization method that allows the evaluation of treatments and biomarkers simultaneously, while providing more patients with potentially more effective treatments according to the patients' marker profiles. The Bayesian design is usually based on a hierarchical model for the endpoint of interests. The model parameters are also random variables modeling the random effects regarding the association of treatments and biomarkers with the outcomes of interest. With the use of hierarchical models, information can be borrowed across different subgroups as a means to increase efficiency.

In the common setting of evaluating two treatments and one binary biomarker, the BAR can be applied to achieve the following three goals: (1) test whether the marker is prognostic or predictive, (2) test whether the new treatment works better than the standard treatment in all patients or in patients within certain marker subsets, and (3) treat patients better in the trial by assigning more patients to the more effective treatment based on the patients' marker status. Most of the frequentist designs can also achieve the first 2 goals.

The BAR enrichment design can be naturally extended to multiple treatments and multiple markers. For a patient with a baseline characteristic following into marker group j, assuming the posterior estimate of effect size in treatment i is δ_{ij}, the randomization ratio to treatment i can be expressed in the form of $\delta_{ij}^{\lambda}/\sum_i \delta_{ij}^{\lambda}$, where λ is the tuning parameter. Note that when $\lambda = 0$, it corresponds to equal randomization. When $\lambda = \infty$, it becomes the "play-the-winner" design, in which the next patient is assigned to the current winner treatment based on the available data, and no randomization is involved. The larger the λ is, the more imbalance the randomization will have.

The BAR enrichment design has been implemented successfully in several high-profile clinical trials in oncology. One example is the Biomarker-integrated approaches of targeted therapy of the lung cancer elimination (BATTLE) trial [56]. The BATTLE project consists of one umbrella trial and four parallel phase II studies with biomarker-based targeted therapies in patients with advanced NSCLC previously treated with chemotherapy but subsequently failed. The main objective of the study was to estimate and test the disease control rate at 8 weeks for each treatment given the patients' tumor biomarker profiles. The Bayesian probit model was used to characterize the disease control rate for each treatment by a marker subgroup with adaptive randomization. Another notable example is the I-SPY 2 (investigation of serial studies to predict your therapeutic response with imaging and molecular analysis 2) phase II trial in the neoadjuvant setting for women with locally advanced breast cancer. It is designed to test investigational agents in combination with standard chemotherapies in a curable patient population. By employing an innovative BAR design, the study aims to test new treatments in half the time, at a fraction of the cost and with significantly fewer participants [58]. Regimens that show a high Bayesian predictive probability of being more effective than the standard therapy will graduate from the trial with their corresponding biomarker signature(s). Regiments will be dropped if they show a low probability of improved efficacy with any biomarker signature. New drugs will enter as those that have undergone testing are graduated or dropped.

One obvious limitation of the BAR design is that adaptive randomization requires a quick turnaround time to learn from the interim data and adjust the randomization rate. As a result, the BAR design is applicable only for trials when the endpoint can be assessed in a relative short period of time.

Korn and Freidlin [59] conducted simulations comparing the outcome-adaptive randomization designs with the fixed 1:1 or 2:1 randomization design in a randomized two-arm setting. The comparisons were done in terms of required sample sizes, the numbers and proportions of patients having an inferior outcome. The authors found no benefits to outcome-adaptive randomization over 1:1 or 2:1 randomization and, as such, recommended using a fixed 2:1 randomization design when a higher proportion of patients being randomly assigned to the experimental treatment is preferred. In a commentary paper, Berry [60] argued that the greatest potential for adaptive randomization is in multi-armed trials, as in the BATTLE and I-SPY 2 studies, despite that in two-arm trials the benefit of adaptive randomization is limited.

11.4.3.2 Bayesian/Frequentist Design for Biomarker Treatment Interaction

In the setting of survival endpoint and only 1 biomarker, Karurui and Simon [61] proposed a two-stage Bayesian design similar to the frequentist designs of Freidlin and Simon [29] and Wang et al. [45]. Specifically, it is a Bayesian version of the adaptive design of Wang et al. [45] where the posterior distribution of treatment effects within the marker-positive and marker-negative strata based on an interim analysis where the first stage data is used to make decisions on patient recruitment and trial progression. It is essentially a hybrid Bayesian/frequentist design that takes advantage of the flexibility of Bayesian methods of incorporating prior confidence in the candidate predictive biomarker, and at the same time controls the type I and II error rates that meet the standards for conventional frequentist phase III trials. At the interim analysis, the posterior probabilities are compared to a prespecified threshold value, and 3 possible actions are taken:

1. Stop the trial
2. Stop recruitment to the marker negative group at the interim stage

3. Continue recruitment of both negative and positive patients.

The Karurui and Simon design enables limiting the number of test negative patients to the test drug if data suggest no benefit. It is also demonstrated that the design offers a number of advantages over the frequentist version of the Wang et al. [45] design.

11.5 Summary

Clinical researchers face increasing challenges and are presented with unique opportunities in the new era of personalized/precision medicine to meet the needs of patients, payers, and the ever increasing costs of health economics. In this chapter, we gave an overview of population enrichment designs that are growing in the statistical literature, with a focus on designs of predictive enrichment strategies so as to increase the power and efficiency to detect an effective therapy with regard to a predictive biomarker in a clinical trial. We categorized the existing designs into classical designs, frequentist adaptive designs, and Bayesian adaptive designs. We also discussed the efficiency of a biomarker enrichment design compared to a traditional all-comers design, which is a function of the prevalence of the biomarker positive population, sensitivity/specificity of the assay, and the relative treatment effect of the biomarker positive group versus the biomarker negative group.

Our focus was on designs that involved one or multiple predictive biomarkers that correlate with clinical efficacy endpoints of interest and the experimental treatment. The case of biomarkers that relate to safety outcomes is an important research area but not covered in this chapter. In addition, prognostic biomarkers, pharmacometric biomarkers, and surrogate biomarkers were out of the scope of this chapter.

References

1. Mandrekar SJ & Sargent D. (2009). Clinical trial designs for predictive biomarker validation: theoretical considerations and practical challenges. *Journal of Clinical Oncology* 27: 4027-4034.

2. Karapetis CS, Khambata-Ford S, Jonker DJ, O'Callaghan CJ, Tu D, Tebbutt NC, Simes RJ, Chalchal H, Shaprio JD, Robitaille S, Price TJ, Shepard L, Au HJ, Langer C, Moore MJ & Zalcberg JR. (2008). K-ras mutations and benefit from cetuximab in advanced colorectal cancer. *New England Journal of Medicine* 359: 1757-1765.

3. Bokemeyer C, Bondarenko I, Makhson A, Hartmann JT, Aparicio J, de Braud F, Donea S, Ludwig H, Schuch G, Stroh C, Loos AH, Zubel A & Koralewski P. (2009). Fluorouracil, leucovorin, and oxaliplatin with and without cetuximab in the first-line treatment of metastatic colorectal cancer. *Journal of Clinical Oncology* 27: 663-671.

4. Van Cutsem E, Köhne CH, Hitre E, Zaluski J, Chang Chien CR, Makhson A, D'Haens G, Pinter T, Lim R, Bodoky G, Roh JK, Folprecht G, Ruff P, Stroh C, Tejpar S, Schlichting M, Nippgen J & Rougier P. (2009). Cetuximab and chemotherapy as initial treatment for metastatic colorectal cancer. *New England Journal of Medicine* 360: 1408-1417.

5. Amado RG, Wolf M, Peeters M, Van Cutsem E, Siena S, Freeman DJ, Juan T, Sikorski R, Suggs S, Radinsky R, Patterson SD & Chang DD. (2008). Wild-type KRAS is required for panitumumab efficacy in patients with metastatic colorectal cancer. *Journal of Clinical Oncology* 26: 1626-1634.

6. Freidlin B, McShane LM & Korn EL. (2010). Randomized clinical trials with biomarkers: design issues Journal of the National Cancer Institute 102: 152-160.

7. Sargent DJ, Conley BA, Allegra C & Collete L. (2005). Clinical trial designs for predictive marker validation in cancer treatment trials. *Journal of Clinical Oncology* 23: 2020-2227.

8. Chapman PB, Hauschild A, Robert C, Haanen JB, Ascierto P, Larkin J, Dummer R, Garbe C, Testori A, Maio M, Hogg D, Lorigan P, Lebbe C, Jouary T, Schadendorf D, Ribas A, O'Day SJ, Sosman JA, Kirkwood JM, Eggermont AMM, Dreno B, Nolop K, Li J, Nelson B, Hou J, Lee RJ, Flaherty KT & McArthur GA. (2011). Improved survival with vemurafenib in melanoma with BRAF V600E mutation. *New England Journal of Medicine* 364: 2507-2516.

9. Romond EH, Perez EA, Bryant J, Suman VJ, Geyer Jr CE, Davidson NE, Tan-Chiu E, Martino S, Paik S, Kaufman PA, Swain SM, Pisansky RM, Fehrenbacher L, Kutteh LA, Vogel VG, Visscher DW, Yothers G, Jenkins RB, Brown AM, Dakhil SR, Mamounas EP, Lingle WL, Klein PM, Ingle JN & Wolmark N. (2005). Trastuzumab plus adjuvant chemotherapy for operable HER2-positive breast cancer. *New England Journal of Medicine* 353: 1673-1684.

10. Simon R & Wang SJ. (2006). Use of genomic signatures in therapeutics development in oncology and other diseases. *The Pharmacogenomics Journal* 6: 166-173.

11. Song Y & Chi GY. (2007). A method for testing a prespecified subgroup in clinical trials. *Statistics in Medicine* 26: 3535-3549.

12. Bauer P. (1991). Multiple testing in clinical trials. Statistics in Medicine 10: 871-890.

13. Albert SR, Sinicrope FA & Grothey A. (2005). N0147: a randomized phase III trial of oxaliplatin plus 5-fluorouracil/leucovorin with or without cetuximab after curative resection of stage III colon cancer. *Clinical Colorectal Cancer* 5: 211-213.

14. Baker SG, Kramer BS, Sargent DJ & Bonetti M. (2012). Biomarkers, subgroup evaluation, and clinical trial design. *Discovery Medicine* 13: 187-192.

15. Baker SG & Freedman LS. (1995). Potential impact of genetic testing on cancer prevention trials, using breast cancer as an example. *Journal of the National Cancer Institute* 87:1137-1144.

16. Janes H, Pepe MS, Bossuyt PM & Barlow WE. (2011). Measuring the performance of markers for guiding treatment decisions. Annals of Internal Medicine 154: 253-259.

17. Song X & Pepe MS. (2004) Evaluating markers for selecting a patient's treatment. *Biometrics* 60: 874-883.

18. Bonetti M & Gelber RD. (2000). A graphical method to assess treatment-covariate interactions using the cox model on subsets of the data. *Statistics in Medicine* 19: 2595-2609.

19. Bonetti M & Gelber RD. (2004). Patterns of treatment effects in subsets of patients in clinical trials. *Biostatistics* 5: 465-481.

20. Cai T, Tian L, Wong PH & Wei LJ. (2011). Analysis of randomized comparative clinical trial data for personalized treatment selections. *Biostatistics* 12: 270-282.

21. Baker SG & Kramer BS. (2005). Statistics for weighing benefits and harms in a proposed genetic substudy of a randomized cancer prevention trial. *Applied Statistics* 54: 941-954.

22. King MC, Wieand S, Hale K, Lee M, Walsh T, Owens K, Tait J, Ford L, Dunn BK, Costantino J, Wickerham L, Wolmark N & Fisher B; National Surgical Adjuvant Breast and Bowel Project. (2001). Tamoxifen and breast cancer incidence among

women with inherited mutations in BRCA1 and BRCA2: National Surgical Adjuvant Breast and Bowel Project (NSABP-P1) Breast Cancer Prevention Trial. *Journal of the American Medical Association* 286: 2251-2256.

23. Cobo M, Isla D, Massuti B, Montes A, Sanchez JM, Provencio M, Vinolas N, Paz-Ares L, Lopez-Vivcanco G, Munoz MA, Felip E, Alberola V, Camps C, Domine M, Sanchez JJ, Sanchez-Ronco M, Danenberg K, Taron M, Gandara D & Rosell R. (2007). Customizing cisplatin based on quantitative excision repair cross-complementing 1 mRNA expression: a phase III trial in non-small-cell lung cancer. *Journal of Clinical Oncology* 25: 2747–2754.
24. Simon R & Maitournam A. (2004). Evaluating the efficiency of targeted designs for randomized clinical trials. *Clinical Cancer Research* 10: 6759-6763.
25. Maitournam A & Simon R. (2005). On the efficiency of targeted clinical trials. *Statistics in Medicine* 24: 329-339.
26. Woodcock J. (2005). FDA introduction comments: clinical studies design and evaluation issues. *Clinical Trials* 2: 273–275.
27. Chow SC, Chang M & Pong A. (2005) Statistical consideration of adaptive methods in clinical development. *Journal of Biopharmaceutical Statistics* 15: 575–591.
28. Gallo P, Chuang-Stein C, Dragalin V, Gaydos B, Krams M & Pinheiro J. (2006). Adaptive design in clinical drug development – an executive summary of the PhRMA Working Group (with discussions). *Journal of Biopharmaceutical Statistics* 16: 275–283.
29. Freidlin B & Simon R. (2005). Adaptive signature design: an adaptive clinical trial design for generating and prospectively testing a gene expression signature for sensitive patients. *Clinical Cancer Research* 11: 7872-7878.
30. Vickers AJ, Kattan MW & Sargent DJ. (2007). Method for evaluating prediction models that apply the results of randomized trials to individual patients. *Trials* 9:14.
31. Foster JC, Taylor JMG & Ruberg SJ. (2011). Subgroup identification from randomized clinical trial data. *Statistics in Medicine* 30: 2867-2880.
32. Jiang W, Freidlin B & Simon R. (2007). Biomarker-adaptive threshold design: a procedure for evaluating treatment with possible biomarker-defined subset effect. *Journal of the National Cancer Institute* 99: 1036-1043.
33. Altman DG, Lausen B, Sauerbrei W & Schumacher M. (1994). Dangers of using "optimal" cutpoints in the evaluation of prognostic factors. *Journal of the National Cancer Institute* 86: 829-835.
34. Tukey J. (1977). Some thoughts on clinical trials, especially problems of multiplicity. *Science* 198: 679-684.
35. Ravaud A, Gardner J, Hawkins R, Von der Maase H, Zantl N, Harper P Rolland F, Audhuy B, Machiels J & El-Hariry I. (2006). Tykerb Renal Cell Cancer Study Group and GSK CoreT. Efficacy of lapatinib in patients with high tumor EGFR expression: results of a phase III trial in advanced renal cell carcinoma (RCC). *ASCO Meeting Abstracts* 24: 4502.
36. Freidlin B, Jiang W & Simon R. (2010). The cross-validated adaptive signature design. *Clinical Cancer Research* 16: 691-698.
37. Molinaro AM, Simon R & Pfeiffer RM. (2005). Prediction error estimation: a comparison of resampling methods. *Bioinformatics* 21: 3301-3307.
38. Bauer P & Köhne K. (1994). Evaluation of experiments with adaptive interim analyses. *Biometrics* 50: 1029–1041.

39. Bauer P & Kieser M. (1999). Combining different phases in the development of medical treatments within a single trial. *Statistics in Medicine* 18:1833–1848.

40. Müller HH & Schäfer H. (2001). Adaptive group sequential designs for clinical trials: combining the advantages of adaptive and classical group sequential approaches. *Biometrics* 57: 886–819.

41. Brannath W, Posch M & Bauer P. (2002). Recursive combination tests. *Journal of the American Statistical Association* 97: 236–244.

42. Schmidli H, Bretz F, Racine A & Maurer W. (2006). Confirmatory seamless phase II/III clinical trials with hypothesis selection at Interim: Applications and practical considerations. *Biometrical Journal* 48: 635–643.

43. Stallard N & Todd S. (2003). Sequential designs for phase III clinical trials incorporating treatment selection. *Statistics in Medicine* 22: 689-703.

44. Royston P, Parmar M K B & Qian W. (2003). Novel designs for multi-arm clinical trials with survival outcomes with an application in ovarian cancer. *Statistics in Medicine* 22: 2239-2256.

45. Wang SJ, O'Neill RT & Hung J. (2007). Approaches to evaluation of treatment effect in randomised clinical trials with genomic subset. *Pharmaceutical Statistics* 6: 227-244.

46. Wang SJ, Hung J & O'Neill, RT. (2009). Adaptive patient enrichment designs in therapeutic trials. *Biometrical Journal* 51: 358–374.

47. Brannath W, Zuber E, Branson M, Bretz F, Gallo P, Posch M & Racine-Poon A. (2009). Confirmatory adaptive designs with Bayesian decision tools for a targeted therapy in oncology. *Statistics in Medicine* 28: 1445–1463.

48. Jenkins M, Stone A & Jennison C. (2011). An adaptive seamless phase II/III design for oncology trials with subpopulation selection using correlated survival endpoints. *Pharmaceutical Statistics* 10: 347–356.

49. Friede T, Parsons N & Stallard N. (2012). A conditional error function approach for subgroup selection in adaptive clinical trials. *Statistics in Medicine* 31: 4309–4320.

50. Bretz F, Schmidli H, Konig F, Racine A & Maurer W. (2006). Confirmatory seamless phase II/III clinical trials with hypothesis selection at interim: General concepts. *Biometrical Journal* 48 (4): 623–634.

51. Hochberg Y. (1988). A sharper Bonferroni procedure for multiple tests of significance. *Biometrika* 75: 800-802.

52. Dunnett CW & Tamhane AC. (1992). A step-up multiple test procedure. *Journal of the American Statistical Association* 87: 162-170.

53. Zaykin D. (2011). Optimally weighted z-test is a powerful method for combining probabilities in meta-analysis. *Journal of Evolutional Biology* 24:1836–1841.

54. Kuan P &Huang B. (2013). A simple and robust method for partially matched samples using the p-values pooling approach. *Statistics in Medicine* 32: 3247-3259.

55. Spiegelhalter DJ, Abrams KR & Myles JP. (2004). *Bayesian Approaches to Clinical Trials and Health-Care Evaluation*. Wiley: Chichester.

56. Zhou X, Liu S, Kim ES, Herbst RS & Lee J. (2008). Bayesian adaptive design for targeted therapy development in lung cancer - a step toward personalized medicine. *Clinical Trials* 5: 181-193.

57. Lee J, Gu X & Liu S. (2010). Bayesian adaptive randomization designs for targeted agent development. *Clinical Trials* 7: 584-596.

58. Barker AD, Sigman CC, Kelloff GJ, Hylton NM, Berry DA & Esserman LJ. (2009). I-SPY 2: an adaptive breast cancer trial design in the setting of neoadjuvant chemotherapy. *Clinical Pharmacology & Therapeutics* 86: 97-100.

59. Korn EL & Freidlin B. (2011). Outcome-adaptive randomization: Is it useful? *Journal of Clinical Oncology* 29: 771-776.

60. Berry DA. (2011). Adaptive clinical trials: the promise and the caution. *Journal of Clinical Oncology* 29: 606-609.

61. Karuri SW & Simon R. (2012). A two-stage Bayesian design for co-development of new drugs and companion diagnostics. *Statistics in Medicine* 31: 901-914.

Authors

Bo Huang, Director of Biostatistics, Pfizer Oncology, Pfizer Inc., Groton, CT, USA.

Jing Wang, Senior Biostatistician, Gilead Sciences, Inc., Foster City, CA, USA.

Sandeep Menon, Vice President and Head of Statistical Research and Consulting Center, Pfizer Inc, Cambridge, MA, USA.

Index

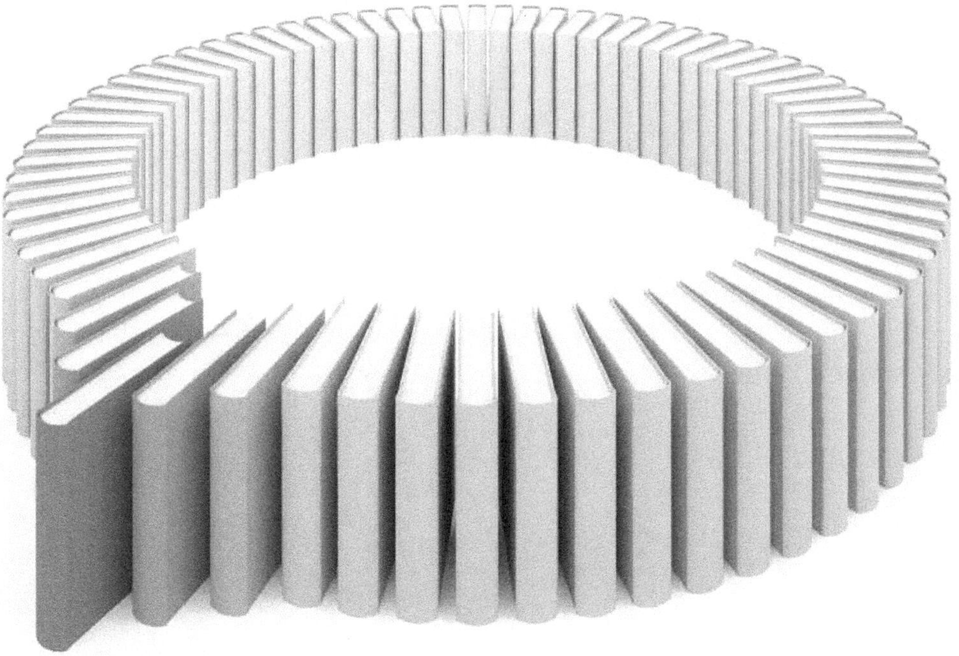

Gain Greater Insight into Your SAS® Software with SAS Books.

Discover all that you need on your journey to knowledge and empowerment.

support.sas.com/bookstore
for additional books and resources.

sas
THE POWER TO KNOW.

SAS and all other SAS Institute Inc. product or service names are registered trademarks or trademarks of SAS Institute Inc. in the USA and other countries. ® indicates USA registration. Other brand and product names are trademarks of their respective companies. © 2013 SAS Institute Inc. All rights reserved. S107969US.0613

www.ingramcontent.com/pod-product-compliance
Lightning Source LLC
LaVergne TN
LVHW061510220926
848485LV00017B/726